ANNALS OF
THE NEW YORK ACADEMY
OF SCIENCES

Volume 886

EDITORIAL STAFF

Executive Editor
BARBARA M. GOLDMAN

Managing Editor
JUSTINE CULLINAN

Associate Editor
ANGELA FINK

The New York Academy of Sciences
2 East 63rd Street
New York, New York 10021

ANTICANCER MOLECULES
STRUCTURE, FUNCTION, AND DESIGN

ANNALS OF THE NEW YORK ACADEMY OF SCIENCES
Volume 886

ANTICANCER MOLECULES[a]
STRUCTURE, FUNCTION, AND DESIGN

Editor
HIROSHI MARUTA

Conference Organizers
NANCY E. KOHL, C. CHANDRA KUMAR, DAVID P. LANE,
WEN-HWA LEE, HIROSHI MARUTA, BERND R. SEIZINGER, AND
PETER TRAXLER

CONTENTS

[a]This volume contains the papers from a conference entitled *Anti-Cancer Proteins and Drugs: Structure, Function and Design*, which was held by the New York Academy of Sciences in New York, New York on November 6–9, 1998.

Financial assistance was received from:

Supporters
- JANSSEN PHARMACEUTICA
- LUDWIG INSTITUTE FOR CANCER RESEARCH — MELBOURNE BRANCH
- NATIONAL CANCER INSTITUTE — NATIONAL INSTITUTES OF HEALTH
- SCHERING-PLOUGH RESEARCH INSTITUTE

Contributors
- AMGEN
- BAYER CORPORATION
- BERLEX LABORATORIES, INC.
- BRISTOL-MYERS SQUIBB PHARMACEUTICAL RESEARCH INSTITUTE
- EISAI CO., LTD.
- ENTREMED, INC.
- GENENTECH, INC.
- GENOME THERAPEUTICS CORP.
- GLAXO-WELLCOME, INC.
- HOECHST MARION ROUSSEL, INC.
- MERCK RESEARCH LABORATORIES
- THE NATIONAL NEUROFIBROMATOSIS FOUNDATION, INC.
- NOVARTIS PRODUKTE AG
- PARKE-DAVIS PHARMACEUTICAL RESEARCH, WARNER-LAMBERT CO.
- VION PHARMACEUTICALS, INC.
- YAKULT HONSHA CO., LTD.
- ZENECA PHARMACEUTICALS

Introduction

HIROSHI MARUTA

Ludwig Institute for Cancer Research, Melbourne, Australia 3050

Conventional cancer therapy, besides surgical removal of malignant tissues, has largely been based on a centuries-old common observation that most malignant cells are growing much faster than the parental normal or benign cell, thereby being more sensitive to radiation and several distinct DNA-damaging drugs (or DNA synthesis inhibitors). However, many normal cells such as bone marrow cells, hair cells, intestinal brush border cells, and germinal cells grow as fast as some of these malignant cells, and therefore these fast growing normal cells are severely damaged by conventional therapeutic approaches. That is the basis of the so-called side effects of conventional chemotherapy.

During the last two decades, however, epoch-making discoveries in molecular oncology, indicating that the development of cancerous tumors is caused by mutations, abnormal expression, or deletion of various genes encoding normal cellular proteins, have opened up new avenues in the treatment of cancer. Gain-of-function mutations of normal mitogenic proteins such as RAS and Src, overexpression of growth factor receptors such as EGF receptor and Neu/ErbB2, and loss-of-function of negative growth regulators/tumor suppressors such as p53 and p21/WAF1 have been shown to play a critical role in malignant transformation and to provide a basis for new and more selective (less harmful) therapeutic approaches.

Since the cloning of the first tumor-suppressor gene, RB, associated with retinoblastoma, new tumor-suppressor genes such as p53 have been cloned, and we now have a much deeper understanding of the structure-function relationship of the corresponding proteins. These genes are potentially useful for genotherapy of cancers. Furthermore, based on our recent understanding, at the molecular level, of various mitogenic signal transduction pathways where many oncogene products such as RAS are critically involved, a new generation of anticancer antibiotics or chemicals, called signal inhibitors, that selectively block one of these mitogenic/oncogenic signaling pathways have been isolated or created by pharmaceutical companies, universities, and academic research institutions. These nonpeptide molecules are potentially useful for the "signaling" chemotherapy of cancers. Furthermore, a few unique viruses, such as the adenovirus mutant ONYX-015 and reovirus, have been developed that selectively kill malignant cells that lack tumor-suppressor p53 or carry oncogenic RAS mutants, respectively.

To discuss the therapeutic potential of these recent discoveries more closely, bringing together leading molecular oncologists from all over the world from both academic institutions and industry, we held a unique conference, sponsored by the New York Academy of Sciences in early November 1998, entitled "Anti-Cancer Proteins and Drugs: Structure, Function and Design" at Rockefeller University. By focusing on the newest anticancer molecules (viruses, genes, proteins/peptides, and chemicals), this conference was designed to promote comprehensive understanding and cooperation between industrial and academic researchers in order to facilitate the design and creation of more effective and selective anticancer molecules in the treatment of cancer. This *Annals* is the proceedings of this conference, including the summaries of oral presentations by 28 distinguished investigators and a poster session covering a variety of anticancer molecules as well as DNA/peptide delivering/ targeting vehicles that are indispensable in the development of effective geno/peptido-therapy of cancer.

In closing this introduction, I would like to express my deep gratitude to the six other enthusiastic coorganizers of this conference who contributed enormously to its success, to the Department of Science and Technology Meetings at the New York Academy of Sciences (headed by Dr. Rashid Shaikh) including the Meeting Coordinator, Renée Wilkerson-Brown, to the more than 20 pharmaceutical/biotechological companies and nonprofit organizations in the list, including the National Cancer Institute, that kindly and enthusiastically supported this conference, and to all the other meeting speakers and attendees. Finally, on behalf of all the contributors to this *Annals*, I thank both Sheila Kane and Angela Fink for their editorial efforts.

Telomerase

A Target for Anticancer Therapy

SERGE P. LICHTSTEINER,[a] JANE S. LEBKOWSKI, AND ALAIN P. VASSEROT

Geron Corporation, 230 Constitution Drive, Menlo Park, California 94025, USA

ABSTRACT: Telomerase is absent in most normal tissues, but is abnormally reactivated in all major cancer types. Telomerase enables tumor cells to maintain telomere length, allowing indefinite replicative capacity. Albeit not sufficient in itself to induce neoplasia, telomerase is believed to be necessary for cancer cells to grow without limit. The presence of telomerase has been detected in virtually all cancer types including the most prevalent cancers of the prostate, breast, lung, colon, bladder, uterus, ovary, and pancreas as well as in lymphomas, leukemias, and melanomas. In addition, data from cancer patients indicate that telomerase levels correlate with clinical outcome in neuroblastomas, leukemias, and prostate, gastric, and breast cancers. Studies using an antisense to the human telomerase RNA component demonstrate that telomerase in human tumor lines can be blocked *ex vivo*. In these experiments, telomerase inhibition led to telomere shortening and cancer cell death, validating telomerase as a target for anticancer therapy. Telomerase is a uniquely appealing target for drug discovery because its dichotomic expression in normal versus cancer cells suggests that no serious side effects would result from a treatment abrogating telomerase activity. A variety of approaches to telomerase inhibition are being investigated and are discussed.

INTRODUCTION

Somatic cells grown in culture reach the end of their replicative capacity after a limited number of population doublings and enter a senescence phase.[1] The phenomenon of replicative senescence in mammalian cells is thought to be governed by the gradual telomeric attrition that occurs after each round of division.[2,3] Telomeres shorten by 50-200 basepairs per division[2,4] due to the inability of eukaryotic polymerases to fully replicate chromosome termini.[5,6] Although the underlying mechanisms are unknown, critically short telomeres are believed to lead ultimately to replicative senescence and growth arrest.[3,7]

Senescence, or mortality stage 1 (M1),[8] can be overcome by blocking the action of p53 and of the pRb family of proteins[9] (FIG. 1). Cells that bypass M1 continue to replicate until mortality stage 2 (M2 or crisis), when telomere length becomes critically short.[8,10] A rare, immortal cell occasionally arises from crisis, a process that is invariably accompanied by the preservation of telomere length. In most cases, telomerase, a ribonucleoprotein complex that synthesizes telomeric repeats, is reactivated.[11,12] Reactivation of telomerase enables cancer cells to maintain telomere

[a]For telecommunication: phone, 650/473-7715; fax, 650/473-7750.
e-mail, slichtsteiner@geron.com

1

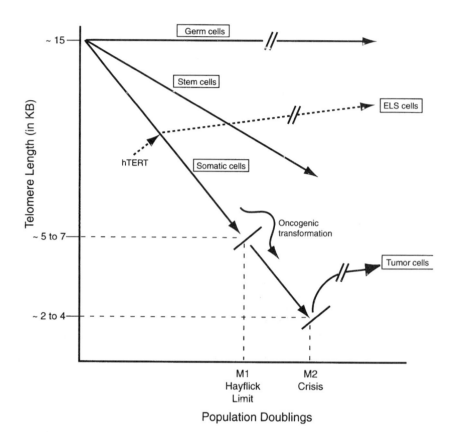

Population Doublings

FIGURE 1. Diagram of the relationship between telomere length, lifespan, immortality, and generation of cancer cells. Germ cells, extended lifespan cells (ELS), and tumor cells have high telomerase activity. Stem cells have moderate telomerase activity. Somatic cells are telomerase-negative. The *dotted line* indicates the effects of expressing hTERT in telomerase-negative somatic cells.

length and to acquire indefinite replicative capacity, or cellular "immortality." While not sufficient in itself to transform a normal cell into a tumor cell, telomerase is believed to be necessary for cancer cells to grow without limit.

The vast majority of normal human cells do not express telomerase activity in detectable amounts. However, cells of the reproductive system express high levels of telomerase and possess very long telomeres.[13] Telomerase can also be detected at low levels in certain hematopoietic, skin, and gastrointestinal cells.[14–17] It is believed that the presence of telomerase in some somatic cells may be required for the continuous self-renewal of stem cell populations. However, these progenitor cells gradually lose telomeric DNA and have a finite replicative capacity, suggesting that a threshold of telomerase activity is required for cellular immortality.[18]

The gene encoding the catalytic component of telomerase (hTERT, human telomerase reverse transcriptase) was recently cloned,[19–21] and after transfer into normal cells, it was shown to confer extended replicative potential.[18] Experiments in fibro-blasts, retinal pigmented epithelial cells, and umbilical cord endothelial cells indicate that this lifespan extension may be indefinite[18] This increased proliferative capacity does not appear to be associated with any signs of transformation, as the response to normal cell cycle checkpoints is maintained and these hTERT-immortalized cells do not form colonies in agarose or tumors in SCID mice.[22]

Approximately 87% of all primary human cancers express telomerase activity,[12,23,24] and gradients of increasing telomerase activity between early (benign) and late stage (malignant) tumors have been observed.[24] These data suggest that telomerase may virtually be a universal target for anticancer therapy.

Experiments using an antisense approach established the validity of telomerase inhibition in cancer therapy; HeLa cells, a cervical carcinoma cell line, that had been transfected with an antisense construct directed against hTR (the RNA component of telomerase), lost telomeric DNA and died after 23–26 doublings.[25] Interestingly, several recent reports have shown that telomerase inhibition by antisense approaches resulted in apoptosis, differentiation, or senescence.[26–28] The exact pathway of growth cessation appears to be determined by the differences in telomere length observed in the various tumor cells tested. These observations suggest that therapies targeting telomerase might become manifest without necessarily requiring extensive telomere shortening.

INHIBITORS OF TELOMERASE

Telomerase catalyzes the addition of TTAGGG DNA repeats to the ends of chromosomes. Minimally, telomerase is composed of hTERT, the protein component, and hTR, the RNA component.[29] hTERT provides enzymatic activity, whereas hTR binds to telomeric DNA and provides the template from which TTAGGG repeats are copied. Although other proteins were reported to be associated with telomerase, none was shown to be necessary for activity. The nature of telomerase allows for the development of inhibitors that target the enzyme at several levels. Some anti-telomerase inhibitors take advantage of the numerous steps required for the biogenesis and function of telomerase (FIG. 2). Telomerase inhibition can potentially be achieved by preventing hTERT and hTR transcription and RNA processing; specifically destroying or blocking regions of hTR and hTERT RNAs; blocking the translation and post-translation modification[s] of hTERT; preventing the assembly of telomerase; inhibiting its active site; preventing translocation into the nucleus; and blocking the natural substrate for telomerase (telomeres). Although some approaches such as specific inhibition of transcription[30] and translation[31] are still in development, others are better established and will be discussed herein (TABLE 1).

With our current knowledge of telomerase biology, apoptosis, differentiation, or senescence is the expected phenotypic result of telomerase inhibition. It is important to note that tumor cells have shorter telomeres than their normal counterparts. Although the molecular mechanisms triggered by telomerase inhibiton are largely unknown, tumors harboring short telomeres are likely to undergo apoptosis, whereas tumors with longer telomeres are predicted to follow a senescence pathway. The selective inhibition of tumor cell growth by telomerase inhibitors will need to be mon-

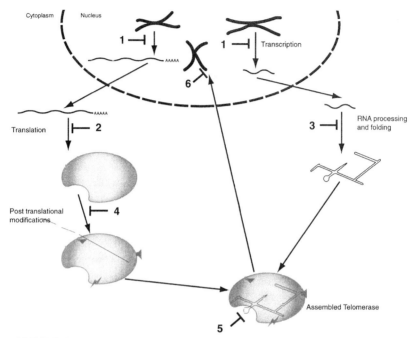

FIGURE 2. Schematic representation of the biogenesis of telomerase and the pathways targeted for inhibition (see text). (1) Inhibition of transcription; (2) translation inhibition by antisense oligonucleotides; (3) oligonucleotide-mediated catalytic breakdown of hTR; (4)post-translational inhibition; (5) inhibition of the assembled enzyme; and (6) inhibition of telomerase by modification of telomeric substrate.

itored *in vitro* and in animal models. No deleterious side effects are expected in most somatic cells, as they lack telomerase, but some effects might be observed in normal telomerase-positive cells.

Biological Inhibition of Telomerase. Fusions between normal cells and tumor cells have been shown to result in senescent hybrid cells with extinguished telomerase activity. These results indicate that the immortal phenotype is recessive.[32] Dissection of this phenomenon by microcell hybrids revealed that several individual chromosomes are capable of repressing telomerase activity and hence inducing senescence.[33] This approach could lead to the identification of biological repressors of telomerase *in vivo*.

Several reports have presented a strong correlation between differentiation and loss of telomerase activity. For instance, treatment of promyelocytic leukemic HL60 cells with retinoic acid[34,36] or vitamin D3[34,36,37] results in differentiation and rapid silencing of telomerase activity. Because of the pleiotropic effects of differentiating agents *in vivo*, their use as anti-telomerase drugs is unlikely. However, studies on the signal transduction mechanisms through which differentiating agents inhibit telomerase have the potential to lead to the design of effective anti-telomerase molecules.

Antisense Approaches. Proof of principle of an antisense approach in telomerase inhibition was first established by overexpression of a full-length antisense hTR in

TABLE 1. Telomerase Inhibitors

Categories	Types of Assays	References
Antisense		
PNA	*In vitro*	38, 39
2'-*O*-methyl-RNA	Tissue culture, *in vitro*	38
DNA and modified DNA	Tissue culture, animals, *in vitro*	26, 38, 39
DNA (2',5' tetra-adenylate)	Tissue culture, animals	27
RNA	Tissue culture	25, 28
Ribozymes	*In vitro*	60, 61
Small molecules		
3'-Azido-deoxythimidine (AZT)	Tissue culture	40–42
Dideoxy GTP	Tissue culture	40
Epigallocatechin gallate	Tissue culture, *in vitro*	43
Amidoanthracene-9,10-dione	Tissue culture	48
2,6-Disubstituted anthraquinone	*In vitro*	47
7-Deaza-deoxypurines	*In vitro*	44
Cationic porphyrin (TMpyP4)	*In vitro*	45
PIPER	*In vitro*	46
Isothiazolones	*In vitro*	49
Proteins		
HIV gp 120	Tissue culture	52
p21[WAF1]	Tissue culture	51
TGF-β1	Tissue culture	52, 53
Dominant-negative hTERT	Tissue culture	57
Rb	Tissue culture	54
Others		
Bisinodolylmaleimide 1	Tissue culture	59
Protein phosphatase 2A	*In vitro*	58
Prostaglandin A1	Tissue culture	53
Vitamin D3	Tissue culture	34, 36, 37
All trans retinoic acid	Tissue culture	34–36

HeLa cells. Transfected cells showed signs of telomeric attrition and began to die after a few passages.[25] In human malignant glioma cells, a similar antisense approach resulted in increased levels of interleukin-1β-converting enzyme [ICE] which led to apoptosis of a subset of cells. Other cells showed signs of reduced growth and invasiveness consistent with a more differentiated state.[28]

Capitalizing on the ability of the RNA component of telomerase to base-pair with telomeric repeats, most of the antisense approaches reported so far have focused on short molecules directed against the template region of hTR. DNA oligonucleotides were used as inhibitors of telomerase but were found to be susceptible to degradation. In addition, short oligonucleotides directed against the template region of hTR are often used as substrate by the telomerase complex (APV and SPL, unpublished data). However, in efforts to identify all accessible regions in hTR, DNA antisense molecules have been designed that completely inhibit enzymatic activity (APV, SPL, and E. M. Atkinson, unpublished data). Modified DNA oligonucleotides have also been used to inhibit telomerase,[26] but in other cases, the same chemistry yielded disappointing results as inhibition was no longer sequence specific.[38]

Peptide nucleic acids (PNA), with their high target avidity, inhibit telomerase with high efficiency (APV and SPL, unpublished data). PNAs represent so far the most potent class of telomerase inhibitors, with reported IC_{50} in the picomolar range.[39] However, protocols to deliver PNAs more efficiently into cells would be useful for the development of clinical applications.

2′-O-methyl-RNA molecules are emerging as powerful inhibitors of telomerase (J.T. Kealey, APV, and SPL, unpublished data). Their chemical structure is similar to that of DNA, which may confer an advantage in substrate recognition by the telomerase complex. In a comparative study, inhibition by 2′-O-methyl-RNA molecules proved to be superior to that afforded by PNAs with identical sequences.[38] The phosphodiester backbone is thought to provide favorable electrostatic contacts with the telomerase complex that would not be present in the amide-based PNA backbone.[38] The availability of protocols for delivery of negatively charged oligonucleotides into cells makes 2′-O-methyl-RNAs promising candidates for initial *in vivo* anti-telomerase studies.

An interesting approach recently surfaced that combines an antisense approach with RNAse L-mediated destruction of the targeted sequences. A 2′,5′ oligoadenylate antisense oligonucleotide directed against a putative single-stranded loop in the hTR sequence resulted in selective degradation of hTR and cellular death after 14 days of treatment. Direct injection of the oligonucleotide into subcutaneous xenografts in mice significantly retarded tumor growth and induced apoptosis in a fraction of tumor cells.[27] Antisense approaches employing a variety of agents have so far targeted hTR with some success, but the recent cloning of the catalytic component of telomerase and a better understanding of the biological molecules involved in its regulation will expand the repertoire of targets available for antisense therapy. Oligonucleotides, with their high sequence specificity and simple design, have the potential to become therapeutically relevant compounds. As support for this approach, successful phase III clinical trials in cytomegalovirus retinitis have resulted in the first antisense treatment to receive FDA approval. Progress in encapsulation methods of short oligonucleotides will be closely monitored to further assess the potential therapeutic value of antisense therapies.

Small Molecules. Small molecules, with molecular weights typically smaller than 1,000, have historically formed the foundation of pharmaceutical drug development. Several small molecules that have been reported to affect telomerase activity include reverse transcriptase inhibitors,[40–42] nucleotide analogs,[40] natural products,[43] G-quartet stabilizers (see below),[44–47] and organic molecules.[48,49] To date, the disclosed potencies are still relatively low, but they provide important information in the development of more potent derivatives that will eventually be of therapeutic value. The recent cloning of the hTERT gene[19–21] and the demonstration that telomerase activity can be reconstituted *in vitro* from its two major components[29] raise new opportunities in the design of screens that will facilitate the development of novel inhibitors of telomerase.

G-Quartet Stabilizers. Mammalian telomeres contain at their ends a 150-base single-stranded 3′ overhang that can form a G-quartet structure.[50] This structure needs to be dissociated in order for telomerase to add TTAGGG repeats. This particular feature of the telomeric end has been exploited to develop molecules that stabilize the G-quartet structure, effectively preventing the enzyme from using it as a substrate. Several G-quartet stabilizers have been described.[44–47] Although it is possible to block telomerase activity, high concentrations of G-quartet stabilizers are necessary.

Proteins. Several reports have demonstrated telomerase inhibition by well-characterized proteins such as p21[WAF1],[51] HIV gp120,[52] TGF β-1,[52,53] and pRb.[54] Human immortalized keratinocytes (HaCaT cells), when transduced with a retrovirus expressing p21[WAF1], have been shown[51] to stop growing and effectively repress telomerase activity. p21[WAF1] interacts with the PCNA/DNA polymerase δ complex.[55] It is tempting to speculate that p21[WAF1] might also bind to telomerase, a specialized polymerase. Interestingly, prostaglandin A1 treatment of cells has been shown to inhibit telomerase,[56] presumably through induction of p21[WAF1].

Uninfected CD34[+] hematopoietic progenitor cells (HPC) from HIV[+] patients have no detectable telomerase activity, whereas the same cells from healthy donors express high levels of the enzyme.[52] When normal CD34[+] cells are treated *in vitro* with gp120 or TGF-β1, telomerase inhibition is observed, the effect being more pronounced with gp120.[52] These factors or other proteins are unlikely to find near-term clinical application in telomerase inhibition because of the difficulties encountered in delivering such agents into cells and because of their potential pleiotropic effects.

The identification of hTERT as the catalytic subunit of the telomerase complex paved the way for the development of dominant negative mutant molecules. Upon reintroduction of such mutants into cells, telomere shortening occurred at a rate comparable to that of telomerase-negative cells. Cells with long telomeres showed an incremental decrease in replicative capacity, whereas cells with short telomeres demonstrated apoptosis.[57]

Further studies aimed at elucidating the mechanisms by which protein regulators affect telomerase activity might also lead to the discovery of new pathways for telomerase inhibition.

Others. A literature survey showed that several additional molecules may have inhibitory effects on telomerase. Of particular interest is the report that *in vitro* treatment of telomerase with phosphatase 2A results in telomerase inhibition.[58] Furthermore, telomerase activity can be immunoprecipitated from 293 cell extracts with anti-phosphoamino acid antibodies (APV and SPL; unpublished data). These results were corroborated by *in vivo* experiments using kinase inhibitors, indicating that the phosphorylation status of telomerase is important for enzymatic function.[59] Interestingly, p21[WAF1], which has been shown to cause telomerase inhibition, is a cyclin-dependent kinase inhibitor. Modulation of phosphorylation is an interesting avenue for telomerase inhibition. However, achieving selective inhibition of telomerase by targeting kinase activities will be a challenge.

CONCLUSION

The most potent and promising inhibitors so far are antisense oligonucleotides (2'-*O*-methyl-RNAs and PNAs); however, improved delivery *in vivo* is desirable.

The development of new, reversible encapsulation particle systems should allow longer survival in the bloodstream, selective delivery through the tumor vasculature and eventual transfer to malignant cells. For small molecule development, the recent cloning and expression of the hTERT gene and the reconstitution of telomerase activity *in vitro* will bolster the development of novel screens for telomerase inhibitors. Further understanding of the molecular interactions important for regulated telomerase activity should provide several targets for rational drug design.

The biogenesis of telomerase is still poorly understood, and future research focused on elucidating the differential regulation of telomerase activity in normal and tumor cells will undoubtedly provide ground for the design of new classes of telomerase inhibitors.

The application of telomerase inhibitors is likely to be effective in numerous clinical settings, including cancer therapy. In particular, the use of telomerase inhibitors after debulking chemotherapy, radiation therapy, and surgical procedures could prevent residual tumor regrowth, for example. Telomerase inhibitors could also conceivably be used to purge hematopoietic cell autografts. Furthermore, application in the treatment of autoimmune diseases can be envisioned.

The development of telomerase-based assays to diagnose and monitor tumor progression in cancer patients is being actively pursued. The combined use of telomerase-based therapeutics and diagnostics should provide innovative regimens for the treatment of cancer patients.

REFERENCES

1. HAYFLICK, L. & P.S. MOORHEAD. 1961. The serial cultivation of human diploid cell strains. Exp. Cell. Res. **25**: 585–621.
2. HARLEY, C.B. *et al.* 1990. Telomeres shorten during ageing of human fibroblasts. Nature **345**: 458–460.
3. DE LANGE, T. *et al.* 1990. Structure and variability of human chromosome ends. Mol. Cell. Biol. **10**: 518–527.
4. HASTIE, N.D. *et al.* 1990. Telomere reduction in human colorectal carcinoma and with ageing. Nature **346**: 866–868.
5. OLOVNIKOV, A.M. 1971. Principle of marginotomy in template synthesis of polynucleotides. Dokl. Akad. Nauk. SSSR **201**: 1496–1499.
6. WATSON, J.D. 1972. Origin of concatemeric T7 DNA. Nat. New Biol. **239**: 197–201.
7. HARLEY, C.B. 1991. Telomere loss: Mitotic clock or genetic time bomb? Mutat. Res. **256**: 271–282.
8. WRIGHT, W.E. *et al.* 1989. Reversible cellular senescence: Implications for immortalization of normal human diploid fibroblasts. Mol. Cell. Biol. **9**: 3088–3092.
9. SHAY, J.W. *et al.* 1991. A role for both Rb and p53 in the regulation of human cellular senescence. Exp. Cell Res. **196**: 33–39.
10. ALLSOPP, R.C. *et al.* 1992. Telomere length predicts replicative capacity of human fibroblasts. Proc. Natl. Acad. Sci. USA **89**: 10114–10118.
11. COUNTER, C.M. *et al.* 1992. Telomere shortening associated with chromosome instability is arrested in immortal cells which express telomerase activity. EMBO J. **11**: 1921–1929.
12. KIM, N.W. *et al.* 1994. Specific association of human telomerase activity with immortal cell lines and cancer. Science **266**: 2011–2015.
13. WRIGHT, W.E. *et al.* 1996. Telomerase activity in human germline and embryonic tissues and cells. Dev. Genet. **18**: 173–179.

14. BROCCOLI, D. *et al.* 1995. Telomerase activity in normal and malignant hematopoietic cells. Proc. Natl. Acad. Sci. USA **92:** 9082–9086.

15. COUNTER, C.M. *et al.* 1995. Telomerase activity in normal leukocytes and in hematologic malignancies. Blood **85:** 2315–2320.

16. TAYLOR, R.S. *et al.* 1996. Detection of telomerase activity in malignant and nonmalignant skin conditions. J. Invest. Dermatol. **106:** 759–765.

17. HIYAMA, E. *et al.* 1996. Telomerase activity in human intestine. Int. J. Oncol. **9:** 453–458.

18. BODNAR, A.G. *et al.* 1998. Extension of life-span by introduction of telomerase into normal human cells. Science **279:** 349–352.

19. NAKAMURA, T.M. *et al.* 1997. Telomerase catalytic subunit homologs from fission yeast and human. Science **277:** 955–959.

20. MEYERSON, M. *et al.* 1997. hEST2, the putative human telomerase catalytic subunit gene, is up-regulated in tumor cells and during immortalization. Cell **90:** 785–795.

21. KILIAN, A. *et al.* 1997. Isolation of a candidate human telomerase catalytic subunit gene, which reveals complex splicing patterns in different cell types. Hum. Mol. Genet. **6:** 2011–2019.

22. LEBKOWSKI, J.S. *et al.* 1998. Expression of telomerase increases the lifespan of primary cells without induction of transformation. Collected Abstracts of the 40th Annual Meeting of the American Society of Hematology (Miami, FL). American Society of Hematology. Westerville, OH.

23. SHAY, J.W. & S. BACCHETTI. 1997. A survey of telomerase activity in human cancer. Eur. J. Cancer **33:** 787–791.

24. SHARMA, S. *et al.* 1997. Preclinical and clinical strategies for development of telomerase and telomere inhibitors. Ann. Oncol. **8:** 1063–1074.

25. FENG, J. *et al.* 1995. The RNA component of human telomerase. Science **269:** 1236–1241.

26. MATA J.E. *et al.* 1997. A hexameric phosphorothioate oligonucleotide telomerase inhibitor arrests growth of Burkitt's lymphoma cells *in vitro* and *in vivo*. Toxicol. Appl. Pharmacol. **144:** 189–197.

27. KONDO, S. *et al.* 1998. Targeted therapy of human malignant glioma in a mouse model by 2–5A antisense directed against telomerase RNA. Oncogene **16:** 3323–3330.

28. KONDO, S. *et al.* 1998. Antisense telomerase treatment: Induction of two distinct pathways, apoptosis and differentiation. FASEB J. **12:** 801–811.

29. WEINRICH, S.L. *et al.* 1997. Reconstitution of human telomerase with the template RNA component hTR and the catalytic protein subunit hTRT. Nature Genet. **17:** 498–502.

30. DICKINSON, L.A. *et al.* 1998. Inhibition of RNA polymerase II transcription in human cells by synthetic DNA-binding ligands. Proc. Natl. Acad. Sci. USA **95:** 12890–12895.

31. WERSTUCK, G. & M.R. GREEN. 1998. Controlling gene expression in living cells through small molecule-RNA interactions. Science **282:** 296–298.

32. WRIGHT, W.E. *et al.* 1996. Experimental elongation of telomeres in immortal human cells extends the lifespan of immortal x normal cell hybrids. EMBO J. **15:** 1734–1741.

33. OHMURA, H. *et al.* 1995. Restoration of the cellular senescence program and repression of telomerase by human chromosome 3. Jpn. J. Cancer Res. **86:** 899–904.

34. SHARMA, H.W. *et al.* 1995. Differentiation of immortal cells inhibits telomerase activity. Proc. Natl. Acad. Sci. USA **92:** 12343–12346.

35. BESTILNY, L.J. *et al.* 1996. Selective inhibition of telomerase activity during terminal differentiation of immortal cell lines. Cancer Res. **56:** 3796–3802.

36. SAVOYSKY, E. *et al.* 1996. Down-regulation of telomerase activity is an early event in the differentiation of HL60 cells. Biochem. Biophys. Res. Commun. **226:** 329–334.
37. XU, D. *et al.* 1996. Suppression of telomerase activity in HL60 cells after treatment with differentiating agents. Leukemia **10:** 1354–1357.
38. PITTS, A.E. & D.R. COREY. 1998. Inhibition of human telomerase by 2′-O-methyl-RNA. Proc. Natl. Acad. Sci. USA **95:** 11549–11554.
39. NORTON, J.C. *et al.* 1996. Inhibition of human telomerase activity by peptide nucleic acids. Nat. Biotechnol. **14:** 615–619.
40. STRAHL, C. & E.H. BLACKBURN. 1996. Effect of reserve transcriptase inhibitors on telomere length and telomerase activity in two immortalized human cell lines. Mol. Cell. Biol. **16:** 53–65.
41. YEGOROV Y.E. *et al.* 1996. Reverse transcriptase inhibitors suppress telomerase function and induce senescence-like processes in cultured mouse fibroblasts. FEBS Lett. **389:** 115–118.
42. MELANA, S.M. *et al.* 1998. Inhibition of cell growth and telomerase activity of breast cancer cells *in vitro* by 3′-azido-3′-deoxythymidine. Clin Cancer Res. **4:** 693–696.
43. NAASANI, I. *et al.* 1998. Telomerase inhibition, telomere shortening, and senescence of cancer cells by tea catechins. Biochem. Biophys. Res. Commun. **249:** 391–396.
44. FLETCHER, T.M. *et al.* 1996. Human telomerase inhibition by 7-deaza-2′-deoxypurine nucleoside triphosphates. Biochemistry **35:** 15611–15617.
45. WHEELHOUSE, R.T. *et al.* 1998. Cationic porphyrins as telomerase inhibitors: The interaction of tetra-(N-methyl-4-pyridyl)porphine with quadruplex DNA. J. Am. Chem. Soc. **120:** 3261–3262.
46. FEDOROFF, O.Y. *et al.* 1998. NMR-based model of a telomerase inhibiting compound bound to G-quadruplex DNA. Biochemistry **37:** 12367–12374.
47. SUN, D. *et al.* 1997. Inhibition of human telomerase by a G-quadruplex-interactive compound. J. Med. Chem. **40:** 2113–2116.
48. PERRY, P.J. *et al.* 1998. 1,4- and 2,6-disubstituted amidoanthracene-9,10-dione derivatives as inhibitors of human telomerase. J. Med. Chem. **41:** 3253–3260.
49. BARE, L.A. *et al.* 1998. Identification of a series of potent telomerase inhibitors using a time-resolved fluorescence-based assay. Drug Dev. Res. **43:** 109–116.
50. BLACKBURN, E.H. & C.W. GREIDER, EDS. 1995. Telomeres. Cold Spring Harbor Press. New York.
51. KALLASSY, M. *et al.* 1998. Growth arrest of immortalized human keratinocytes and suppression of telomerase activity by p21^{WAF1} gene expression. Mol. Carcinog. **21:** 26–36.
52. VIGNOLI, M. *et al.* 1998. Impaired telomerase activity in uninfected haematopoietic progenitors in HIV-1-infected patients. AIDS **12:** 999–1005.
53. ZHU, X. *et al.* 1996. Cell cycle-dependent modulation of telomerase activity in tumor cells. Proc. Natl. Acad. Sci. USA **93:** 6091–6095.
54. XU, H.J. *et al.* 1997. Reexpression of the retinoblastoma protein in tumor cells induces senescence and telomerase inhibition. Oncogene **15:** 2589–2596.
55. LUO, Y. *et al.* 1995. Cell-cycle inhibition by independent CDK and PCNA binding domains in p21Cip1. Nature **375:** 159–161.
56. FRANZESE, O. *et al.* 1998. Effect of prostaglandin A1 on proliferation and telomerase activity of human melanoma cells *in vitro*. Melanoma Res. **8:** 323–328.
57. ROBINSON, M. *et al.* 1998. hTERT inhibition in human immortal cells. Collected Abstracts of the Geron Symposium No. 2: Telomerase and Telomere Dynamics in Cancer and Aging (Maui, HI). Geron Corporation. Menlo Park, CA.
58. LI, H. *et al.* 1997. Protein phosphatase 2A inhibits nuclear telomerase activity in human breast cancer cells. J. Biol. Chem. **272:** 16729–16732.

59. KU, W.C. *et al.* 1997. Inhibition of telomerase activity by PKC inhibitors in human nasopharyngeal cancer cells in culture. Biochem. Biophys. Res. Commun. **241:** 730–736.
60. KANAZAWA, Y. *et al.* 1996. Hammerhead ribozyme-mediated inhibition of telomerase activity in extracts of human hepatocellular carcinoma cells. Biochem. Biophys. Res. Commun. **225:** 570–576.
61. WAN, M.S. *et al.* 1998. Synthetic 2′-O-methyl-modified hammerhead ribozymes targeted to the RNA component of telomerase as sequence-specific inhibitors of telomerase activity. Antisense Nucleic Acid Drug Dev. **8:** 309–317.

A Paradigm for Cancer Treatment Using the Retinoblastoma Gene in a Mouse Model

ALEXANDER YU. NIKITIN,[a] DANIEL J. RILEY,[b] AND WEN-HWA LEE[a,c]

[a]Department of Molecular Medicine/Institute of Biotechnology, and
[b]Department of Medicine, The University of Texas Health Science Center, San Antonio,
Texas 78245-3207, USA

ABSTRACT: Discovery of tumor suppressor genes has provided a rational approach to cancer prevention and treatment. Loss of retinoblastoma susceptibility gene (*Rb*) function is a rate-limiting event in the development of human and mouse cancers. Establishment of animal models of cancer associated with Rb deficiency allowed us to develop and test long-awaited approaches to genetic correction for treating tumors *in vivo*. Recent studies demonstrated that (1) prevention of carcinogenesis is achieved by correction of gene copy number in *Rb*[+/−] mice, and (2) reconstitution of *Rb* gene functions is sufficient for suppression of neoplasia in immunocompetent mice. These results fulfill a promise of cancer treatment by reconstitution of tumor suppressor function.

RB AS A PROTOTYPE OF A TUMOR SUPPRESSOR

The discovery and characterization of the *RB* gene is a milestone in understanding cancer as a genetic disease. The original hypothesis that cancer is the result of chromosomal, presumably recessive, defects is attributed to Theodor Boveri.[1] In a largely unnoticed paper, Charles and Luce-Clausen were the first to present current terminology.[2,3] After performing statistical analyses of carcinogen-induced formation of mouse papilloma, they hypothesized in 1942:

> The first step towards the abnormal condition is mutation of some particular gene which is essential to normal differentiation of new skin cells. If normal and abnormal forms of the gene are represented by P and p respectively, the cell is Pp at this stage in contrast to the normal cells around it which are PP. The Pp cell still gives rise to a normal cell lineage because it still contains one normal P. The abnormal physiology which produces a papilloma is established when the second allele mutates, so that the cell is pp. Thereafter it forms only daughter cells which become papillomatous.

A large breakthrough in the development of the tumor suppressor gene paradigm emerged in studies of retinoblastoma, a childhood eye tumor that occurs in inherited and sporadic forms. By comparing relative incidence, multiplicity, and age at diagnosis of unilateral and bilateral retinoblastoma, Knudson[4] showed convincing evidence that in addition to a primary mutation, either germinal or somatic, only one additional somatic mutation is required for carcinogenesis. Comings[5] subsequently

[c]To whom requests for reprints should be addressed: Institute of Biotechnology, The University of Texas Health Science Center, 15355 Lambda Drive, San Antonio, Texas 78245-3207. Phone, 210/567-7351; fax, 210/567-7377.
e-mail, leew@uthscsa.edu

extended Knudson's hypothesis by proposing that the two "hits" inactivated both alleles of a single gene responsible for suppressing retinoblastoma formation.

In addition to its role in predisposition to the cancer, the concept of tumor suppressor genes promises suppression of established tumors. Experimental support of this idea was provided by Harris and colleagues.[6] Using a cell-fusion approach, they demonstrated that the phenotype of normal cells is dominant over the pertinent properties of neoplastic cells. This work implied that carcinogenesis may require the loss of function of tumor suppressive factors, presumably products of genes. Remarkably, such a model predicted that reconstitution of tumor suppressor gene function could abrogate carcinogenesis. The genetic basis for tumor retardation was further indicated by suppression of the malignant phenotype after the introduction of a single wild-type chromosome.[7]

Isolation of the *RB* gene[8–10] provided the opportunity to test the cancer suppression hypothesis using molecular methods. Using retrovirus–mediated gene transfer, we demonstrated that tumorigenic properties of cells deficient for RB can be suppressed by reintroduction of the normal *RB* gene.[11] These results gave direct evidence that **suppression of the malignant phenotype can be achieved by a single gene**. RB-mediated suppression was observed not only in retinoblastoma cells but also in other RB-deficient cells, such as those derived from osteosarcomas,[11] leukemias,[12] carcinoma of the prostate,[13] bladder,[12,14–16] mammary gland,[17] and lung.[16,18] Importantly, similar results were observed in experiments with other common human tumor suppressor genes, p53[17,19–21] and DCC.[22] Thus, the molecular foundation for the modern concept of tumor suppression had been laid.

NEOPLASIA ASSOCIATED WITH RB DEFICIENCY CAN BE PREVENTED AND TREATED BY GENE RECONSTITUTION *IN VIVO*

Advances in animal modeling allowed initiation of studies to evaluate RB as a potential tumor suppressor *in vivo*. In 1992, three groups including ours simultaneously established mouse lines with inactivated *Rb* gene.[23–25] As in humans with germ-line mutations, $Rb^{+/-}$ mice develop Rb-deficient tumors with nearly complete penetrance. However, the predominant tumors identified in $Rb^{+/-}$ mice, instead of developing from retinoblasts, derive from melanotroph precursor cells located in the intermediate lobe of the pituitary gland.[26–29] Although these melanotroph tumors are not perfect models of human cancer (to be described), they have allowed evaluation of assertions made earlier in human studies of neoplasia associated with RB deficiency.

Complete inactivation of *Rb* is required for initiation of carcinogenesis in animals with a single wild-type copy of the gene. The remaining wild-type copy of *Rb* is consistently absent in the earliest atypical cells, as directly demonstrated by microdissection-polymerase chain reaction (PCR) and immunohistochemical analyses in tumors from $Rb^{+/-}$ mice.[30] Accordingly, in $Rb^{-/-}/Rb^{+/+}$ chimeras, $Rb^{-/-}$ melanotroph progenitors undergo malignant transformation at an accelerated rate.[31,32] Moreover, tumor formation is prevented in $Rb^{+/-}$ mice carrying the human *RB* minigene with a separate integration place (TgRB).[25,33] The $Rb^{+/-}$ TgRB mice can be rescued from their malignant phenotype by as little as 5–10% of exogenous human *RB* transgene

TABLE 1. Neoplasia in moribund and 120-day-old (P120) $Rb^{+/-}$ mice

	Frequency (%)	
Neoplasia	Moribund	$P120^a$
Melanotroph tumor of pituitary intermediate lobe	100 (41/41)^b	100 (17/17)
Tumor of pituitary anterior lobe	22 (9/41)	18 (7/39)
C-cell thyroid carcinoma	95 (36/38)	86 (6/7)
Parathyroid adenoma	8 (3/39)	ND^c
Lung metastases of thyroid C-cell carcinoma	68 (26/38)	0 (0/8)
Neuroendocrine hyperplasia of lung	11 (4/38)	ND
Adrenal pheochromocytoma	71 (22/31)	77 (7/9)
Islet of Langerhans hyperplasia	41 (7/17)	ND

^{a}Both invasive tumors and foci of early atypical proliferation are included.
^{b}Numbers in parentheses indicate number of mice with tumor out of total number of mice.
^{c}Not determined.

expression.[27] By contrast, $Rb^{-/-}$ TgRB mice expressing human RB in amounts equal to endogenous Rb developed tumors at the same frequency as did $Rb^{+/-}$ mice.[27] Thus, Rb gene dosage (i.e., the number of unlinked gene copies), not protein amount, imposes the critical threshold for carcinogenesis. **Taken together, these results formally confirmed the genetic role of Rb in the prevention of cancer.**

Detailed characterization of spontaneous melanotroph carcinogenesis in $Rb^{+/-}$ mice provided us with the necessary information to test the ability of RB to suppress tumor growth in immunocompetent animals. In addition, early transgenic experiments demonstrated that expression of an RB minigene driven by a fragment of the human RB promoter is functionally adequate for tumor suppression, indicating its potential for use in gene therapy. Based on these studies, direct transfer of the RB gene to RB-deficient neoplastic cells was performed *in vivo*. The stereotactic delivery of adenovirus containing an RB minigene into the pituitary intermediate gland resulted in slower tumor cell proliferation and reconstitution of growth–inhibitory innervation.[34] In agreement with these observations, single adenoviral injection during either the earliest, P35, or the later, P180, stages of carcinogenesis significantly prolonged the lifespan of treated animals by a mean of ~20% compared with that of controls. Thus, the potential of RB gene therapy was demonstrated *in vivo*.

In humans the intermediate lobe of the pituitary gland is rudimentary, and melanotroph tumors are very rare.[35] Furthermore, relatively few cell types are regulated to proliferate or differentiate by immediate contact with inhibitory nerve terminals similar to melanotrophs. The difficulty in extrapolating experimental results to human pathology prompted us to evaluate the tumor phenotype of $Rb^{+/-}$ mice in greater detail. In earlier studies of $Rb^{+/-}$ mice and $Rb^{-/-}/Rb^{+/+}$ chimeras, other neuroendocrine tumors such as C-cell thyroid carcinomas[28,29,31,36] and hyperplasia of the adrenal medulla,[31,36] were observed in addition to the predominant melanotroph tumors.[28,29,31,32] Our recent results, based on careful morphologic analyses with three-dimensional reconstruction of target organs, demonstrated that $Rb^{+/-}$ mice contain C-cell thyroid and parathyroid tumors, adrenal pheochromocytomas, and α-glycoprotein hormone subunit (α-GSU) containing pituitary anterior lobe tumors by the time of their death. Pancreatic Langerhans islets and neuroendocrine cells in lungs also become pathologically hyperplastic (TABLE 1).[37] Notably, $Rb^{+/-}$ mice surviving over 380 days develop metastases in lung and liver in 84% (21 of 25 animals) and 10% (3 of 30 animals) of cases, respectively. By using a panel of cell-type specific markers, including calcitonin, α-melanocyte stimulating hormone, parathyroid hormone, and α-GSU, thyroid C-cells (calcitonin-secreting cells) have been identified as a source of metastatic disease.

Sequential morphologic studies of C-cell carcinomas, adrenal pheochromocytomas, and anterior lobe tumors identified a narrow developmental time period, postnatal days 35–120 (P35–P120), for the appearance of early atypical cells in each target tissue[37] (TABLE 1). In each case, early atypical cells contained no wild-type *Rb*. Therefore, all tumors begin development at about the same time, and loss of the wild-type *Rb* is critical in each case. These results suggest that Rb deficiency is associated with the syndrome of multiple neuroendocrine neoplasia.

The importance of these findings is threefold. First, unlike melanotroph tumors, other neuroendocrine tumors are common in humans. Either Rb deficiency or loss of heterozygosity for the *Rb* locus was described in neuroendocrine tumors of the lung, small cell lung carcinomas (95%), and parathyroid carcinomas (16%), as well as in some of C-cell thyroid carcinomas and anterior pituitary tumors[38–41,42] (our preliminary observations). Second, high frequency and relatively synchronous development of metastases make this model particularly attractive for studies of metastatic processes and the role of Rb in them. Third, identification of the syndrome of multiple neuroendocrine neoplasia in $Rb^{+/-}$ mice indicates the intriguing possibility of defective RB-mediated signaling pathways in human MEN syndromes. Interestingly, Rb-deficient tumors in $Rb^{+/-}$ mice contain activating mutations in the *ret* gene, the hallmark of MEN tumors.[43]

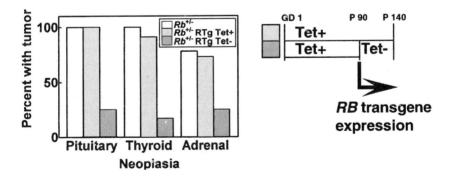

FIGURE 1. Suppression of neuroendocrine carcinogenesis by tetracycline-regulated expression of an *RB* transgene in $Rb^{+/-}$ mice ($Rb^{+/-}$ RTg). Animals treated with tetracycline from fertilization until either P90 (Tet-; $n = 12$) or P140 (Tet+; $n = 11$) were sacrificed on P140 and scored for tumors, including foci of early atypical proliferation. Fisher's exact test *P* values (Tet- vs. Tet+) are 0.0003, 0.0006, and 0.0391 for melanotroph, thyroid C-cell, and adrenal medullar neoplasia, respectively. No significant difference in the frequencies of tumors was observed between $Rb^{+/-}$ mice (*white bars*) and RTg (*RBp-tTA; hCMV*-1p-RB*) mice continuously treated with tetracycline (*light grey bars*, Tet+).

Identification and characterization of multiple neuroendocrine neoplasia in $Rb^{+/-}$ allowed direct testing of the hypothesis that the tumor suppressive effect of RB reconstitution is a more general phenomenon *in vivo*. As a first step in determining whether tumor suppression might be achieved in other Rb-negative cells, we crossed RTg*RB* transgenic mice,[37] in which expression of the *RB* transgene can be repressed by tetracycline administration, with $Rb^{+/-}$ mice. When tetracycline was continuously administered, the resulting $Rb^{+/-}$ RTg*RB* mice expressed only endogenous Rb[37] and manifested the expected spectrum of neuroendocrine tumors. Termination of tetracycline treatment on P90 resulted in expression of the *RB* transgene and a marked decrease in the number of animals that developed these varied tumors (FIG. 1 and ref. 37). These results indicate that RB-mediated suppression of Rb-deficient tumors *in vivo* is not limited to melanotrophs.

Although a critical role for the *RB* gene in the initial stages of carcinogenesis is well established, the impact of RB deficiency on tumor progression remains mostly uncharacterized. A few studies indicate that RB might contribute to cell properties relative to metastasis such as cell adhesion,[44] invasion,[45,46] and motility.[47] Recent studies demonstrated regulation of expression of E-cadherin, a homophilic cell adhesion molecule, by RB.[48] Most human RB-deficient tumors, such as small cell lung carcinoma, are detected at relatively late stages and exhibit pronounced metastatic potential. It is therefore clinically beneficial to know whether RB deficiency remains critical for tumor progression.

Carcinogenesis is thought to be a multistage process in which the accumulation of genetic alterations results in selection of the most autonomous and, by extension, the most malignant cell clones.[49–52] In agreement with human studies (reviewed in refs. 53–55), mouse models suggest that additional genetic and/or epigenetic changes must occur to promote progression of tumors associated with Rb deficiency. Based on the limited period of intensive melanotroph proliferation during perinatal development, loss of the last wild-type copy of *Rb* was deduced to occur within the 6-week period between gestational day (GD) 14 and postnatal day (P) 35. Indeed, sequential analyses of melanotroph carcinogenesis allowed identification of the earliest $Rb^{-/-}$ atypical cells already on P35.[30] However, detectable melanotroph tumors develop only after long latency periods, that is, by P300.[26,28,29,56] Requirements for additional factors promoting carcinogenesis were also demonstrated by such observations as more rapid tumor formation in $Rb^{+/-}$ mice treated with *N*-ethyl-*N*-nitrotrosourea,[56] the influence of genomic imprinting on melanotroph carcinogenesis,[57] and the cooperative tumorigenic effects of germline mutations in *Rb* and p53.[29,58] Gene therapy of tumors at advanced stages may thus require the targeting of multiple genes. Carcinogenesis in the salivary gland, for example, may be abrogated by termination of SV40 large T-antigen expression only until a certain stage has been achieved.[59]

To address these concerns, the effects of Rb reconstitution were studied in the model of spontaneous metastasis in $Rb^{+/-}$ mice.[37] Since DNA can be efficiently delivered to metastatic cells by intravenous injections of lipid-entrapped polycation-condensed DNA (LPD),[60–62] we adapted this method to deliver LPD complexes containing *RB* cDNA under the control of the *RB* promoter. This therapeutic approach was sufficient to significantly reduce the proliferative activity of metastatic cells in $Rb^{+/-}$ mice compared with that apparent in untreated animals or in mice treated with Lpds containing either *LacZ* (β-galactosidase), *Luc* (luciferase), or H209 RB inactive mutant[63] constructs. Furthermore, after repeated LPD-RB administration, metastatic spread was reduced from 84 to 12%.[37] These results indicate that introduction of RB reduces both the proliferation of metastatic cells and their colonization in the lung. **Thus, reconstitution of Rb function is sufficient for suppression of even advanced stages of carcinogenesis despite the substantial period of time that elapses between tumor initiation and the development of metastatic potential, during which numerous genetic alterations can accumulate.** These observations should contribute significantly to the development of the next generation of gene therapy for primary treatment of RB-deficient disseminated tumors in clinical settings.

FUTURE ANIMAL MODELS AND GENE THERAPEUTIC APPROACHES

In addition to human tumors with neuroendocrine and neuroepithelial phenotypes, such as small cell lung carcinoma, parathyroid carcinoma, C-cell carcinoma, and retinoblastoma, inactivation of the *RB* gene is found in tumors of the mammary and prostate glands, kidney, and bladder, as well as some soft tissue sarcomas and leukemias (reviewed in ref. 55). Even more significantly, numerous upstream regulators and downstream effectors of the RB protein are known to be oncogenes and tumor suppressor genes (for reviews see refs. 64–66). As just discussed, growth of RB-deficient tumors can be suppressed by RB reconstitution even in the most advanced stages. Unfortunately, available $Rb^{+/-}$ mice and $Rb^{-/-}/Rb^{+/+}$ chimeras die prematurely from brainstem compression by melanotroph tumors. Consequently, complete evaluation and treatment of advanced stages of other tumors are virtually impossible in these mice. Available mouse models also do not adequately recapitulate non-neuroendocrine forms of human RB-deficient neoplasia. Therefore, the efficacy of *RB* gene therapy in the cell type-specific context of the whole organism remains unclear.

To address these issues we are developing more mouse systems by refining current models and by creating new ones.[67] The next generation of mouse models is based on integration of Cre-*loxP* systems[68–70] and tetracycline-mediated gene regulation.[71–74] These systems will allow conditional regulation of gene function in specific cell types. Development of animal models that closely parallel human cancer will provide the most rigorous proof of RB-mediated tumor suppression *in vivo* and allow testing of therapeutically relevant approaches to rational gene targeting.

ACKNOWLEDGMENTS

This work was supported by National Institutes of Health Grants CA58318 and EY05758 and McDermott Endowment Funds.

REFERENCES

1. BOVERI, T. 1929. The Origin of Malignant Tumors. Williams & Williams. Baltimore.

2. CHARLES, D.R. & E.M. LUCE-CLAUSEN. 1942. The kinetics of papilloma formation in Benzpyrene-treated mice. Cancer Res. **2:** 261–263.
3. WUNDERLICH, V. & M.F. RAJEWSKY. 1995. "Tumour suppressor gene" concept of carcinogenesis. Lancet **345:** 1570–1571.
4. KNUDSON, A.G. 1971. Mutation and cancer: Statistical study of retinoblastoma. Proc. Natl. Acad. Sci. USA **68:** 820–823.
5. COMINGS, D.E. 1973. A general theory of carcinogenesis. Proc. Natl. Acad. Sci. USA **70:** 3324–3328.
6. HARRIS, H., O.J. MILLER, G. KLEIN, P. WORST & T. TACHIBANA. 1969. Suppression of malignancy by cell fusion. Nature **223:** 363–368.
7. WEISSMAN, B.E., P.J. SAXON, S.R. PASQUALE, G.R. JONES, A.G. GEISER & E.J. STANBRIDGE. 1987. Introduction of a normal human chromosome 11 into a Wilms' tumor cell line controls its tumorigenic expression. Science **236:** 175–180.
8. FRIEND, S.H., R. BERNARDS, S. ROGELJ, R.A. WEINBERG, J.M. RAPAPORT & D.M.D. ALBERT. 1986. A human DNA segment with properties of the gene that predisposes to retinoblastoma and osteosarcoma. Nature **323:** 643–646.
9. LEE, W.H., R. BOOKSTEIN, F. HONG, L.J. YOUNG, J.Y. SHEW & E.Y. LEE. 1987. Human retinoblastoma susceptibility gene: Cloning, identification, and sequence. Science **235:** 1394–1399.
10. FUNG, Y.K., A.L. MURPHREE, A. T'ANG, J. QIAN, S.H. HINRICHS & W.F. BENEDICT. 1987. Structural evidence for the authenticity of the human retinoblastoma gene. Science **236:** 1657–1661.
11. HUANG, H.J., J.K. YEE, J.Y. SHEW, P.L. CHEN, R. BOOKSTEIN, T. FRIEDMANN, E.Y.-P. LEE & W.H. LEE. 1988. Suppression of the neoplastic phenotype by replacement of the RB gene in human cancer cells. Science **242:** 1563–1566.
12. PAGLIARO, L.C., D. ANTELMAN, D.E. JOHNSON, T. MACHEMER, E.A. MCCULLOCH, E.J. FREIREICH, S.A. STASS, H.M. SHEPARD, D. MANEVAL & J.U. GUTTERMAN. 1995. Recombinant human retinoblastoma protein inhibits cancer cell growth. Cell Growth Differ. **6:** 673–680.
13. BOOKSTEIN, R., J.Y. SHEW, P.L. CHEN, P. SCULLY & W.H. LEE. 1990. Suppression of tumorigenicity of human prostate carcinoma cells by replacing a mutated RB gene. Science **247:** 712–715.
14. GOODRICH, D.W., Y. CHEN, P. SCULLY & W.-H. LEE. 1992. Expression of the retinoblastoma gene product in bladder carcinoma cells associates with a low frequency of tumor formation. Cancer Res. **52:** 1968–1973.
15. TAKAHASHI, R., T. HASHIMOTO, H.J. XU, S.X. HU, T. MATSUI, T. MIKI, H. BIGO-MARSHALL, S.A. AARONSON & W.F. BENEDICT. 1991. The retinoblastoma gene functions as a growth and tumor suppressor in human bladder carcinoma cells. Proc. Natl. Acad. Sci. USA **88:** 5257–5261.
16. XU, H.J., Y. ZHOU, J. SEIGNE, G.S. PERNG, M. MIXON, C. ZHANG, J. LI, W.F. BENEDICT & S.X. HU. 1996. Enhanced tumor suppressor gene therapy via replication-deficient adenovirus vectors expressing an N-terminal truncated retinoblastoma protein. Cancer Res. **56:** 2245–2249.
17. WANG, N.P., H. TO, W.H. LEE & E.Y. LEE. 1993. Tumor suppressor activity of RB and p53 genes in human breast carcinoma cells. Oncogene **8:** 279–288.
18. ANTELMAN, D., T. MACHEMER, B.G. HUYGHE, H.M. SHEPARD, D. MANEVAL & D.E. JOHNSON. 1995. Inhibition of tumor cell proliferation *in vitro* and *in vivo* by exogenous p110RB, the retinoblastoma tumor suppressor protein. Oncogene **10:** 697–704.
19. CHEN, P.-L., Y. CHEN, R. BOOKSTEIN & W.-H. LEE. 1990. Genetic mechanisms of tumor suppression by the human p53 gene. Science **250:** 1576–1580.
20. BAKER, S.J., S. MARKOWITZ, E.R. FEARON, J.K. WILLSON & B. VOGELSTEIN. 1990. Suppression of human colorectal carcinoma cell growth by wild-type p53. Science **249:** 912–915.

21. CASEY, G., M. LO-HSUEH, M.E. LOPEZ, B. VOGELSTEIN & E.J. STANBRIDGE. 1991. Growth suppression of human breast cancer cells by the introduction of a wild-type p53 gene. Oncogene **6:** 1791–1797.

22. GOYETTE, M.C., K. CHO, C.L. FASCHING, D.B. LEVY, K.W. KINZLER, C. PARASKEVA, B. VOGELSTEIN & E.J. STANBRIDGE. 1992. Progression of colorectal cancer is associated with multiple tumor suppressor gene defects but inhibition of tumorigenicity is accomplished by correction of any single defect via chromosome transfer. Mol. Cell. Biol. **12:** 1387–1395.

23. CLARKE, A.R., E.R. MAANDAG, M. VAN ROON, N.M. VAN DER LUGT, M. VAN DER VALK, A. BERNS & H. TE RIELE. 1992. Requirement for a functional Rb-1 gene in murine development. Nature **359:** 328–330.

24. JACKS, T., A. FAZELI, E.M. SCHMITT, R.T. BRONSON, M.A. GOODELL & R.A. WEINBERG. 1992. Effects of an *Rb* mutation in the mouse. Nature **359:** 295–300.

25. LEE, E.Y., C.Y. CHANG, N. HU, Y.C. WANG, C.C. LAI, K. HERRUP, W.H. LEE & A. BRADLEY. 1992. Mice deficient for Rb are nonviable and show defects in neurogenesis and haematopoiesis. Nature **359:** 288–294.

26. HU, N., A. GUTSMANN, D.C. HERBERT, A. BRADLEY, W.H. LEE & E.Y. LEE. 1994. Heterozygous Rb-1 delta 20/+mice are predisposed to tumors of the pituitary gland with a nearly complete penetrance. Oncogene **9:** 1021–1027.

27. CHANG, C.Y., D.J. RILEY, E.Y. LEE & W.H. LEE. 1993. Quantitative effects of the retinoblastoma gene on mouse development and tissue-specific tumorigenesis. Cell Growth Differ. **4:** 1057–1064.

28. HARRISON, D.J., M.L. HOOPER, J.F. ARMSTRONG & A.R. CLARKE. 1995. Effects of heterozygosity for the Rb-1t19neo allele in the mouse. Oncogene **10:** 1615–1620.

29. WILLIAMS, B.O., L. REMINGTON, D.M. ALBERT, S. MUKAI, R.T. BRONSON & T. JACKS. 1994. Cooperative tumorigenic effects of germline mutations in Rb and p53. Nature Genet. **7:** 480–484.

30. NIKITIN, A.Y. & W.H. LEE. 1996. Early loss of the retinoblastoma gene is associated with impaired growth inhibitory innervation during melanotroph carcinogenesis in $Rb^{+/-}$ mice. Genes Dev. **10:** 1870–1879.

31. WILLIAMS, B.O., E.M. SCHMITT, L. REMINGTON, R.T. BRONSON, D.M. ALBERT, R. WEINBERG & T. JACKS. 1994. Extensive contribution of Rb-deficient cells to adult chimeric mice with limited histopathological consequences. EMBO J. **13:** 4251–4259.

32. ROBANUS-MAANDAG, E.C., M. VAN DER VALK, M. VLAAR, C. FELTKAMP, J. O'BRIEN, M. VAN ROON, N. VAN DER LUGT, A. BERNS & H. TE RIELE. 1994. Developmental rescue of an embryonic-lethal mutation in the retinoblastoma gene in chimeric mice. EMBO J. **13:** 4260–4268.

33. BIGNON, Y.J., Y. CHEN, C.Y. CHANG, D.J. RILEY, J.J. WINDLE, P.L. MELLON & W.H. LEE. 1993. Expression of a retinoblastoma transgene results in dwarf mice. Genes Dev. **7:** 1654–1662.

34. RILEY, D.J., A.Y. NIKITIN & W.-H. LEE. 1996. Adenovirus-mediated retinoblastoma gene therapy suppresses spontaneous pituitary melantroph tumors in $Rb^{+/-}$ mice. Nature Med. **2:** 1316–1321.

35. LAMBERTS, S.W.J. *et al.* 1982. Adrenocorticotropin-secreting pituitary adenomas originate from the anterior or the intermediate lobe in Cushing's disease: Difference in the regulation of hormone secretion. J. Clin. Endocrinol. Metab. **54:** 286–291.

36. YAMASAKI, L., R. BRONSON, B.O. WILLIAMS, N.J. DYSON, E. HARLOW & T. JACKS. 1998. Loss of E2F-1 reduces tumorigenesis and extends the lifespan of Rb1(+/−) mice. Nature Genet. **18:** 360–364.

37. NIKITIN, A.Y., M.I. JUÁREZ-PÉREZ, S. LI, L. HUANG & W.-H. LEE. 1999. RB-mediated suppression of multiple neuroendocrine neoplasia and lung metastases in $Rb^{+/-}$ mice. Proc. Natl. Acad. Sci. USA **96:** 3916–3921.

38. CRYNS, V.L., A. THOR, H.J. XU, S.X. HU, M.E. WIERMAN, A.L. VICKERY, JR., W.F. BENEDICT & A. ARNOLD. 1994. Loss of the retinoblastoma tumor-suppressor gene in parathyroid carcinoma. N. Engl. J. Med. **330:** 757–761.
39. BATES, A.S., W.E. FARRELL, E.J. BICKNELL, A.M. MCNICOL, A.J. TALBOT, J.C. BROOME, C.W. PERRETT, R.V. THAKKER & R.N. CLAYTON. 1997. Allelic deletion in pituitary adenomas reflects aggressive biological activity and has potential value as a prognostic marker. J. Clin. Endocrinol. Metabol. **82:** 818–824.
40. PEI, L., S. MELMED, B. SCHEITHAUER, K. KOVACS, W.F. BENEDICT & D. PRAGER. 1995. Frequent loss of heterozygosity at the retinoblastoma susceptibility gene (RB) locus in aggressive pituitary tumors: Evidence for a chromosome 13 tumor suppressor gene other than RB. Cancer Res. **55:** 1613–1616.
41. PEARCE, S.H., D. TRUMP, C. WOODING, M.N. SHEPPARD, R.N. CLAYTON & R.V. THAKKER. 1996. Loss of heterozygosity studies at the retinoblastoma and breast cancer susceptibility (BRCA2) loci in pituitary, parathyroid, pancreatic and carcinoid tumours. Clin. Endocrinol. **45:** 195–200.
42. YOSHIMOTO, K., H. ENDO, M. TSUYUGUCHI, C. TANAKA, T. KIMURA, H. IWAHANA, G. KATO, T. SANO & M. ITAKURA. 1998. Familial isolated primary hyperparathyroidism with parathyroid carcinomas: clinical and molecular features. Clin. Endocrinol. **48:** 67–72.
43. COXON, A.B., J.M. WARD, J. GERADTS, G.A. OTTERSON, M. ZAJAC-KAYE & F.J. KAYE. 1998. RET cooperates with RB/p53 inactivation in a somatic multi-step model for murine thyroid cancer. Oncogene **17:** 1625–1628.
44. DAY, M.L., R.G. FOSTER, K.C. DAY, X. ZHAO, P. HUMPHREY, P. SWANSON, A.A. POSTIGO, S.H. ZHANG & D.C. DEAN. 1997. Cell anchorage regulates apoptosis through the retinoblastoma tumor suppressor/E2F pathway. J. Biol. Chem. **272:** 8125–8128.
45. LI, J., S.X. HU, G.S. PERNG, Y. ZHOU, K. XU, C. ZHANG, J. SEIGNE, W.F. BENEDICT & H.J. XU. 1996. Expression of the retinoblastoma (RB) tumor suppressor gene inhibits tumor cell invasion in vitro. Oncogene **13:** 2379–2386.
46. MARTEL, C., F. HARPER, S. CEREGHINI, V. NOE, M. MAREEL & C. CREMISI. 1997. Inactivation of retinoblastoma family proteins by SV40 T antigen results in creation of a hepatocyte growth factor/scatter factor autocrine loop associated with an epithelial-fibroblastoid conversion and invasiveness. Cell Growth Differ. **8:** 165–178.
47. VALENTE, P., A. MELCHIORI, M.G. PAGGI, L. MASIELLO, D. RIBATTI, L. SANTI, R. TAKAHASHI, A. ALBINI & D.M. NOONAN. 1996. RB1 oncosuppressor gene overexpression inhibits tumor progression and induces melanogenesis in metastatic melanoma cells. Oncogene **13:** 1169–1178.
48. BATSCHE, E., C. MUCHARDT, J. BEHRENS, H.C. HURST & C. CREMISI. 1998. RB and c-Myc activate expression of the E-cadherin gene in epithelial cells through interaction with transcription factor AP-2. Mol. Cell. Biol. **18:** 3647–3658.
49. NOWELL, P.C. 1976. The clonal evolution of tumor cell populations. Science **194:** 23–28.
50. FIALKOW, P.J. 1974. The origin and development of human tumors studied with cell markers. N. Engl. J. Med. **291:** 26–35.
51. FEARON, E.R. & B. VOGELSTEIN. 1990. A genetic model for colorectal tumorigenesis. Cell **61:** 759–767.
52. KINZLER, K.W. & B. VOGELSTEIN. 1997. Cancer-susceptibility genes. Gatekeepers and caretakers. Nature **386:** 761–763.
53. HAMEL, P.A., R.A. PHILLIPS, M. MUNCASTER & B.L. GALLIE. 1993. Speculations on the roles of RB1 in tissue-specific differentiation, tumor initiation, and tumor progression. FASEB J. **7:** 846–854.

54. KNUDSON, A.G. 1993. Antioncogenes and human cancer. Proc. Natl. Acad. Sci. USA **90:** 10914–10921.

55. BOOKSTEIN, R. & W.H. LEE. 1991. Molecular genetics of the retinoblastoma suppressor gene. Crit. Rev. Oncogen. **2:** 211–227.

56. RILEY, D.J., C.C. LAI, C.Y. CHANG, D. JONES, E.Y. LEE & W.H. LEE. 1994. Susceptibility to tumors induced in mice by ethylnitrosourea is independent of retinoblastoma gene dosage. Cancer Res. **54:** 6097–6101.

57. NIKITIN, A.Y., D.J. RILEY & W.H. LEE. 1997. Earlier onset of melanotroph carcinogenesis in mice with inherited mutant paternal allele of the retinoblastoma gene. Cancer Res. **57:** 4274–4278.

58. HARVEY, M., H. VOGEL, E.Y. LEE, A. BRADLEY & L.A. DONEHOWER. 1995. Mice deficient in both p53 and Rb develop tumors primarily of endocrine origin. Cancer Res. **55:** 1146–1151.

59. EWALD, D., M. LI, S. EFRAT, G. AUER, R.J. WALL, P.A. FURTH & L. HENNIGHAUSEN. 1996. Time-sensitive reversal of hyperplasia in transgenic mice expressing SV40 T antigen. Science **273:** 1384–1386.

60. LI, S. & L. HUANG. 1997. In vivo gene transfer via intravenous administration of cationic lipid- protamine-DNA (LPD) complexes. Gene Ther. **4:** 891–900.

61. LI, S., M. BRISSON, Y. HE & L. HUANG. 1997. Delivery of a PCR amplified DNA fragment into cells: A model for using synthetic genes for gene therapy. Gene Ther. **4:** 449–454.

62. Liu, F., H. Qi, L. Huang & D. Liu. 1997. Factors controlling the efficiency of cationic lipid-mediated transfection in vivo via intravenous administration. Gene Ther. **4:** 517–523.

63. BIGNON, Y.J., J.Y. SHEW, D. RAPPOLEE, S.L. NAYLOR, E.Y. LEE, J. SCHNIER & W.-H. LEE. 1990. A single Cys706 to Phe substitution in the retinoblastoma protein causes the loss of binding to SV40 T antigen. Cell Growth Differ. **1:** 647–651.

64. RILEY, D.J., E.Y. LEE & W.H. LEE. 1994. The retinoblastoma protein: more than a tumor suppressor. Annu. Rev. Cell. Biol. **10:** 1–29.

65. CHEN, P.L., D.J. RILEY & W.H. LEE. 1995. The retinoblastoma protein as a fundamental mediator of growth and differentiation signals. Crit. Rev. Eukar. Gene Express. **5:** 79–95.

66. JACKS, T. & R.A. WEINBERG. 1998. The expanding role of cell cycle regulators. Science **280:** 1035–1036.

67. UTOMO, A.R.H., A.Y. NIKITIN & W.-H. LEE. 1999. Temporal, spatial, and cell type-specific control of Cre-mediated DNA recombination in transgenic mice. Nature Biotechnol. In press.

68. STERNBERG, N., D. HAMILTON & R. HOESS. 1981. Bacteriophage P1 site-specific recombination. II. Recombination between loxP and the bacterial chromosome. J. Mol. Biol. **150:** 487–507.

69. SAUER, B. & N. HENDERSON. 1988. Site-specific DNA recombination in mammalian cells by the Cre recombinase of bacteriophage P1. Proc. Natl. Acad. Sci. USA **85:** 5166–5170.

70. GU, H., J.D. MARTH, P.C. ORBAN, H. MOSSMANN & K. RAJEWSKY. 1994. Deletion of a DNA polymerase beta gene segment in T cells using cell type-specific gene targeting. Science **265:** 103–106.

71. GOSSEN, M. & H. BUJARD. 1992. Tight control of gene expression in mammalian cells by tetracycline-responsive promoters. Proc. Natl. Acad. Sci. USA **89:** 5547–5551.

72. GOSSEN, M., S. FREUNDLIEB, G. BENDER, G. MULLER, W. HILLEN & H. BUJARD. 1995. Transcriptional activation by tetracyclines in mammalian cells. Science **268:** 1766–1769.

73. FURTH, P.A., L. ST ONGE, H. BÖGER, P. GRUSS, M. GOSSEN, A. KISTNER, H. BUJARD & L. HENNIGHAUSEN. 1994. Temporal control of gene expression in transgenic mice by a tetracycline-responsive promoter. Proc. Natl. Acad. Sci. USA **91:** 9302–9306.
74. KISTNER, A., M. GOSSEN, F. ZIMMERMANN, J. JERECIC, C. ULLMER, H. LUBBERT & H. BUJARD. 1996. Doxycycline-mediated quantitative and tissue-specific control of gene expression in transgenic mice. Proc. Natl. Acad. Sci. USA **93:** 10933–10938.

Trichostatin and Leptomycin

Inhibition of Histone Deacetylation and Signal-Dependent Nuclear Export

MINORU YOSHIDA[a] AND SUEHARU HORINOUCHI

Department of Biotechnology, Graduate School of Agriculture and Life Sciences, The University of Tokyo, Bunkyo-ku, Tokyo 113, Japan

ABSTRACT: Trichostatin A (TSA), an inhibitor of the eukaryotic cell cycle and an inducer of morphological reversion of transformed cells, inhibits histone deacetylase (HDAC) at nanomolar concentrations. Recently, trapoxin, oxamflatin, and FR901228, antitumor agents structurally unrelated to TSA, were found to be potent HDAC inhibitors. These inhibitors activate expression of p21Waf1 and 16INK4A in a p53-independent manner. Changes in the expression of these cell cycle regulators by an increase in histone acetylation may be responsible for cell cycle arrest and antitumor activity by HDAC inhibitors. The target molecule of leptomycin B (LMB), a potent antitumor agent, was genetically and biochemically identified as CRM1, a protein reported as being required for chromosome structure control. We showed that CRM1 was a receptor for the nuclear export signal (NES) and that LMB inhibited nuclear export of proteins. Using LMB, we identified a novel NES in fission yeast transcription factor Pap1, the function of which is abolished by oxidative stress in a manner conserved in eukaryotes.

INTRODUCTION

Eukaryotic cells receive a variety of positive and negative signals from external (growth factors, stresses, etc.) and internal (DNA damages, microtubule integrity, etc.) conditions. These signals are eventually transduced to the nucleus by importing the regulatory protein(s) into the nucleus. It is therefore important to understand the mechanisms by which the regulatory proteins are imported and exported over the nuclear envelope. The signals mediated by the regulatory proteins that are imported into the nucleus are transferred to some specific transcription factors that direct transcription of a subset of genes. Accumulating evidence suggests that histone acetylation is necessary for the signal-mediated induction of gene expression.

Identification of target molecules of antitumor drugs sometimes provides new insights into cancer therapy. *Streptomyces* produces a variety of metabolites, some of which are employed as chemical probes for analysis of coordinated mechanisms to control cellular responses in higher eukaryotes as well as drugs for therapeutics including anticancer agents. We isolated trichostatin A (TSA) and leptomoycin B

[a]Address for correspondence: Minoru Yoshida, Department of Biotechnology, Graduate School of Agriculture and Life Sciences, University of Tokyo, Yayoi 1-1-1, Bunkyo-ku, Tokyo 113, Japan. Phone, +81-3-5841-5124; fax, +81-3-5841-5337.
e-mail, ayoshida@mail.ecc.u-tokyo.ac.jp

(LMB) from *Streptomyces* metabolites as inducers of leukemia cell differentiation and morphologic abnormalities in fungi, respectively. TSA and LMB blocked the cell cycle at both G1 and G2 phases. We have identified histone deacetylase (HDAC) and CRM1/exportin as the targets of TSA and LMB, respectively. The importance of these proteins in signal transduction and signal-mediated gene expression is discussed.

HISTONE DEACETYLASE: THE TARGET OF TRICHOSTATIN A

TSA was originally isolated from *Streptomyces hygroscopicus* as an antifungal antibiotic active against *Trichophyton*[1,2] (FIG. 1). About 10 years later, very potent activities of TSA in inducing differentiation of Friend murine erythroleukemia (MEL) cells and inhibiting cell proliferation of mammalian cells were found.[3] The skeletal structure of TSA possesses a chiral center at the 6 position. Natural TSA was *R* configuration, whereas its antipode (*S*)-TSA was biologically inactive.[4] A low effective concentration and strict structural specificity of (*R*)-TSA suggest the presence of a specific target molecule to which (*R*)-TSA binds.[5]

A clue to understanding the target of TSA was incidentally obtained from analysis of the modification of histones. Acid urea Triton (AUT) gel electrophoresis which can separate core histone molecules with different extents of acetylation revealed that the histones in the cells treated with TSA were acetylated to an unusually high extent. Pulse-chase experiments revealed that histone hyperacetylation induced by TSA was due not to increased acetylation but to decreased deacetylation of histones. *In vitro* experiments using partially purified HDAC from mouse mammary tumor cells (FM3A) showed that TSA was a potent inhibitor with a K_i value of 3.4 nM, which almost corresponded to the *in vivo* effective concentrations of TSA. Furthermore, we derived a TSA-resistant mutant cell line, named TR303, from FM3A and found that the HDAC from the mutant cells possessed the markedly increased K_i value of 31 nM, indicating that the enzyme itself had changed to being resistant to TSA. This genetic evidence clearly indicated that HDAC is the primary target of TSA.[6] TSA at nanomolar concentrations causes an increase in the acetylation of all histones that are naturally acetylated *in vivo*. The very potent activity of TSA with high specificity allows its use as a well-defined biochemical probe for histone acetylation instead of butyrate.[7]

Identification of HDAC as the target of TSA led to the hypothesis that HDAC is essential for the cell cycle progression and is involved in oncogenesis. This was further supported by the discovery of another inhibitor of HDAC, whose structure is different from that of TSA. Trapoxins A and B, novel cyclic tetrapeptides (FIG. 1), were isolated from fungal metabolites as agents inducing morphologic reversion of v-*sis*-transformed NIH3T3 cells.[8] Since TSA was also reported to possess similar activity in inducing morphologic reversion of v-*sis*-transformed cells, we examined the similarity between the molecular action of these agents. Trapoxin A (TPX) caused the accumulation of highly acetylated core histones in a variety of mammalian cells. *In vitro* experiments using partially purified HDAC showed that a low concentration of TPX irreversibly inhibited deacetylation of acetylated histone molecules, in contrast to the reversible inhibition by TSA. Kinetic analysis indicates that TPX is classified

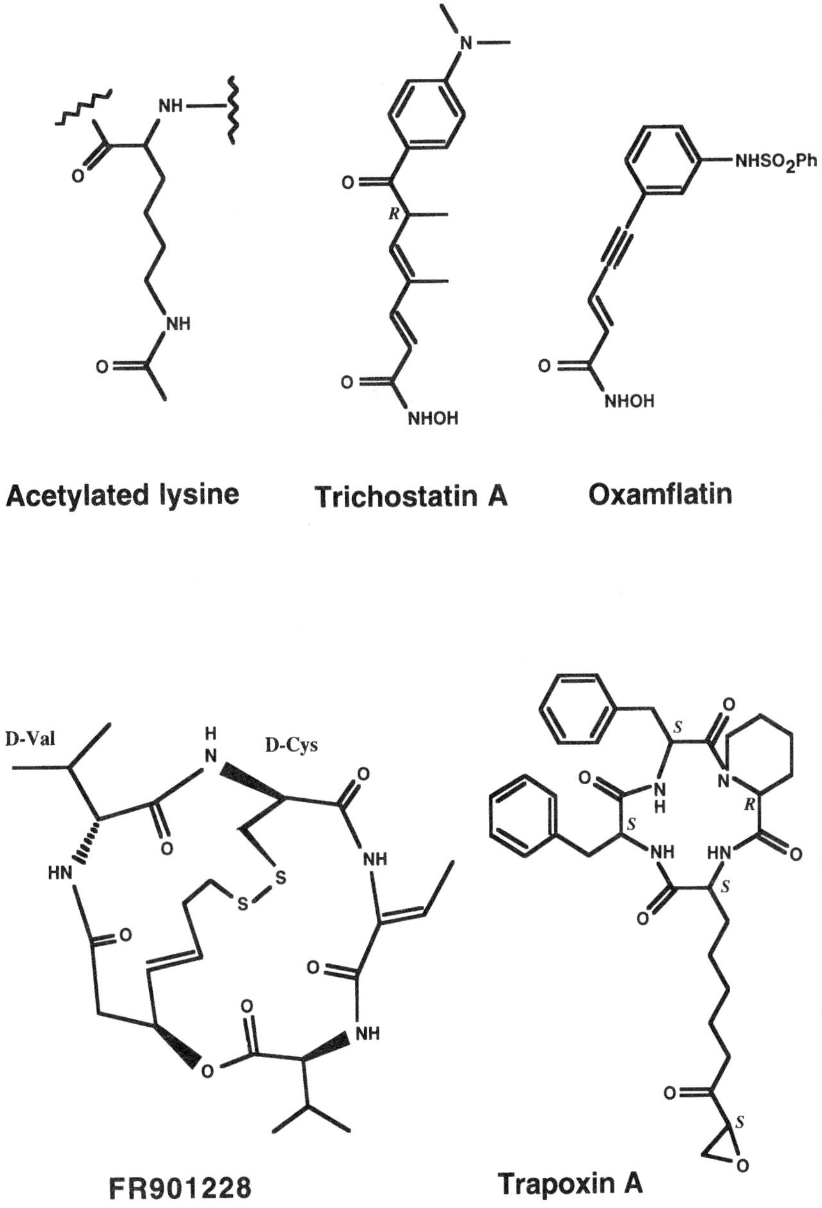
Acetylated lysine
Trichostatin A
Oxamflatin
D-Val
D-Cys
FR901228
Trapoxin A

FIGURE 1. Structures of HDAC inhibitors.

as a "slow-binding inhibitor." TPX contains an unusual amino acid, 2-amino-8-oxo-9,10-epoxy-decanoic acid (AOE), which may act as a lysine substrate mimic (FIG. 1). Thus, TPX is a new additional member of specific inhibitors of HDAC.[9] Interest-

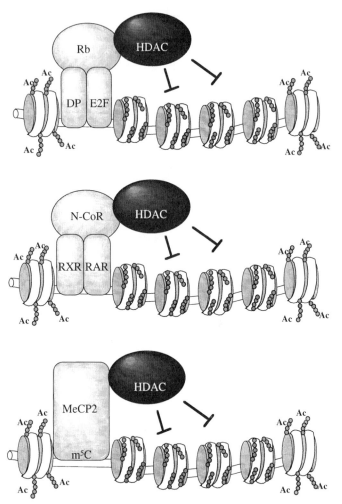

FIGURE 2. Transcriptional repression by HDAC recruited to the specific DNA sequences.

ingly, all the biologic activities of TPX were almost identical to those of TSA, indicating the importance of HDAC in the cell cycle and in cell differentiation.

Recently, several histone acetyltransferases (HATs) were cloned and were found to be identical or related to the transcriptional coactivators. These findings imply that HATs are complexed with other proteins and recruited by sequence-specific transcription factors to the promoter and/or enhancer regions, which are directly involved in transcriptional "on" signals.[10] Conversely, the hypothesis that core histone deacetylation leads to transcriptional repression was shown to be partly consistent with the observation that a mammalian HDAC, HDAC1, is related to the yeast RPD3,[11] which is required for full repression as well as full activation of gene expression. Search of the yeast genome database revealed that at least three other ho-

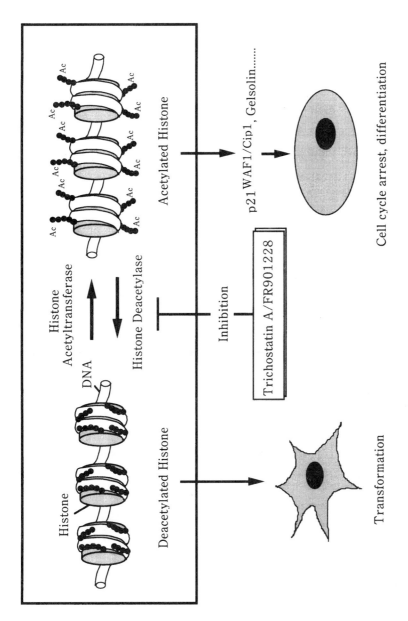

FIGURE 3. A model for the cell cycle arrest and antitumor activity induced by HDAC inhibitors.

mologs, HOS1, HOS2, and HOS3, in addition to two known HDAC genes, RPD3 and HDA1, are present in yeast; however, their enzymatic activity is yet unidentified. These results suggest that HDAC genes constitute a gene family like HAT genes. Mammalian HDAC also forms large protein complexes. The affinity-purified HDAC1 was complexed with RbAp48,[11] whereas HDAC2, also known as mRPD3, was identified as a binding protein for YY1, a sequence-specific DNA-binding protein that acts as both a repressor and an activator.[12] More recently, HDAC complexes were found to be associated with several sequence-specific DNA binding repressors, such as E2F-pRb,[13,14] nuclear receptors without ligands,[15,16] and methylated CpG binding protein (MeCP2).[17] Inhibition of HDAC activity by TSA or TPX alleviated the transcriptional repression directed by the DNA-bound repressors. Thus, HDAC can be recruited by the sequence-specific transcriptional repressors to promoters, which causes deacetylation of core histones, leading to gene-specific or chromatin region-specific transcriptional repression (FIG. 2).

TSA INDUCES ELEVATED EXPRESSION OF P21 AND GELSOLIN

All known HDAC inhibitors induce G1 cell cycle arrest and morphologic changes in various cell lines.[9,18-20] However, it is unclear how the induced hyperacetylation leads to this arrest. Recent studies have shown that HAT acts as a transcriptional co-activator, whereas HDAC acts as the corepressor.[10] Therefore, it seems reasonable that HDAC inhibitors exhibit various biologic activities by directly affecting the transcription of some endogenous genes. We analyzed the expression of several en-dogenous genes mainly related to cell cycle control by reverse transcriptase-poly-merase chain reaction (RT-PCR) or Western blotting. Both mRNA and the protein levels of Cdc2, Cdk2, Cdk4, and Cdk6 were unchanged upon treatment of HeLa cells with 0.5 µg/ml of TSA for 24 hours. On the other hand, gelsolin, cyclin E, p21Waf1/Cip1, and p16INK4A were obviously upregulated. By contrast, cyclins A and D1 were downregulated in a dose-dependent manner. The induction of p21 by TSA was independent of p53. Deletion analysis of the p21 promoter region showed that sev-eral Sp1 binding elements adjacent to the TATA box are necessary for the TSA-in-duced p21 expression. The p21 level correlated well with cell cycle arrest rather than accumulation of acetylated histone species, suggesting that p21 induction is involved in the TSA-induced cell cycle arrest. In addition to p21, gelsolin expression was also activated by TSA in a dose-dependent manner.[21] We further analyzed the expression of other actin regulatory proteins, such as α-actinin, cofilin, and profilin, by Western blotting. No protein other than gelsolin was affected by TSA. These results suggest that the drastic changes in the intracellular protein levels of a small subset of the im-portant regulators of the cell cycle and cell morphology are associated with the cell cycle arrest and morphologic changes caused by HDAC inhibitors (FIG. 3).

CLINICAL POSSIBILITY OF HDAC INHIBITORS

Molecular analyses of human diseases have suggested that changes in acetylation may play a role in the uncontrolled cell growth of cancer. For example, BRCA2, a breast cancer suppressor gene, encodes HAT.[22] One copy of the CBP gene was mutated in the Rubinstein-Taybi syndrome, which is accompanied by unusual incidence of neoplasms.[23] These findings suggest that some HATs are involved in tumor suppression and that inhibition of HDAC results in antitumor effects.

The potent activity of TSA or TPX in inducing cell cycle arrest and subsequent apoptotic cell death suggests its potential usefulness in cancer chemotherapy. However, TSA and TPX *per se* were not sufficiently effective in experimental tumor models, probably because of their instability. Recently, a promising antitumor agent was found to be a new HDAC inhibitor. FR901228 (FIG. 1) was isolated from *Chromobacterium violaceum* as an agent inducing morphologic reversion of H-*ras*-transformed NIH3T3 cells.[24–26] FR901228 also strongly inhibited proliferation of tumor cells *in vitro* by arresting cell cycle transition at G1 and G2. In addition, FR901228 greatly enhanced transcription from the SV40 promoter, as does TSA.[27] FR901228 inhibited HDAC partially purified from cells in a dose-dependent manner.[20] Thus, FR901228, a cyclic depsipeptide lacking both AOE and a hydroxamate group, is a novel inhibitor of HDAC, structurally distinct from known inhibitors. Since the antitumor activity of FR901228 against xenografted human solid tumors was remarkable,[26] the antitumor potential of FR901228 is further evaluated at the National Cancer Institute (Bethesda, Maryland). FR901228 is now undergoing clinical trials for cancer therapy. Identification of FR901228 as an HDAC inhibitor with potent antitumor activity implies that HDAC is an attractive target for cancer therapy and that the potential activity of TSA, TPX derivatives, and short-chain fatty acids may be improved by chemical modification.

CRM1/EXPORTIN 1: THE TARGET OF LEPTOMYCIN B (LMB)

Leptomycins A and B (FIG. 4) were originally discovered during the course of screening for antifungal antibiotics.[28] The chemical structures of these compounds are unsaturated long-chain fatty acids with a terminal δ-lactone ring.[29] Leptomycin B (LMB) was the major active compound that inhibited fungal growth. A characteristic feature of these compounds is their ability to induce morphologic abnormalities

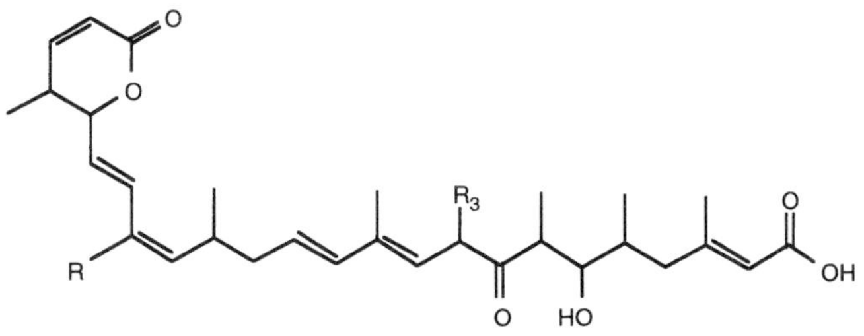

Leptomycin A   (LMA, R=CH$_3$)
Leptomycin B   (LMB, R=CH$_2$CH$_3$)

FIGURE 4. Structures of leptomycins.

in yeast and fungi such as cell elongation of the fission yeast *Schizosaccharomyces pombe*.[30] LMB also causes *in vitro* G1 cell cycle arrest in various mammalian cells at nanomolar concentrations and *in vivo* antitumor activity against several murine experimental tumors[31,32] Following the discovery of LMB, several related compounds were isolated as potent antitumor agents.

Potent antiproliferative activity of LMB against both lower and higher eukaryotes suggests that the target molecule of LMB is highly conserved in eukaryotes and plays an important role in cell cycle control. To approach the target, we took advantage of the fission yeast molecular genetic system, because *S. pombe* is one of the most sensitive organisms to LMB. We isolated an LMB-resistant gene from an LMB-resistant mutant of *S. pombe*, which conferred LMB resistance on wild-type *S. pombe*. The gene thus cloned was a mutant of *crm1+*, which had originally been reported as a gene essential for chromosome region maintenance. Cold-sensitive *crm1* mutants were isolated during visual screening by means of DAPI staining, which showed deformed filamentous or fragmented nuclear structures at the restrictive temperature.[33] The *crm1+* gene encodes a 115- kD protein that is essential for proliferation of *S. pombe* and is localized in the nucleus and its periphery. Crm1 is involved in the regulation of not only nuclear structure but also specific gene activity; the *crm1* mutants produce an increased amount of p25 whose expression is regulated by an AP-1-like transcription factor. Genetic analysis demonstrated that Crm1 was a negative regulator of Pap1, the *S. pombe* AP-1 homolog.[34,35] Treatment of wild-type *S. pombe* with LMB caused abnormal nuclear morphology and p25 overproduction, which were almost identical to the terminal phenotypes of *crm1* mutants. Taken together, we propose that Crm1 or its regulatory cascade is the cellular target of LMB.[36] However, the molecular function of Crm1 was still unclear.

We next cloned cDNA encoding a functional mammalian homolog of Crm1.[37] The cloned cDNA, named human CRM1 (hCRM1), complemented the *S. pombe crm1* mutation and caused growth inhibition and morphologic abnormalities in *S. pombe* when overproduced. The mammalian *CRM1* gene was ubiquitously transcribed in all the tissues tested, and its transcription level in cultured cells was regulated during the cell cycle. hCRM1 expressed in mammalian cells localized preferentially in the nuclear envelope. Recently, Wolff *et al.*[38] reported that LMB inhibited nuclear export of the human immunodeficiency virus type 1 (HIV-1) Rev protein and Rev-dependent mRNA. Rev contains an NES that may be recognized by the host nuclear export machinery.[39] This finding raised the possibility that mammalian CRM1 is involved in nuclear export of proteins and that the cell cycle arrest of mammalian cells by LMB is ascribable to inhibition of the mammalian CRM1 function.

CRM1/EXPORTIN 1 IS ESSENTIAL FOR NUCLEAR EXPORT OF PROTEINS

We showed that LMB inhibited nuclear export of not only HIV-1 Rev but also other cellular proteins such as MAPKK and PKIα, when GFP-fusion proteins bearing NESs were injected into the nucleus.[40,41] These results indicate that LMB is a general nuclear export inhibitor. To confirm that CRM1 is the target of LMB, we tested whether LMB binds directly to hCRM1.[41] A biotinylated derivative of LMB binds to a protein that reacts with an anti-hCRM1 antibody but not in the presence of 100-fold excess LMB. Microinjection of a purified anti-hCRM1 antibody as well as LMB specifically inhibited nuclear export of NES-containing proteins. Furthermore, the fission yeast *crm1* mutant was defective in the nuclear export of NES-fused proteins but not in the import of NLS-fused proteins. Interestingly, the protein containing both the NES and the NLS that would shuttle between the nucleus and the cytoplasm was highly accumulated in the nucleus in the *crm1* mutant cells or the cells treated with LMB. Finally, we showed interaction of CRM1 with NES by employing the immobilized NES and HeLa cell extracts. This association was disrupted by adding LMB or the purified anti-hCRM1 antibody.[41] These results together with those by others show that CRM1, like importin β for import, is an essential factor for nuclear export of proteins in all eukaryotes.[40–44] Thus, CRM1 has been called exportin 1.

A model for nuclear protein import and export is illustrated in FIGURE 5. The import of proteins into the nucleus occurs through nuclear pore complexes (NPC) which allow diffusion of small molecules and can accommodate the active transport of particles as large as several million daltons in weight.[45,46] The active import is energy dependent and is conferred by virtue of the NLS, which is rich in basic amino acids. Translocation of the NLS-bearing protein into the nucleoplasm is mediated by the saturable import machinery that recognizes basic NLSs.[47] The import receptor for the NLS was identified as a heterodimeric complex of importin α and importin β (also known as karyopherin α and β, or PTACs). Importin α recognizes and binds basic NLSs, whereas importin β mediates docking of the cargo-importin complex

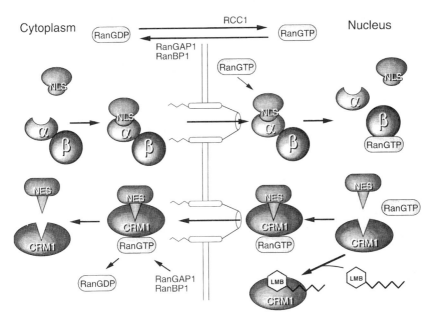

FIGURE 5. A model for nucleocytoplasmic transport and molecular action of LMB.

with the NPC in a temperature-independent manner. Translocation into the nucleoplasm is mediated by the Ran GTPase cycle and requires energy in the form of GTP hydrolysis.[48,49] Importin β binds directly to the NPC and Ran-GTP. In turn, Ran-GTP binding to importin β dissociates the importin α-β heterodimer.[50,51] Ran-GTP binds to the amino terminus of importin β, whereas importin α binds to the carboxy-terminal region of importin β. Release of importin α upon Ran-GTP binding to importin β is therefore probably explained by a conformational change in importin β. CRM1/exportin 1 shares low but significant homology to importin β.[52,53] CRM1/exportin 1 conveys NES-bearing proteins through the NPC in a Ran-GTP–dependent manner.the GTP hydrolysis that may occur in the cytoplasm likely dissociates the cargo-CRM1/exportin 1 complex. In contrast to the import system mediated by the importin heterodimer, CRM1/exportin 1 alone can associate with both a cargo and a Ran-GTP (FIG. 5). LMB binds to CRM1/exportin 1, thereby inhibiting cargo loading and subsequent nuclear export.

ROLE FOR LMB AS A CHEMICAL PROBE

Increased evidence suggests that many signaling molecules have the NLS or the NES, or both, by which they relocalize in response to various stimuli. For instance, unstimulated MEK binds and anchors MAPK in the cytoplasm by its NES. The phosphorylated, activated MAPK can be released from MEK and enter the nucleus, but it is still unclear how MAPK dissociates from the complex.[40,54] An NES in cyclin B1[55,56] is inactivated by phosphorylation of the amino-terminal region of the protein, which allows nuclear translocation of cyclin B1/Cdc2 complex upon the onset of mitosis.[57] Recently, we showed that Pap1, an *S. pombe* bZip transcription factor, contained both an NLS and an NES, whose transcriptional activity was negatively regulated by CRM1/exportin 1-dependent cytoplasmic localization. Surprisingly, the nuclear export of Pap1 was abolished by a subset of oxidants, suggesting that the Pap1 NES is sensitive to oxidative stress. The oxidative stress response of the Pap1 NES is conserved through evolution, as GFP-fused proteins bearing the Pap1 NES expressed in mammalian cells responded to the oxidants. Thus, LMB played and will continue to play a particularly important role in identifying NES-bearing proteins.

The mechanisms by which LMB induces G1 and/or G2 arrest of the cell cycle and the antitumor effects are still unclear. CAN/Nup214, the product of a human oncogene associated with myeloid leukemia that is activated by translocation (6;9) with other genes,[58] was shown to be complexed with CRM1/exportin 1.[59] CAN/Nup214 is a member of nucleoporins, the components of the NPC.[60] This finding suggests that nucleocytoplasmic transport itself is one of the targets of oncogenesis. Inhibition of the nuclear export of some regulatory proteins involved in cell cycle control and oncogenesis is likely responsible for the cell cycle arrest and tumor suppression by LMB and its derivatives. One candidate may be p53, in which we recently found an NES that allows shuttling of p53 between the nucleus and the cytoplasm. Identification of the substrate proteins responsible for cell cycle arrest and antitumor activity is obviously important for future development of antitumor agents.

CONCLUSIONS

TSA is shown to be a specific inhibitor of HDAC and LMB as an inhibitor of CRM1/exportin 1. TSA and LMB will continue to play an important part in understanding the roles of these proteins in cell cycle control and oncogenesis. Our study suggests that the cycles of histone acetylation/deacetylation and protein nuclear import/export will be potential targets for anticancer drugs. However, it is still unclear how many isozymes are present in human cells and how different their substrate specificities are. Perhaps isozyme-specific inhibitors may be more effective as chemotherapeutic drugs. In addition, we have not yet seen what happens if cellular HAT activity or protein nuclear import is inhibited. Inhibitors of HAT or protein import would also be extremely useful in understanding their roles in cell cycle control and oncogenesis.

REFERENCES

1. Tsuji, N., M. Kobayashi, K. Nagashima et al. 1976. A new antifungal antibiotic, trichostatin. J. Antibiot. **29**: 1–6.
2. Tsuji, N. & M. Kobayashi. 1978. Trichostatin C, a glucopyranosyl hydroxamate. J. Antibiot. **31**: 939–944.
3. Yoshida, M., S. Nomura & T. Beppu. 1987. Effects of trichostatins on differentiation of murine erythroleukemia cells. Cancer Res. **47**: 3688–3691.
4. Mori, K. & K. Koseki. 1988. Synthesis of trichostatin A, a potent differentiation inducer of Friend leukemic cells, and its antipode. Tetrahedron **44**: 6013–6020.
5. Yoshida, M., Y. Hoshikawa, K. Koseki et al. 1990. Structural specificity for biological activity of trichostatin A, a specific inhibitor of mammalian cell cycle with potent differentiation-inducing activity in Friend leukemia cells. J. Antibiot. **43**: 1101–1106.
6. Yoshida, M., M. Kijima, M. Akita et al. 1990. Potent and specific inhibition of mammalian histone deacetylase both in vivo and in vitro by trichostatin A. J. Biol. Chem. **265**: 17174–17179.
7. Yoshida, M., S. Horinouchi & T. Beppu. 1995. Trichostatin A and trapoxin: Novel chemical probes for the role of histone acetylation in chromatin structure and function. BioEssays **17**: 423–430.
8. Itazaki, H., K. Nagashima, K. Sugita et al. 1990. Isolation and structural elucidation of new cyclotetrapeptides, trapoxins A and B, having detransformation activities as antitumor agents. J. Antibiot. **43**: 1524–1532.
9. Kijima, M., M. Yoshida, K. Sugita et al. 1993. Trapoxin, an antitumor cyclic tetrapeptide, is an irreversible inhibitor of mammalian histone deacetylase. J. Biol. Chem. **268**: 22429–22435.
10. Grunstein, M. 1997. Histone acetylation in chromatin structure and transcription. Nature **389**: 349–352.
11. Taunton, J., C.A. Hassig & S.L. Schreiber. 1996. A mammalian histone deacetylase related to the yeast transcriptional regulator Rpd3p. Science **272**: 408–411.
12. Yang, W., C. Inouye, Y. Zeng et al. 1996. Transcriptional repression by YY1 is mediated by interaction with the mammalian homolog of the yeast global regulator RPD3. Proc. Natl. Acad. Sci. USA **93**: 12845–12850.
13. Magnaghi, J.L., R. Groisman, I. Naguibneva et al. 1998. Retinoblastoma protein represses transcription by recruiting a histone deacetylase. Nature **391**: 601–605.
14. Brehm, A., E.A. Miska, D.J. McCance et al. 1998. Retinoblastoma protein recruits histone deacetylase to repress transcription. Nature **391**: 597–601.
15. Nagy, L., H.Y. Kao, D. Chakravarti et al. 1997. Nuclear receptor repression mediated by a complex containing SMRT, mSin3A, and histone deacetylase. Cell **89**: 373–380.

16. CHEN, H., R.J. LIN, R.L. SCHILTZ et al. 1997. Nuclear receptor coactivator ACTR is a novel histone acetyltransferase and forms a multimeric activation complex with P/CAF and CBP/p300. Cell **90:** 569–580.

17. NAN, X., H.H. NG, C.A. JOHNSON et al. 1998. Transcriptional repression by the methyl-Cpg-binding protein Mecp2 involves a histone deacetylase complex. Nature **393:** 386–389.

18. FALLON, R.J. & R.P. COX. 1979. Cell cycle analysis of sodium butyrate and hydroxyurea, inducers of ectopic hormone production in HeLa cells. J. Cell. Physiol. **100:** 251–262.

19. YOSHIDA, M. & T. BEPPU. 1988. Reversible arrest of proliferation of rat 3Y1 fibroblasts in both the G1 and G2 phases by trichostatin A. Exp. Cell Res. **177:** 122–131.

20. NAKAJIMA, H., Y.B. KIM, H. TERANO et al. 1998. FR901228, a potent antitumor antibiotic, is a novel histone deacetylase inhibitor. Exp. Cell Res. **241:** 126–133.

21. HOSHIKAWA, Y., H.J. KWON, M. YOSHIDA et al. 1994. Trichostatin A induces morphological changes and gelsolin expression by inhibiting histone deacetylase in human carcinoma cell lines. Exp. Cell Res. **214:** 189–197.

22. SIDDIQUE, H., J.P. ZOU, V.N. RAO et al. 1998. The BRCA2 is a histone acetyltransferase. Oncogene **16:** 2283–2285.

23. PETRIJ, F., R.H. GILES, H.G. DAUWERSE et al. 1995. Rubinstein-Taybi syndrome caused by mutations in the transcriptional co-activator CBP. Nature **376:** 348–351.

24. UEDA, M., H. NAKAJIMA, Y. HORI et al. 1994. FR901228, a novel antitumor bicyclic depsipeptide produced by *Chromobacterium violaceum* No. 968. I. Taxonomy, fermentation, isolation, physico-chemical and biological properties, and antitumor activity. J. Antibiot. **47:** 301–310.

25. SHIGEMATSU, N., H. UEDA, S. TAKASE et al. 1994. FR901228, a novel antitumor bicyclic depsipeptide produced by *Chromobacterium violaceum* No. 968. II. Structure determination. J. Antibiot. **47:** 311–314.

26. UEDA, H., T. MANDA, S. MATSUMOTO et al. 1994. FR901228, a novel antitumor bicyclic depsipeptide produced by *Chromobacterium violaceum* No. 968. III. Antitumor activities on experimental tumors in mice. J. Antibiot. **47:** 315–323.

27. SCHLAKE, T., W.D. KLEHR, M. YOSHIDA et al. 1994. Gene expression within a chromatin domain: the role of core histone hyperacetylation. Biochemistry **33:** 4197–4206.

28. HAMAMOTO, T., S. GUNJI, H. TSUJI et al. 1983. Leptomycins A and B, new antifungal antibiotics. I. Taxonomy of the producing strain and their fermentation, purification and characterization. J. Antibiot. **36:** 639–645.

29. HAMAMOTO, T., H. SETO & T. BEPPU. 1983. Leptomycins A and B, new antifungal antibiotics. II. Structure elucidation. J. Antibiot. **36:** 646–650.

30. HAMAMOTO, T., T. UOZUMI & T. BEPPU. 1985. Leptomycins A and B, new antifungal antibiotics. III. Mode of action of leptomycin B on *Schizosaccharomyces pombe*. J. Antibiot. **38:** 1573–1580.

31. YOSHIDA, M., M. NISHIKAWA, K. NISHI et al. 1990. Effects of leptomycin B on the cell cycle of fibroblasts and fission yeast cells. Exp. Cell Res. **187:** 150–156.

32. KOMIYAMA, K., K. OKADA, S. TOMISAKA et al. 1985. Antitumor activity of leptomycin B. J. Antibiot. **38:** 427–429.

33. ADACHI, Y. & M. YANAGIDA. 1989. Higher order chromosome structure is affected by cold-sensitive mutations in a *Schizosaccharomyces pombe* gene crm1+ which encodes a 115-kD protein preferentially localized in the nucleus and at its periphery. J. Cell Biol. **108:** 1195–1207.

34. TODA, T., M. SHIMANUKI, Y. SAKA et al. 1992. Fission yeast pap1-dependent transcription is negatively regulated by an essential nuclear protein, crm1. Mol. Cell. Biol. **12:** 5474–5484.

35. KUMADA, K., M. YANAGIDA & T. TODA. 1996. Caffeine-resistance in fission yeast is caused by mutations in a single essential gene, crm1+. Mol. Gen. Genet. **250:** 59–68.

36. NISHI, K., M. YOSHIDA, D. FUJIWARA et al. 1994. Leptomycin B targets a regulatory cascade of crm1, a fission yeast nuclear protein, involved in control of higher order chromosome structure and gene expression. J. Biol. Chem. **269:** 6320–6324.

37. KUDO, N., S. KHOCHBIN, K. NISHI et al. 1997. Molecular cloning and cell cycle-dependent expression of mammalian CRM1, a protein involved in nuclear export of proteins. J. Biol. Chem. **272:** 29742–29751.

38. WOLFF, B., J.-J. SANGLIER & Y. WANG. 1997. Leptomycin B is an inhibitor of nuclear export: inhibition of nucleo-cytoplasmic translocation of the human immunodeficiency virus type 1 (HIV-1) Rev protein and Rev-dependent mRNA. Chem. Biol. **4:** 139–147.

39. FISCHER, U., J. HUBER, W.C. BOELENS et al. 1995. The HIV-1 Rev activation domain is a nuclear export signal that accesses an export pathway used by specific cellular RNAs. Cell **82:** 475–483.

40. FUKUDA, M., S. ASANO, T. NAKAMURA et al. 1997. CRM1 is responsible for intracellular transport mediated by the nuclear export signal. Nature **390:** 308–311.

41. KUDO, N., B. WOLFF, T. SEKIMOTO et al. 1998. Leptomycin B inhibition of signal-mediated nuclear export by direct binding to CRM1. Exp. Cell Res. **242:** 540–547.

42. FORNEROD, M., M. OHNO, M. YOSHIDA et al. 1997. CRM1 is an export receptor for leucine-rich nuclear export signals. Cell **90:** 1051–1060.

43. OSSAREH-NAZARI, B., F. BACHELERIE & C. DARGEMONT. 1997. Evidence for a role of CRM1 in signal-mediated nuclear protein export. Science **278:** 141–144.

44. STADE, K., C.S. FORD, C. GUTHRIE et al. 1997. Exportin 1 (Crm1p) is an essential nuclear export factor. Cell **90:** 1041–1050.

45. DWORETZKY, S.I., R.E. LANFORD & C.M. FELDHERR. 1988. The effects of variations in the number and sequence of targeting signals on nuclear uptake. J. Cell Biol. **107:** 1279–1287.

46. ROUT, M.P. & S.R. WENTE. 1994. Pores for thought: nuclear pore complex proteins. Trends Cell Biol. **4:** 357–365.

47. DINGWALL, C. & R.A. LASKEY. 1991. Nuclear targeting sequences - a consensus? Trends Biochem. Sci. **16:** 478–481.

48. GÖRLICH, D. & I.W. MATTAJ. 1996. Nucleocytoplasmic transport. Science **271:** 1513–1518.

49. MELCHIOR, R. & L. GERACE. 1995. Mechanisms of nuclear protein import. Curr. Opin. Cell Biol. **7:** 310–318.

50. GÖRLICH, D., N. PANTE, U. KUTAY et al. 1996. Identification of different roles for RanGDP and RanGTP in nuclear protein import. EMBO J. **15:** 5584–5594.

51. REXACH, M. & G. BLOBEL. 1995. Protein import into nuclei: Association and dissociation reactions involving transport substrate, transport factors, and nucleoporins. Cell **83:** 683–692.

52. GÖRLICH, D., F. VOGEL, A.D. MILLS et al. 1995. Distinct functions for the two importin subunits in nuclear protein import. Nature **377:** 246–248.

53. MOROIANU, J., M. HIJIKATA, G. BLOBEL et al. 1995. Mammalian karyopherin α1b and α2b heterodimers: α1 or α2 subunit binds nuclear localization sequence and β subunit interacts with peptide repeat containing nucleoporins. Proc. Natl. Acad. Sci. USA **92:** 6532–6536.

54. FUKUDA, M., I. GOTOH, Y. GOTOH et al. 1996. Cytoplasmic localization of mitogen-activated protein kinase kinase directed by its NH2-terminal, leucine-rich short amino acid sequence, which acts as a nuclear export signal. J. Biol. Chem. **271:** 20024–20028.

55. HAGTING, A., C. KARLSSON, P. CLUTE et al. 1998. MPF localization is controlled by nuclear export. EMBO J. **17:** 4127–4138.
56. TOYOSHIMA, F., T. MORIGUCHI, A. WADA et al. 1998. Nuclear export of cyclin B1 and its possible role in the DNA damage- induced G2 checkpoint. EMBO J. **17:** 2728–2735.
57. YANG, J., E.S. BARDES, J.D. MOORE et al. 1998. Control of cyclin B1 localization through regulated binding of the nuclear export factor CRM1. Genes Dev. **12:** 2131–2143.
58. VON LINDERN, M., S. VAN BAAL, J. WIEGANT et al. 1992. Can, a putative oncogene associated with myeloid leukemogenesis, may be activated by fusion of its 3' half to different genes: Characterization of the set gene. Mol. Cell. Biol. **12:** 3346–3355.
59. FORNEROD, M., J.VAN DEURSEN, S.VAN BAAL et al. 1997. The human homologue of yeast CRM1 is in a dynamic subcomplex with CAN/Nup214 and a novel nuclear pore component Nup88. EMBO J. **16:** 807–816.
60. FORNEROD, M., J. BOER, S. VAN BAAL et al. 1996. Interaction of cellular proteins with the leukemia specific fusion proteins DEK-CAN and SET-CAN and their normal counterpart, the nucleoporin CAN. Oncogene **13:** 1801–1808.

The Dual Role of Cytoskeletal Anchor Proteins in Cell Adhesion and Signal Transduction

AVRI BEN-ZE'EV[a]

Department of Molecular Cell Biology, The Weizmann Institute of Science, Rehovot, 76100, Israel

ABSTRACT: β-Catenin and plakoglobin are homologous proteins having a dual role in cell adhesion and in transactivation together with LEF/TCF transcription factors. Overexpression of plakoglobin suppresses tumorigenicity, whereas increased β-catenin levels are considered oncogenic. We compared the nuclear translocation and transactivation by β-catenin and plakoglobin. Overexpression of each protein resulted in nuclear translocation and formation of structures that also contained LEF-1 and vinculin with β-catenin, but not with plakoglobin. Transfection of LEF-1 translocated endogenous β-catenin, but not plakoglobin into the nucleus. Chimeras of the Gal4 DNA-binding domain and the transactivation domains of either plakoglobin or β-catenin were equally potent in transactivation, but induction of LEF-1–responsive transcription was higher with β-catenin. Overexpression of wt plakoglobin or mutant β-catenin lacking the transactivation domain induced nuclear accumulation of the enodogenous β-catenin and LEF-1–responsive transactivation. The nuclear localization and constitutive β-catenin–dependent transactivation in SW480 cancer cells were inhibited by overexpressing cadherin or α-catenin. Moreover, transfecting the cytoplasmic tail of cadherin inhibited transactivation, by competition with LEF-1 in the nucleus for β-catenin binding. The results indicate that (1) plakoglobin and β-catenin differ in nuclear translocation and complexing with LEF-1 and vinculin, (2) LEF-1–dependent transactivation is mainly driven by β-catenin, (3) cadherin and α-catenin can sequester β-catenin, inhibit its transcriptional activity, and antagonize its oncogenic action.

INTRODUCTION

The form and structure of complex tissues and the interactions between their constituent cells are major features that distinguish unicellular from multicellular organisms.[1–4] Therefore, investigation of the mechanisms that determine the organization of the cytoskeleton and its linkage via cytoskeletal anchor proteins to cell adhesion sites is important for our understanding of how genetic information is translated into the three-dimensional organization and function of cells in tissues. Changes in cytoarchitecture are characteristic of cell motility, growth activation, differentiation, and cell transformation.[5–8] Malignant transformation is often associated with altered cytoskeletal organization and adhesion, and "anchorage dependence" and "contact inhibition of growth" are disrupted in many cancer cells. In our laboratory, we are studying the regulation of cytoskeletal anchor proteins that link the cytoskeleton to

[a]Address for correspondence: phone, 972-8-934-2422; fax, 972-8-946-5261.
e-mail, Lgbenzev@weizmann.weizmann.ac.il

cell adhesion receptors, with particular emphasis on the role of changes in the expression of these anchor proteins in cell structure and function. Our experiments are addressing the possible regulatory (signaling) role of changes in the levels of these junctional plaque proteins in important cellular processes such as motility, growth, transformation, and gene expression.

TARGETED MODULATION OF VINCULIN EXPRESSION AND ITS EFFECT ON CELL BEHAVIOR

Our earlier studies have indicated that changes in the assembly and expression of cytoskeletal and junctional plaque proteins are important parts of the programs leading to cell differentiation and growth activation.[9–17] Since these architectural proteins are considered constitutive components of the cell and belong to the class of abundant and stable proteins, we examined their long-range effect on cells, when their expression was stably altered by molecular and classical genetic approaches.

Elimination of Vinculin Expression by Gene Disruption via Homologous Recombination

To study the role of vinculin in cell behavior, we targeted the vinculin genes in F9 embryonal carcinoma and in embryonic stem (ES) cells.[18] The vinculin-null F9 and ES cells displayed a significantly reduced rate of adhesion to ECM or fibronectin, and their spreading on the substrate, in long-term cultures, was reduced. These cells also displayed a reduced ability to extend lamellipodia, and time lapse video microscopy showed that they extend unstable filopodia. Under favorable conditions for adhesion, however, the vinculin-null F9 cells were able to form focal adhesions that appeared indistinguishable from those of wild-type F9 cells, by transmission electron microscopy (EM) and interference reflection microscopy. Fluorescence labeling for actin, talin, α-actinin, paxillin, and phosphotyrosinated proteins showed essentially the same organization for control and vinculin-null F9 cells. Quantitative digitized microscopic analysis indicated that the assembly of α-actinin, talin, and paxillin in focal adhesion of vinculin-null cells was higher than that in control F9 cells.[19] These results demonstrated that whereas vinculin has an important role in determining cell shape, adhesion and surface protrusive activity, alternative molecular mechanisms for adhesion plaque assembly are present in the absence of vinculin.

Modulation of Vinculin Expression Affects Cell Motility

We examined the motile properties of F9 vinculin (–/–) cells. The motility of vinculin-null F9 cells was elevated about 2.5-fold compared to that of wild-type F9. This increase in motility was also observed in F9 cells that were induced to differentiate into parietal endoderm with retinoic acid and cAMP.[18] Such cells are known to have increased motility, but when compared to vinculin-containing parietal endoderm cells, the vinculin-null cells exhibited a higher locomotion.

In parallel with studies employing a genetic approach to control vinculin expression in cells, we also isolated 3T3 cells either that stably overexpress transfected chicken vinculin[20] or in which vinculin expression was decreased to varying degrees (down to ~10% of control levels), by stably expressing an antisense vinculin cDNA.[21] 3T3 cells overexpressing vinculin displayed a significant increase in the number and size of focal adhesions and stress fibers.[22] The motility of such cells was decreased dramatically, although the level of exogenous vinculin constituted only ~20% of the endogenous protein.[20] On the basis of the cooperative model suggested for the assembly of focal adhesions in numerous studies, we hypothesize that a relatively modest increase in vinculin level could lead to massive recruitment into focal adhesions of other molecules known to bind vinculin (including vinculin itself, α-actinin, actin, talin, and paxillin). This could then lead to clustering of integrin receptors and stabilization of a stronger adhesion to the substrate, which would result in decreased motility.[23] We also examined the effect of reduced vinculin expression in 3T3 cells expressing antisense vinculin and found that cells expressing low vinculin levels are poorly spread and display fewer and smaller adhesion plaques compared to controls.[21] Furthermore, the motility of such cells was increased, supporting our results with vinculin knockout F9 cells. Because vinculin, when stably overexpressed in 3T3 cells, conferred an opposite phenotype (i.e., decreased motility and increased focal adhesion assembly),[20,22] this implies that vinculin may have an important role in regulating cell motility.

VINCULIN, α-ACTININ, AND THE TRANSFORMED PHENOTYPE

3T3 cells in which the level of vinculin was suppressed by antisense transfection, as just described, displayed numerous morphologic properties characteristic of transformed fibroblasts, including reduced adhesion and spreading on the substrate, poorly organized microfilaments, and fewer and smaller adhesion plaques, when compared to nontransformed 3T3 cells. In addition, such cells became anchorage independent (i.e., formed large colonies in soft agar with high efficiency), a property closely correlated with the tumorigenic ability of transformed fibroblasts, thus more closely linking changes in vinculin expression to cell transformation.

Suppression of α-Actinin Expression Confers Tumorigenicity in 3T3 Cells

In vitro binding studies have suggested that actin filaments are linked to the β₁ integrin receptor via talin, vinculin, and α-actinin or by direct binding of a specific domain on α-actinin to β₁ integrin.[24] Our studies with vinculin knockout cells are consistent with this view, as they have shown α-actinin assembled into the adhesion plaques of vinculin-null F9 cells.[19] We also transfected α-actinin into 3T3 cells and found a decrease in cell motility in cells overexpressing this protein.[25] Antisense transfection experiments with α-actinin cDNA yielded stable clones in culture, and these showed that cells with reduced α-actinin levels were capable of forming tumors in nude mice. The extent of α-actinin suppression correlated with the time required for tumor formation (the more extensive the decrease in α-actinin expression, the faster the tumors appeared).[25] Taken together, the antisense transfection studies with vinculin and α-actinin suggest that these submembranal cytoskeletal plaque proteins can act as effective suppressors of tumorigenicity.

Suppression of Tumorigenicity in Cancer Cells by Transfection with Vinculin or α-Actinin cDNAs

The phenotype of tumor cells is characterized by conspicuous changes in cell morphology, anchorage dependence, and microfilament structure. Whereas alterations in both cell structure and growth are inherent in transformed cells, the relationships between these two are not completely understood. We have addressed the question of whether changes in cell adhesion are responsible for the loss of adhesion-dependent growth control, by modulating in tumor cells the expression of vinculin or α-actinin, and analyzed their effect on the transformed phenotype.

Transfection of vinculin into SV40-transformed 3T3 cells (SVT2) that express reduced levels of vinculin or into a malignant metastatic adenocarcinoma cell line that expresses no vinculin, showed that restoration of vinculin to the level found in 3T3 cells resulted in increased adhesiveness to the substrate and stress fiber formation.[26] In addition, the ability of these cells to grow in soft agar was reduced, and when injected into syngeneic and nude mice, their tumorigenicity was completely suppressed when high levels of vinculin were expressed.[26] Similar results were obtained with transfecting α-actinin into SVT2 cells that have a greatly reduced level of this protein.[27] Upon transfection of cytoplasmic α-actinin, the tumorigenicity of the cells was inhibited in correlation with the level of expression of the transgene. These results suggest that junctional plaque proteins that mediate the structural link of the actin-cytoskeleton to cell adhesion sites can act as effective suppressors of the tumorigenic ability of cells transformed by oncogenes. The mechanisms underlying this new role for junctional plaque proteins is not known, but it could be exerted by influencing the assembly of adhesion plaques and the actin-cytoskeleton, which are suggested to be involved in adhesion-mediated signaling.[8]

PLAKOGLOBIN AND β-CATENIN: JUNCTIONAL PLAQUE PROTEINS AT CELL-CELL CONTACT SITES THAT ARE INVOLVED IN REGULATING TUMORIGENESIS

Cell-cell adhesion, together with cell-ECM adhesion, plays an important role in developing tissues and patterns of morphogenesis. In cultured cells, "contact inhibition of growth" is characteristic of nontransformed cells and is usually lost during cell transformation. Plakoglobin is a major component of the submembranal plaque of both adherens junctions and desmosomes in mammalian cells and links members of the cadherin cell-cell receptor family to the cytoskeleton[28] (FIG. 1A). Plakoglobin is closely related to the *Drosophila* segment polarity gene *armadillo* that has a role in the transduction of transmembrane signals elicited by the Wg/Wnt pathway that regulate cell fate in both flies and vertebrates.[29] Like its close homolog β-catenin, plakoglobin can associate with the tumor suppressor adenomatous polyposis coli (APC) protein that is linked to human colon cancer, and to members of the LEF/TCF family of transcription factors[30–34] (FIG. 1A).

We have studied the effect of plakoglobin overexpression, and the cooperation between plakoglobin and N-cadherin, on the morphology and tumorigenic ability of cells either lacking or expressing cadherin and α- and β-catenin.[35] Overexpression of plakoglobin in SV40-transformed 3T3 (SVT2) cells that possess cadherin and α- and β-

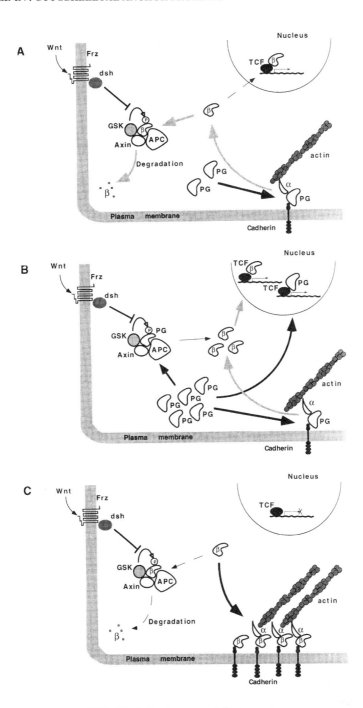

FIGURE 1. *See legend on following page.*

catenin suppressed the tumorigenicity of the cells in syngeneic mice. Transfection with N-cadherin conferred an epithelial phenotype on the cell culture, but it had no significant effect on the tumorigenicity of the cells. Cotransfection of plakoglobin and N-cadherin into SVT2 cells, however, was considerably more effective in tumor suppression than was plakoglobin overexpression alone. Transfection of plakoglobin into a human renal carcinoma cell line that expresses neither cadherins nor plakoglobin, or α- and β-catenin, resulted in dose-dependent suppression of tumor formation by these cells in nude mice.[35] Plakoglobin, in these cells, did not exhibit junctional localization, was diffusely distributed in the cytoplasm, and mostly localized in the nucleus. These results suggest that plakoglobin suppresses the tumorigenicity of cells in the presence of or independently of the cadherin-catenin complex while localized in the nucleus.

Regulation of β–Catenin Levels and Localization by Overexpression of Plakoglobin and Inhibition of the Ubiquitin-Proteasome System

β-Catenin and plakoglobin, which are closely related structurally, belong to the Armadillo family of proteins and are mainly localized at the submembrane plaques of cell-cell adherens junctions where they form independent complexes with classical cadherins and α-catenin to establish the link with the actin-cytoskeleton.[30] In addition to its role in junctional assembly, β-catenin has been shown to play an essential role in signal transduction by the Wnt pathway which results in its translocation into the nucleus[36,37] (FIG. 1A). To study the relation between plakoglobin expression and the level of β-catenin, and the localization of these proteins in the same cell, we employed tumor cell lines that express N-cadherin, and α- and β-catenin, but no plakoglobin or desmosomal components. Individual clones expressing various levels of plakoglobin were established by stable transfection. Plakoglobin overexpression resulted in a dose-dependent decrease in the level of β-catenin in each clone.[38] Induction of plakoglobin expression increased the turnover of β-catenin without affecting RNA levels, suggest-

---

FIGURE 1. The different molecular interactions of β-catenin in Wnt signaling and cell adhesion. When Wnt signaling is activated, by binding of Wnt to the Frizzled (Frz) family of receptors, the disheveled (dsh) protein is recruited to the membrane area. Activated dsh inhibits glycogen synthase kinase (GSK) action that normally phosphorylates (P) and directs β-catenin (β), together with adenomatosis polyposis coli (APC) and axin, to degradation by the ubiquitin-proteasome system. Decreased degradation of β-catenin results in its accumulation, nuclear translocation, and association with LEF/TCF transcription factors leading to activation of gene expression. In addition to Wnt signaling, β-catenin is part of the adhesion system that links cadherins via α-catenin (α) to the actin-cytoskeleton. By varying the level of β-catenin partners in the adhesion system (plakoglobin [PG], cadherin, and α-catenin), its role in signaling can be affected.[38-40] (A) A moderate increase in plakoglobin level leads to the displacement of β-catenin from cell-cell junctions by competition for cadherin binding, resulting in enhanced turnover of β-catenin in cells containing an APC/GSK/Axin-competent degradation system.[38] (B) Massive overexpression of plakoglobin results in effective competition with β-catenin for both cadherin- and APC-binding, accumulation of β-catenin, and its nuclear translocation.[38,39] In the nucleus, plakoglobin may either displace β-catenin from complexing with TCF or allow transactivation by β-catenin, if β-catenin complexes with TCF are more stable than those with plakoglobin. (C) Overexpression of cadherin or α-catenin results in the recruitment to cell-cell junctions and stabilization of "free" cytoplasmic and nuclear β-catenin[39,40] and inhibition of transactivation and β-catenin-mediated signaling (modified from ref. 30).

ing posttranslational regulation of β-catenin (FIG. 1B). In plakoglobin overexpressing cells, both β-catenin and plakoglobin were localized at cell-cell junctions. Stable transfection of mutant plakoglobin molecules showed that deletion of the N-cadherin binding domain, but not the α-catenin binding domain, abolished β-catenin downregulation. Inhibition of the ubiquitin-proteasome pathway in such plakoglobin-overexpressing cells blocked the decrease in β-catenin levels and resulted in the accumulation of both β-catenin and plakoglobin in the nucleus[38] (FIG. 1B). These results suggest that (1) plakoglobin substitutes effectively for β-catenin in its association with N-cadherin in adherens junctions, (2) extrajunctional β-catenin is rapidly degraded by the proteasome-ubiquitin system, but (3) excess β-catenin and plakoglobin translocate into the nucleus.

Differential Nuclear Translocation and Transactivation Potential of β-Catenin and Plakoglobin

β-Catenin and plakoglobin have a dual role in the cell: they function in cell adhesion by linking cadherins to the cytoskeleton and also in signaling by transactivation together with LEF/TCF transcription factors.[31–34] We therefore compared the nuclear translocation and transactivation abilities of β-catenin and plakoglobin in mammalian cells.[39] Overexpression of each of the two proteins in MDCK cells resulted in their nuclear translocation and formation of nuclear aggregates. The β-catenin–containing nuclear structures also contained LEF-1 and vinculin, whereas plakoglobin was inefficient in recruiting these molecules into the nucleus, suggesting that its interaction with LEF-1 and vinculin is significantly weaker. Moreover, transfection of LEF-1 translocated endogenous β-catenin, but not plakoglobin into the nucleus. Chimeras consisting of the Gal4 DNA-binding domain and the transactivation domains of either plakoglobin or β-catenin were equally potent in transactivating a Gal4-responsive reporter, whereas activation of LEF-1–responsive transcription was significantly higher with β-catenin than with plakoglobin. Overexpression of wild-type plakoglobin or mutant β-catenin that lacked the transactivation domain induced the accumulation of endogenous β-catenin in the nucleus and LEF-1–responsive transactivation[39] (FIG. 1B). We further showed that the constitutive β-catenin–dependent transactivation in SW480 colon carcinoma cells and the nuclear localization of β-catenin can be inhibited by overexpressing N-cadherin or α-catenin in these cells[39] (FIG. 1C). These results indicate that (1) plakoglobin and β-catenin differ in their nuclear translocation and complexing with LEF-1 and vinculin, (2) LEF-1–dependent transactivation is preferentially driven by β-catenin, (3) the cytoplasmic partners of β-catenin, cadherin and α–catenin, can sequester β-catenin to the cytoplasm and inhibit its transcriptional activity, while vinculin can colocalize with β-catenin in the nucleus.

Inhibition of β-Catenin–Mediated Transactivation by Cadherin Derivatives

We studied the effect of N-cadherin, its cytoplasmic domain and a transmembrane chimeric molecule containing the cadherin cytoplasmic tail, on the level and localization of β-catenin and its ability to induce LEF-1–responsive transactivation.[40] These cadherin derivatives formed complexes with β-catenin and protected it from degradation by the ubiquitin/proteasome system (FIG. 1C). N-cadherin directed β-catenin into adherens junctions, the chimeric transmembrane protein and the associated β-catenin were diffusely distributed on the membrane, while the free cytoplasmic domain of N-cadherin colocalized with β-catenin in the nucleus. Cotransfection of β-catenin and LEF-1 induced transactivation of a synthetic LEF-1 reporter gene. In CHO cells (which lack cadherins and do not express detectable levels of β-catenin) cotransfection of the N-cadherin–derived molecules blocked β-catenin–driven transactivation. Expression of N-cadherin and the IL-2 receptor/cadherin chimera in SW480 cells (which express high levels of β-catenin in the nucleus) relocated β-catenin from the nucleus to the plasma membrane and reduced β-catenin–directed transactivation[40] (FIG. 1C). The cytoplasmic tail of N- or E-cadherin colocalized with β-catenin in the nucleus and suppressed the constitutive LEF-1–mediated transactivation by blocking β-catenin–LEF-1 interaction. Moreover, the 72 C-terminal amino acids of cadherin stabilized β-catenin and inhibited its transactivation potential in colon cancer cells.[40] These results indicate that β-catenin binding to the cadherin cytoplasmic tail either in the membrane or the nucleus can inhibit β-catenin degradation and efficiently block its transactivation capacity. Cadherin derivatives thus may be useful in effectively antagonizing the oncogenic transcription mediated by excess β-catenin.

CONCLUSIONS AND PERSPECTIVES

The network of molecular interactions involving β-catenin and plakoglobin displays an intriguing complexity that at present is only partially understood. Major issues for future research include:

Differential transcriptional specificity of β-catenin and plakoglobin: While both proteins appear to be potent transactivators interacting with LEF/TCF transcription factors, their specificity in binding and regulating the target genes in mammalian cells is unknown. As signaling by β-catenin and plakoglobin is suggested to result from their transactivation potential, unraveling the nature of their target genes is of utmost importance. The recent discovery that the c-*MYC* promoter is a target for the β-catenin/TCF pathway[41] is an exciting new direction for such research.

Cadherin-catenin relationships: Cadherin could play a dual role in regulating catenin-mediated signaling. On the one hand, it can stabilize these proteins (especially β-catenin; FIG. 1C), yet most of such stabilized molecules are transcriptionally inactive, being membrane-bound with their LEF/TCF-binding site blocked (FIG. 1C). A related key question is the physiologic condition(s) that can confer a regulated release of catenins from junctions and their controlled transport into the nucleus.

β-Catenin–vinculin relationships: The nuclear translocation and colocalization of vinculin with β-catenin may provide an alternative explanation for the effects observed in cells where vinculin levels are altered. In addition to affecting adhesion and motility, vinculin complexes formed with β-catenin in the nucleus may affect the transactivation mediated by β-catenin and thus influence β-catenin's oncogenic action.

β-Catenin-plakoglobin relationships: Being very similar and sharing molecular partners, changes in the relative levels of the two proteins may trigger a variety of indirect responses. For example, overexpression of plakoglobin can release β-catenin from junctions and target it to degradation (in cells containing an active APC-related turnover system; FIG. 1A) or to transactivation when the APC-degradation pathway is defective or inhibited by Wnt signaling (FIG. 1B). Excess plakoglobin may compete with β-catenin for APC binding and thus block its degradation (FIG. 1B). Other shared molecular partners for β-catenin and plakoglobin such as α-catenin and transcription factors of the LEF/TCF family can bind to both molecules. Competition between the two molecules on the binding to α-catenin and LEF/TCF may also have very different effects on catenin signaling.

Better understanding of these aspects and their physiologic relevance depends on direct characterization of the affinities of the two proteins towards their different cytoplasmic and nuclear partners and the cellular mechanisms that may selectively modulate such interactions.

ACKNOWLEDGMENTS

I thank past and present members of our laboratory and in collaborating laboratories that contributed to the work described in this review. The studies from the author's laboratory were supported by grants the USA-Israel Binational Foundation, the German-Israeli Foundation for Scientific Research and Development, the Forchheimer Center for Molecular Genetics, and the Cooperation Program in Cancer Research between DKFZ and IMOSA. A.B.-Z. holds the Lunenfeld-Kunin Chair in Cell Biology and Genetics.

REFERENCES

1. TAKEICHI, M. 1995. Morphogenetic roles of classic cadherins. Curr. Opin. Cell Biol. **7:** 619–627.
2. GUMBINER, B.M. 1996. Cell adhesion: The molecular basis of tissue architecture and morphogenesis. Cell **84:** 345–357.
3. BEN-ZE'EV, A. 1986. The relationship between cytoplasmic organization, gene expression and morphogenesis. Trends Biochem. Sci. **11:** 478–481.
4. BEN-ZE'EV, A. 1991. Animal cell shape changes and gene expression. BioEssays **13:** 207–212.
5. BEN-ZE'EV, A. 1985. The cytoskeleton in cancer cells. Biochim. Biophys. Acta **780:** 197–212.
6. BEN-ZE'EV, A. 1986. Regulation of cytoskeletal protein synthesis in normal and cancer cells. Cancer Rev. **4:** 91–116.
7. RAZ, A. & A. BEN-ZE'EV. 1987. Cell-contact and architecture of malignant cells and their relationship to metastasis. Cancer Metastasis Rev. **6:** 3–21.
8. BEN-ZE'EV, A. 1997. Cytoskeletal and adhesion proteins as tumor suppressors. Curr. Opin. Cell Biol. **9:** 99–108.
9. BEN-ZE'EV, A. 1990. Application of two-dimensional gel electrophoresis in the study of cytoskeletal protein regulation during growth activation and differentiation. Electrophoresis **11:** 191–200.
10. BEN-ZE'EV, A. 1987. The role of changes in cell shape and contacts in the regulation of cytoskeleton expression during differentiation. J. Cell Sci. Suppl. **8:** 293–312.
11. BEN-ZE'EV, A. & A. AMSTERDAM. 1986. Regulation of cytoskeletal proteins involved in cell contact formation during differentiation of granulosa cells on ECM. Proc. Natl. Acad. Sci. USA **83:** 2894–2898.
12. BEN-ZE'EV, A., G.S. ROBINSON, N.L.R. BUCHER & S.R. FARMER. 1988. Cell-cell and cell-matrix interactions differentially regulate the expression of hepatic and

cytoskeletal genes in primary cultures of rat hepatocytes. Proc. Natl. Acad. Sci. USA. **85:** 2161–2165.

13. RODRÍGUEZ FERNÁNDEZ, J.L. & A. BEN-ZE'EV. 1989. Regulation of fibronectin, integrin and cytoskeleton expression in differentiating adipocytes: Inhibition by extracellular matrix and polylysine. Differentiation **42:** 65–74.

14. BEN-ZE'EV, A., R. REISS, R. BENDORI & B. GORODECKI. 1990. Transient induction of vinculin gene expression in 3T3 fibroblasts stimulated by serum growth factors. Cell Regul. **1:** 621–636.

15. BEN-ZE'EV, A., J.L.F RODRÍGUEZ, G. BAUM & B. GORODECKI. 1990. Regulation of cell contacts, cell configuration and cytoskeletal gene expression in differentiating systems. *In* Mechanisms of Differentiation. P. Fisher, Ed.: Vol. **II,** 143–173. CRC Press. Boca Raton, FL.

16. BAUM, G., B-S. SUH, A. AMSTERDAM & A. BEN-ZE'EV. 1990. Regulation of tropomyosin expression in transformed granulosa cell lines with steroidogenic ability. Dev. Biol. **142:** 115–128.

17. GLÜCK, U., J.L. RODRÍGUEZ FERNÁNDEZ, R. PANKOV & A. BEN-ZE'EV. 1992. Induction of adherens junction protein expression in growth-activated 3T3 cells and in regenerating liver. Exp. Cell Res. **202:** 477–486.

18. COLL, J.-L., A. BEN-ZE'EV, R.M. EZZELL, J.L. RODRÍGUEZ FERNÁNDEZ, H. BARIBAULT, R.G. OSHIMA & E.D. ADAMSON. 1995. Targeted disruption of vinculin genes in F9 and ES cells changes cell morphology, adhesion and locomotion. Proc. Natl. Acad. Sci. USA **92:** 9161–9165.

19. VOLBERG, T., B. GEIGER, Z. KAM, R. PANKOV, I. SIMCHA, H. SABANAY, J.-L. COLL, E. ADAMSON & A. BEN-ZE'EV. 1995. Focal adhesion formation by F9 embryonal carcinoma cells after vinculin gene disruption. J. Cell Sci. **108:** 2253–2260.

20. RODRÍGUEZ FERNÁNDEZ, J.L., B. GEIGER, D. SALOMON & A. BEN-ZE'EV. 1992. Overexpression of vinculin suppresses cell motility in Balb/C 3T3 cells. Cell Motil. Cytoskel. **22:** 127–134.

21. RODRÍGUEZ FERNÁNDEZ, J.L., B. GEIGER, D. SALOMON & A. BEN-ZE'EV. 1993. Suppression of vinculin expression by antisense transfection confers changes in cell morphology, motility, and anchorage dependent growth. J. Cell Biol. **122:** 1285–1294.

22. GEIGER, B., D. GINSBERG, O. AYALON, T. VOLBERG, J.L. RODRÍGUEZ FERNÁNDEZ, Y. YARDEN, & A. BEN-ZE'EV. 1992. Cytoplasmic control of cell adhesion. *In* Cold Spring Harbor Symp. Quant. Biol. **57:** 631–642.

23. BEN-ZE'EV, A., J.L. RODRÍGUEZ FERNÁNDEZ, U. GLÜCK, D. SALOMON & B. GEIGER. 1994. Changes in adhesion plaque protein levels regulate cell motility and tumorigenicity. Adv. Exp. Med. Biol. **358:** 147–157.

24. OTEY, C.A., F.M. PAVALKO & K. BURRIDGE. 1990. An interaction between α-actinin and the β_1 integrin subunit *in vitro*. J. Cell Biol. **111:** 721–729.

25. GLÜCK, U. & A. BEN-ZE'EV. 1994. Modulation of α-actinin levels affects cell motility and confers tumorigenicity in 3T3 cells. J. Cell Sci. **107:** 1773–1782.

26. RODRÍGUEZ FERNÁNDEZ, J.L., B. GEIGER, D. SALOMON, I. SABANAY, M. ZÖLLER & A. Ben-Ze'ev. 1992. Suppression of tumorigenicity in transformed cells after transfection with vinculin cDNA. J. Cell Biol. **119:** 427–438.

27. GLÜCK,U., D.J. KWIATKOWSKI & A. BEN-ZE'EV. 1993. Suppression of tumorigenicity in simian virus 40-transformed 3T3 cells transfected with α-actinin cDNA. Proc. Natl. Acad. Sci. USA **90:** 383–387.

28. COWIN, P., H.P. KAPPRELL, W.W. FRANKE, J. TAMKUN & R.O. HYNES. 1986. Plakoglobin: A protein common to different kinds of intercellular adhering junctions. Cell **46:** 1063–1073.

29. PEIFER, M. & E. WIESCHAUS. 1990. The segment polarity gene *armadillo* encodes a functionally modular protein that is the *Drosophila* homolog of human plakoglobin. Cell **63:** 1167–1176.

30. BEN-ZE'EV, A. & B. GEIGER. 1998. Differential molecular interactions of β-catenin and plakoglobin in adhesion, signaling and cancer. Curr. Opin. Cell Biol. **10:** 629–639.
31. MOLENAAR, M., M. VAN DE WETERING, M. OOSTERWEGEL, J. PETERSON-MADURO, S. GODSAVE, V. KORINEK, J. ROOSE, O. DESTREE & H. CLEVERS. 1996. XTcf-3 transcription factor mediates β-catenin-induced axis formation in *Xenopus* embryos. Cell **86:** 391–399.
32. HUBER, O., R. KORN, J. MCLAUGHLIN, M. OHSUGI, B.G. HERRMANN & R. KEMLER. 1996. Nuclear localization of β-catenin by interaction with transcription factor LEF-1. Mech. Dev. **59:** 3–11.
33. MERRIAM, J.M., A.B. RUBENSTEIN & M.W. KLYMKOWSKY. 1997. Cytoplasmically anchored plakoglobin induces a wnt-like phenotype in *Xenopus*. Dev. Biol. **185:** 67–81.
34. BEHRENS, J., J.P. VON KRIES, M. KUHL, L. BRUHN, D. WEDLICH, R. GROSSCHEDL & W. BIRCHMEIER. 1996. Functional interaction of β-catenin with the transcription factor LEF-1. Nature **382:** 638–642.
35. SIMCHA, I., B. GEIGER, S. YEHUDA-LEVENBERG, D. SALOMON & A. BEN-ZE'EV. 1996. Suppression of tumorigenicity by plakoglobin: An augmenting effect of N-cadherin. J. Cell Biol. **133:** 199–206.
36. BROWN, J. & R.T. MOON. 1998. Wnt signaling: Why is everything so negative? Curr. Opin. Cell Biol. **10:** 182–187.
37. WILLERT, K. & R. NUSSE. 1998. β-catenin: A key modulator of Wnt signaling. Curr. Opin. Gen. Cell Biol. **8:** 95–102.
38. SALOMON, D., P. SACCO, S. GUHA ROY, I. SIMCHA, K.R. JOHNSON, M.J. WHEELOCK & A. BEN-ZE'EV. 1997. Regulation of β-catenin levels and localization by overexpression of plakoglobin and inhibition of the ubiquitin-proteasome system. J. Cell Biol. **139:** 1325–1335.
39. SIMCHA, I., M. SHTUTMAN, D. SALOMON, J. ZHURINSKY, E. SADOT, B. GEIGER & A. BEN-ZE'EV. 1998. Differential nuclear translocation and transactivation potential of β-catenin and plakoglobin. J. Cell Biol. **141:** 1433–1448.
40. SADOT, E., I. SIMCHA, M. SHTUTMAN, A. BEN-ZE'EV & B. GEIGER. 1998. Inhibition of β-catenin-mediated transactivation by cadherin derivatives. Proc. Natl. Acad. Sci. USA. **95:** 15339–15344.
41. HE, T.-C., A.B. SPARKS, H. HERMEKING, L. ZAWEL, L.T. DA COSTA, P.J. MORIN, B. VOGELSTEIN & K.W. KINZLER. 1998. Identification of c-*MYC* as a target of the APC pathway. Science **281:** 1509–1512.

Cytoskeletal Tumor Suppressors That Block Oncogenic RAS Signaling

HIROSHI MARUTA,[a] HONG HE, ANJALI TIKOO, AND MSA NUR-E-KAMAL

Ludwig Institute for Cancer Research, Melbourne, Australia 3050

ABSTRACT: Several distinct peptides or drugs that block the Rho family GTPases-mediated pathways were found to suppress RAS-induced malignant phenotype. They include (1) C3 enzyme that selectively inactivates Rho, (2) ACK42, a peptide that blocks the interaction of CDC42 with its effectors such as ACKs, (3) PAK18, a peptide that blocks the activation of PAK and membrane ruffling, and (4) actin-binding drugs, chaetoglobosin K (CK) and MKT-077, that block membrane ruffling by capping and bundling actin filaments, respectively.

INTRODUCTION

Oncogenic RAS mutants cause a dramatic change in actin cytoskeleton by activating Rho family G proteins including Rho, Rac, and CDC42, which are essential for RAS transformation.[1-3] Rac is known to act downstream of PI-3 kinase, which is activated by RAS directly.[4] We therefore examined the anti-RAS cancer potentials of several distinct molecules that control the function of these GTPases or their effectors. We found that the following three distinct molecules are capable of suppressing RAS transformation: (1) the bacterial exotoxin C3 which selectively inactivates Rho by ADP-ribosylation, (2) ACK42-WR, the 42 amino acid fragment of a Tyr-kinase called ACK-1 conjugated with a cell-permeable peptide vector of 16 amino acids called WR/penetratin, that binds only CDC42 in the GTP-bound form,[5] and (3) PAK18-WR, the 18 amino acid fragment of a Rac/CDC42-activated Ser/Thr kinase called PAK conjugated with WR, that binds the PIX SH3 domain.[5] Thus, we are currently determining the 3-dimensional structure of PAK18 and ACK42 to design their peptidomimetics which are useful for the chemotherapy of RAS-associated cancers. In addition, we found that a unique F-actin capping antibiotic called chaetoglobosin K (CK) and an F-acting cross-linking dye called MKT-077 suppress RAS transformation,[6,7] as does overexpression of several F-actin capping/severing/cross-linking proteins such as tensin, gelsolin, and HS1.

RESULTS AND DISCUSSION

C3 Selectively Inhibits the Growth of Ras Transformants

Although it still remains to be clarified how Ras activates Rho through the SH3 domain of Ras GAP of 120 kD,[8] it has been established that Rho GTPases, in par-

---

[a]Corresponding author: fax, 613-9341-3104.
e-mail, hiroshi.maruta@ludwig.edu.au

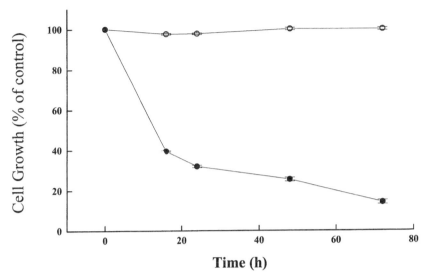

Time (h)

FIGURE 1. Effects of C3 on the growth of normal and Ras-transformed cells. Normal (*open circle*) and v-Ha-Ras transformed (*closed circle*) NIH 3T3 cells were cultured in the standard medium containing 5% fetal calf serum (FCS) in the presence or absence of 50 μg/ml C3, with 10 μl of lipofectamin. Their growth in the presence of C3 compared with that in the control (no C3) is shown with time (hrs). C3 inhibits the growth of Ras transformants, but not of normal cells.

ticular RhoB, are essential for Ras transformation.[1] For instance, the farnesyltransferase (FTase) inhibitor L-739,749 (Merck) strongly inhibits farnesylation of RhoB, prior to that of Ras GTPases, in v-Ha-Ras transformed NIH 3T3 fibroblasts, and rapidly reverses malignant phenotypes to normal by restoring the anchorage dependency and contact inhibition of growth as well as flat morphology and actin stress fibers.[1] Because the C3 selectively inactivates Rho by ADP-ribosylation in the effector domain,[9] we determined the selective toxicity of C3 towards Ras transformants by comparing its effect on the growth of normal and v-Ha-Ras transformed NIH 3T3 cells. Although recombinant C3 alone has no effect on growth of both cell types (probably because of its poor penetration through the plasma membranes), in the presence of 10 μl of lipofectamin (a positively charged liposome), C3 (50 μg/ml) strongly inhibits the growth of Ras transformants, but it has no effect on the growth of parental normal cells (FIG. 1). These observations indicate that C3 is a specific growth inhibitor for Ras transformants.

ACK42 Suppresses Ras Transformation

Although it has been shown that Ras transformation is suppressed by the dominant negative N17 mutant of CDC42[3] which inactivates CDC42 by sequestering its upstream activators, CDC42 GDP-dissociation stimulators (GDSs), the possibility still remains that this mutant could also inactivate Rho or Rac by sequestering a few GDSs which bind Rho or Rac, in addition to CDC42, such as DBL, OST, and Tiam-

TABLE 1. ACK42 suppresses colony formation of v-Ha-Ras transformants in soft agar[a]

	Colonies (n)[b]			
Clone (n)	Small	Large	Total	Suppression (%)
Parental v-Ha-Ras cells	650	320	970	0
pMV7 alone transfectants	720	270	990	0
ACK42 transfectants				
Clone 1	50	0	50	95
Clone 2	10	0	10	99
Clone 3	80	0	80	92
Clone 4	0	0	0	100
Clone 5	5	0	5	95.5
Clone 6	0	0	0	100
Clone 7	20	0	20	98

[a]10^3 cell (parental, pMV7 alone transfected or ACK2 overexpressing v-Ha-Ras transformants) were plated in soft agar. After 20 days of incubation the number of colonies was counted under a microscope.
[b]Size of colonies: large, more than 30 cells per colony; small, less than 30 cells per colony.

1.[10] To clarify this point, we need a CDC42-specific inhibitor. ACK-1 is the CDC42-binding Tyr-kinase of 1091 amino acids (FIG. 2), and the minimum CDC42 binding domain (residues 504–545) binds only CDC42 in the GTP-bound form.[11]

Thus, this 42 amino acid fragment, called ACK42, would serve as a CDC42-specific inhibitor that blocks the interactions of CDC42 with any of its effectors such as the ACK family of Tyr kinases (ACK-1 and ACK-2), the F-actin severing protein N-WASP, the PAK family of Ser/Thr kinases, and CDC42 GAPs including p190-A and n-Chimerin.[10] We previously showed that overexpression of ACK42 in PC12 cells

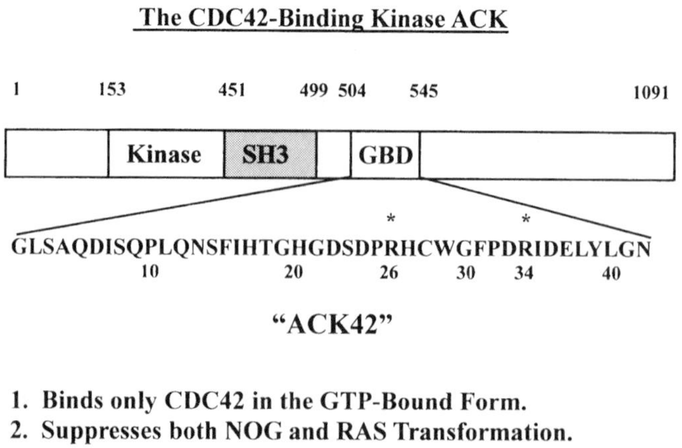

The CDC42-Binding Kinase ACK

FIGURE 2. Structure of ACK-1 and sequence of its CDC42-binding domain (GBD/ACK42).

completely blocks NGF/Ras-induced neurite outgrowth (NOG), indicating that CDC42 is essential for NOG.[12] Here we demonstrate that overexpression of ACK42 almost completely suppresses Ras transformation, that is, the anchorage-independent growth in soft agar (TABLE 1). Furthermore, we have generated a cell-permeable derivative of ACK42, called WR-ACK42, by conjugating ACK42 with a cell-permeable peptide vector of 16 amino acids called WR, a penetratin consisting of only Arg and Trp residues.[13] Under the conditions in which the vector WR alone has no effect on the growth of Ras transformants, WR-ACK42 conjugate (5 μM) strongly inhibits the growth of Ras transformants.

These observations suggest the possibility that some ACK42 peptidominetics, that is, chemicals mimicking ACK42, would be potentially useful for the treatment of Ras-associated cancers. We are currently determining the 3-dimensional structure of the ACK42 bound to CDC42/GTP complex, conducting a systematic mutational analysis of ACK42 to identify the critical residues of ACK42 responsible for its binding to CDC42, and are screening for the high-affinity mutants of ACK42 that bind CDC42 much more tightly and therefore serve as more potent CDC42 inhibitors.

CDC42 is mainly involved in the formation of actin microspikes in fibroblasts and cytokinesis.[14,15] Recently it was shown that N-WASP, a CDC42-activated F-actin severing protein, is also required for microspike formation.[16] Because neurites of PC12 cells consist of actin filaments and look like gigantic microspikes, it is con-

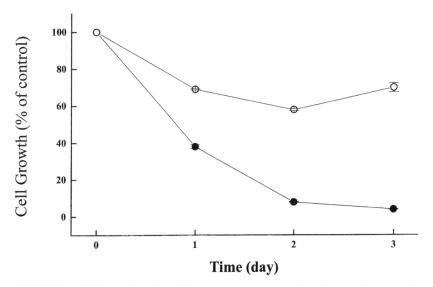

Time (day)

FIGURE 3. Effects of PAK18-WR on the growth of normal and Ras-transformed cells. Normal (*open circle*) and v-Ha-Ras transformed (*closed circle*) NIH 3T3 cells were cultured in the standard medium containing 10% FCS in the presence or absence of 10 μM PAK18-WR, that is, **RRWRRWWRRWWRRWRR-PPVIAPRPEHTKSVYTRS**. Their growth in the presence of PAK18-WR compared with that in the control (no PAK18-WR) is shown with time (days). PAK18-WR strongly inhibits the growth of Ras transformants, but only weakly the normal cell growth. PAK18 or WR alone has no effect on their growth.

ceivable that N-WASP is also required for NOG. Overexpressing of an antisense 'N-WASP RNA, we are currently examining whether N-WASP is essential for both NOG of PC12 cells and Ras transformation.

PAK18 Selectively Inhibits the Growth of Ras Transformants

PAK is a CDC42/Rac-activated Ser/Thr kinase, and its Pro-rich domain of 18 amino acids, called PAK18, binds the SH3 domain of another protein called PIX/ Cool.[17] The PIX-PAK interaction was shown to be essential for membrane ruffling of PC12 cells.[18] Because Ras/Rac-induced membrane ruffling is required for Ras transformation of fibroblasts,[19] we examined the effect on the v-Ha-Ras transformants of a cell-permeable derivative of PAK18, called WR-PAK18. Under conditions in which the WR alone has little effect on the growth of normal cells, the WR-PAK18 conjugate (10 μM) strongly inhibits the growth of Ras transformants (FIG. 3). The parental normal cells are much more resistant to the action of the WR-PAK18. A mutant of PAK18-WR, which no longer binds PIX due to the replacement of Arg7 by Ala in PAK18, has no effect on the growth of Ras transformants.

These findings clearly indicate that PIX-PAK interaction (leading to activation of Rac and eventual membrane ruffling) is essential for Ras transformation and suggest the possibility that some PAK18 peptidomimetics would also be useful in the treatment of Ras-associated cancers. The anti-Ras cancer drug SCH51344 (Schering–Plough) blocks the downstream of Rac,[19] but its direct target still remains to be identified, whereas PAK18 binds PIX to block the upstream of Rac. To understand more precisely the nature of the PIX-PAK interaction, we are currently determining the 3-dimensional structure of PAK18 bound to the SH3 domain of PIX and also generating the high-affinity mutants of PAK18 that bind PIX much more tightly, in an attempt to improve the anti-cancer potential of PAK18.

F-actin Cappers, Tensin and CK, Suppress Ras Transformation

Rac GTPase was reported to activate PI-4/PI-5 kinases which produces PIP2 (phosphatidylinositol 4, 5 bisphosphate), and PIP2 in turn inactivates several F-actin capping proteins, such as tensin and gelsolin that cap the plus ends of actin filaments, induces uncapping of actin filaments, and stimulates actin polymerization.[20] We showed previously that HS1 sequesters PIP2 and suppresses Ras transformation,[21] suggesting that PIP2-induced uncapping of actin filaments is essential for Ras transformation. In fact, gelsolin, which caps the plus end of actin filament, suppresses Ras transformation.[22] However, because gelsolin is a multifunctional protein that severs actin filaments as well as binding PIP2, it is not clear which function of gelsolin actually contributes to the suppression of Ras transformation. Therefore, we examined the effect on Ras transformation of tensin, an F-actin capping protein of 1744 amino acids that does not sever actin filaments.[23] Overexpression of chicken tensin almost completely suppresses the anchorage-independent growth of v-Ha-Ras transformed NIH 3T3 cells (TABLE 2). This finding supports the notion that F-actin capping is sufficient for suppressing Ras transformation.

To prove it more directly, we used a unique F-actin capping antibiotic, chaetoglobosin K (CK) (for the structure, see FIG. 4), that was isolated from a plant fungus called *Diplodia macrospora* almost two decades ago by Cutler and his colleagues.[24]

TABLE 2. Tensin suppresses v-Ha-RAS–induced malignancy[a]

	Colonies (n)[b]				
Clone	Large	Medium	Small	Total	(%)
Vector alone	334	160	130	624	(100.0)
Tensin transfectants					
Clone 02	0	0	0.5	0.5	(0.1)
Clone 05	0	0	0.5	0.5	(0.1)
Clone 11	0	1	0.5	1.5	(0.2)
Clone 03	0	0.5	2.5	3	(0.5)
Clone 07	0	1	13.5	14.5	(2.3)
Average	0	0.5	3.6	4.1	(0.6)

[a]10^3 cell (vector alone transfected or tensin overexpressing v-Ha-Ras transformants) were plated in soft agar. After 18 days of incubation, the number of colonies formed in each plate was counted.
[b]Size of colonies: large, more than 100 cells per colony; medium, 10–100 cells per colony; small, less than 10 cells per colony.

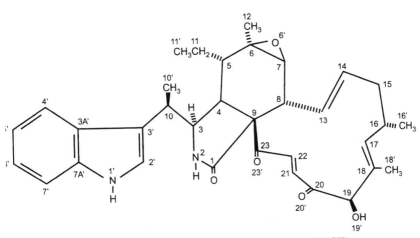

FIGURE 4. Chemical structure of chaetoglobosin K (CK).

CK (2 μM) caps the plus end of the actin filament and blocks membrane ruffling as do many other cytochalasins, but unlike other cytochalasins, CK does not cause either rounding-up of cells or contraction of actin cables, suggesting that CK has so far the least "side" effects among the more than 24 distinct cytochalasins, all of which are plus-end F-actin cappers.[25] We found that 2 μM CK is sufficient to block almost completely the anchorage-independent growth of v-Ha-Ras transformed NIH 3T3 cells (FIG. 5).

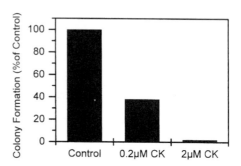

FIGURE 5. Effect of CK on the anchorage-independent growth of Ras transformants. 10^3 Ras transformants were cultured in soft agar in the presence of various concentrations of CK for 3 weeks, and the number of colonies formed was counted.

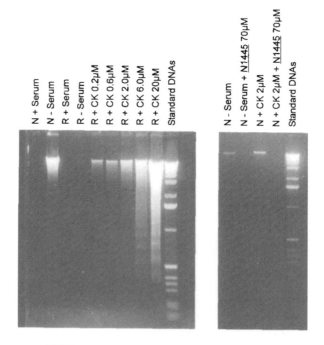

ICE Inhibitor Blocks CK-Induced Apoptosis

FIGURE 6. Caspase-1 inhibitor N1445 rescues normal cells from CK-induced apoptosis. The DNA leakage from nuclei in 1% Triton X-100 lysate of cells could be detected by agarose gel electrophoresis as an early sign of apoptosis after normal NIH 3T3 cells (N) were incubated in the absence of serum (–) for 24 hours or in the presence of 2 μM CK (+) and 10% FCS for 48 hours. However, incubation of these cells with 70 μM N1445 abolishes the apoptosis (DNA leakage) caused by either serum withdrawal or CK treatment.

TABLE 3. Suppression by CK of the colony-forming ability of v-Ha-RAS transformants in the presence of N1445[a]

	Colonies (n)[b]			
	Large	Small	Total	Suppression (%)
Control				
No CK added: +N1445 (µM)				
0	486	93	579	0
2.3	413	129	592	0
7.0	456	111	567	0
23	454	129	583	0
70	244	67	311	47
2 µM CK added: +N1445 (µM)				
0	0	12	12	98
2.3	0	21	21	97
7.0	0	15	15	98
23	0	2	2	100

[a]10^3 cells of v-Ha-Ras transformants were incubated in soft agar containing 2 µM of CK in the presence of the indicated concentrations of N1445. After 18 days the number of colonies formed in each dish was counted.
[b]Size of colonies: large, more than 30 cells per colony; small, less than 30 cells per colony. Each value is the average of data from triplicated assay. Standard deviation of each was less than 5%.

THE ICE/CASPASE-1 INHIBITOR N1445 ABOLISHES CK-INDUCED APOPTOSIS

CK, however, causes apoptosis of Ras transformants and, to a lesser extent, of parental normal cells (FIG. 6). Because tensin does not cause apoptosis, CK-induced apoptosis is not due to its F-actin capping activity per se. To abolish this undesirable apoptotic effect of CK, we screened for a specific caspase inhibitor that blocks CK-induced apoptosis and found that the drug N1445 (Bachem), an inhibitor of ICE/caspase-1, at 50–70 µM completely abolishes the apoptosis of normal cells caused by either CK or serum starvation (FIG. 6). The Ser/Thr kinase PKB/AKT, which is activated by an end-product of PI-3 kinase, is required for normal cell survival.[26] To understand the more detailed role of CK and N1445 in apoptosis, we examined their effects on the PKB, using histone 2B as a substrate. CK treatment reduced kinase activity, whereas N1445 was a potent activator of PKB in normal cells (FIG. 7). Thus, N1445 could overcome the inhibitory effect of CK on the PKB. Interestingly, N1445 does not affect the anti-Ras tumor suppressor activity of CK (TABLE 3). These findings suggest an anti-cancer drug potential of the CK-N1445 combination in the treatment of Ras-associated cancers. We are currently examining the effect of this combination therapy on the development of Ras-induced tumors in nude mice.

1 2 3 4

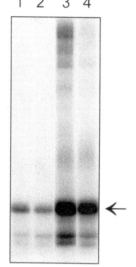

FIGURE 7. Opposite effects of CK and N1445 on PKB/
AKT kinase activity. Normal NIH 3T3 cells were cultured in
the standard medium for 24 hours in the absence (*lane 1*) or
presence (*lane 2*) of 2 μM CK alone, 50 μM N1445 alone
(*lane 3*), or both drugs (*lane 4*). Cells were disrupted with 1%
NP-40, and each cleared supernatant (3 mg proteins) was immunoprecipitated with an antibody against PKB, and the
PKB kinase activity of each pellet was assayed with histone
2B as a substrate in the presence of [gamma-^{32}P] ATP. Phosphorylated histone 2B (*arrow*) was separated from other proteins by SDS PAGE and visualized by autoradiography.

For details of the anti-Ras action of the novel F-actin cross-linking drug MKT-
077, see the poster entitled "The anti-RAS cancer drug MKT-077 is an F-actin cross-
linker" by Maruta *et al.* in this volume.

REFERENCES

1. LEBOWITZ, P.F., J.P. DAVIDE & G.C. PRENDERGAST. 1995. Evidence that farnesylation
   inhibitors suppress Ras transformation by interfering with Rho activity. Mol. Cell
   Biol. **15:** 6613–6622.
2. QUI, R.G., J. CHEN, D. KIRN, F. MCCORMICK & M. SYMONS. 1995. An essential role
   for Rac in Ras transformation. Nature **374:** 457–459.
3. QUI, R.G., A. ABO, F. MCCORMICK & M. SYMONS. 1997. CDC42 regulates anchorage-
   independent growth and is necessary for Ras transformation. Mol. Cell Biol. **17:**
   3449–3458.
4. RODRIGUEZ-VICIANA, P., P. WARNE, A. KHWAJA, B. MARTE, P. DAS, M. WATERFIELD,
   A. RIDLEY & J. DOWNWARD. 1997. Role of PI-3 kinase in cell transformation and
   control of the actin cytoskeleton by Ras. Cell **89:** 457–467.
5. MARUTA, H., H. HE, A. TIKOO, T. VUONG & MSA NUR-E-KAMAL. 1999. G. Proteins,
   phosphoinositides, and actin-cytoskeleton in the control of cancer growth. Microsc.
   Res. Tech **47:** 61–66.
6. TIKOO, A., H. CUTLER, S.H. LO, L.B. CHEN & H. MARUTA. 1999. Treatment of TAS-
   induced cancers by the F-actin cappers, tensin, and chaetoglobosin K, in combination with the caspase-1 inhibitor N1445. Cancer J. (Sci. Amer.) **5:** 293–300.
7. MARUTA, H., A. TIKOO, R. SHAKRI, L. ZUGARO, Y. HIROKOWA, T. SHISHIDO, B. BOW-
   ERS, L.H. YE, K. KOHAMA & R. SIMPSON. 1999. The anti-cancer drug MKT-077
   cross-links actin filaments and binds HSC70 chaperone ATPase in v-Ha-Ras transformants. Cancer Res. **59:** in press.
8. LEBLANC, V., B. TOCQUE & I. DELUMEAU. 1998. Ras GAP controls Rho-mediated
   cytoskeletal rearrangement through its SH3 domain. Mol Cell Biol. **18:** 5567–5578.

9. SEKINE, A., M. FUJIWARA & S. NARUMIYA. 1989. Asn residue in the Rho is the modification site for Botulinum ADP-ribosyltransferase C3. J. Biol. Chem. **264:** 8602–8605.

10. MARUTA, H. 1998. GTPase regulators: Gaps, Gdss & Gdis. *In* G proteins, Cytoskeleton & Cancer. H. Maruta & K. Kohama, Eds. :151–170. Landes Bioscience. Austin, TX.

11. MANSER, E., T. LEUNG, H. SALIHUDDIN, L. TAN & L. LIM. 1993. A non-receptor Tyr kinase that inhibits the GTPase activity of CDC42. Nature **363:** 364–367.

12. NUR-E-KAMAL, MSA., J.M. KAMAL, M.M. QURESHI & H. MARUTA. 1999. The CDC42-specific inhibitor derived from ACK-1 blocks v-Ha-Ras-induced transformation. Oncogene **18**. In press.

13. DEROSSI, D., G. CHASSAING & A. PROCHIANTZ. 1998. Trojan peptides; the penetratin system for intracellular delivery. Trends Cell Biol. **8:** 84–87.

14. HALL, A. 1998. Rho GTPases and actin cytoskeleton. Science **279:** 558–560.

15. DRECHSEL, D.N., A.A. HYMAN, A. HALL & M. GLOTZER. 1996. A requirement for Rho & CDC42 during cytokinesis in Xenopus embryos. Curr. Biol. **7:** 12–23.

16. MIKI, H., T. SASAKI, Y. TAKAI & T. TAKENAWA. 1998. Induction of filopodium formation by a WASP-related actin-depolymerizing protein N-WASP. Nature **391:** 93–96.

17. MANSER, E., T.H. LOO, C.G. KOH, Z.S. ZHAO, X.Q. CHEN, L. TAN, I. TAN, T. LEUNG & L. LIM. 1998. PAK kinases are directly coupled to the PIX family of Gdss. Mol. Cell **1:** 183–192.

18. OBERMEIER, A., S. AHMED, E. MANSER, S.C. YEN, C. HALL & L. LIM. 1998. PAK promotes morphological changes by acting upstream of Rac. EMBO J. **17:** 4328–4339.

19. WALSH, A.B., M. DHANASEKARAN, D. BAR-SAGI & C.C. KUMAR. 1997. SCH51344-induced reversal of RAS-transformation is accompanied by the specific inhibition of the RAS/Rac-dependent cell morphology pathway. Oncogene **15:** 2553–2560.

20. HARTWIG, J.G., G. BOKOCH, C. CARPENTER, P. JANMEY, L. TAYLOR, A. TOKER & T. STOSSEL. 1995. Thrombin receptor ligation and activated Rac uncap actin filament barbed ends through phosphoinositide synthesis. Cell **82:** 643–653.

21. HE, H., T. WATANABE, X. ZHAN, C. HUANG, E. SCHUURING, K. FUKAMI, T. TAKENAWA, C.C. KUMAR, R. SIMPSON. & H. MARUTA. 1998. Role of PIP2 in Ras/Rac-induced disruption of the cortactin-actomyosin II complex and malignant transformation. Mol. Cell Biol. **18:** 3829–3837.

22. MUELLAUER, L., H. FUJITA, A. SHIZAKI & N. KUZUMAKI. 1993. Tumor-suppressive function of mutated gelsolin in Ras-transformed cells. Oncogene **8:** 2531–2536.

23. LO, S.H., E. WEISBERG & L.B. CHEN. 1994. Tensin: A potential link between cytoskeleton and signal transduction. BioEssays **16:** 817–823.

24. CUTLER, H., F. CRUMLEY, R.COX, R. COLE, J. DORNER, J. SPRINGER, F. LATTERELL, J. THEAN & A. ROSSI. 1980. Chaetoglobosin K: A new plant growth inhibitor and toxin from *Diplodia macrospora*. J. Agric. Food Chem. **28:** 139-142.

25. YAHARA, I., F. HARADA, S. SEKITA, K. YOSHIHIRA & S. NATORI. 1982. Correlation between effects of 24 different cytochalasins on cellular structures and events and those on actin in vitro. J. Cell Biol. **92:** 69–78.

26. MARTE, B.M. & J. DOWNWARD. 1997. PKB/AKT: Connecting PI-3 kinase to cell survival and beyond. Trends Biochem. Sci. **22:** 355–358.

Antiangiogenic Domains Shared by Thrombospondins and Metallospondins, a New Family of Angiogenic Inhibitors

M. LUISA IRUELA-ARISPE,[a] FRANCISCA VÁZQUEZ, AND
MARIA ASUNCIÓN ORTEGA

Department of Molecular, Cell and Developmental Biology and Molecular Biology Institute, University of California, Los Angeles, California 90095, USA

ABSTRACT: The growth of solid tumors has been shown to depend on neovascularization. By understanding the mechanisms that control the neovascular response, it may be possible to design therapeutic strategies to selectively prevent or halt pathologic vascular growth and restrain cancer progression. Thrombospondin-1 is an extracellular matrix protein that among several functions suppresses capillary growth in angiogenesis assays. We have demonstrated that within the context of the mammary gland TSP1 can modulate normal development of blood vessels. Expression of TSP1 in transgenic animals under the control of the MMTV promoter was associated with a 50–72% reduction in capillary growth. In addition, TSP1 reduced tumor size in transgenic overexpressors. The data suggest an important role for TSP1 in modulating vascular growth in both normal and pathologic tissues. The antiangiogenic region of TSP1 has been mapped to the type I (properdin) repeats. To identify novel proteins with such a domain, we have cloned two cDNAs (METH-1 and METH-2) which also have antiangiogenic properties. In addition to carboxyterminal thrombospondin-like domains they also contain metalloproteinase and disintegrin sequences. Expression of both proteins is broad but nonoverlapping. Recombinant fragments from these sequences have strong antiangiogenic potential in the CAM and cornea pocket assays. At the same molar ratio, METH-1 and METH-2 are about 20-fold more potent than TSP1. We predict that these proteins are likely endogenous modulators of vascular growth with relevant therapeutic potential in cancer and other disease states.

INTRODUCTION

Reduction or suppression of tumorigenicity can be accomplished at multiple levels: by direct cell cycle regulation, targeted cellular ablation, control of signal transduction, and/or inhibition of angiogenesis.[1–6] Several investigators have implicated tumor suppressor genes in cell cycle regulation or signal transduction pathways, and considerable effort is being made to identify the critical points in cell transformation that might be sensitive to pharmacologic control. A parallel line of investigation has focused on understanding the regulation of vascular growth. It is recognized that an

[a]Address for correspondence: Luisa Iruela-Arispe, Ph.D., Molecular Biology Institute—UCLA, 611 Circle Drive East, Los Angeles, CA 90095. Phone, 310/794–5763; fax, 310/794–5766.

e-mail, arispe@mbi.ucla.edu

increase in the vascular supply plays a central role in tumor progression and metastasis.[5,7-9] In most tumors, angiogenesis has been acknowledged as a significant indicator of tumor progression that is independent of axillary lymph node status.[9-11] Angiogenesis therapy has recently gained recognized value as a means to suppress tumor growth and metastasis.[6] Several inhibitors and antagonists of VEGF function are currently being tested in clinical trials, and initial evaluations have instigated high levels of enthusiasm (Keystone Symposia, Steamboat, 1998). In this chapter, we provide a general background on angiogenesis inhibitors and introduce a new family of proteins, named metallospondins, that display significant angioinhibitory properties.

ANGIOGENESIS AND THE GROWTH OF TUMORS

The growth of solid tumors strictly depends on new blood vessel formation (reviewed in ref. 5). This relationship between tumor growth and angiogenesis was initially proposed by Folkman and colleagues[12] three decades ago. Thirty years later, their initial observations have gained solid acceptance, and the vascular-density–tumor size relationship has been validated in a variety of tumors including breast carcinoma,[11] melanoma,[13] and brain tumors[14] among others. In fact, the degree of tumor angiogenesis has been identified as a significant and independent prognostic indicator and a requirement for the expansion and metastatic progression of malignant disease.[9,10]

The possibility that tumor progression could be regulated by pharmacologic and/ or genetic suppression of blood vessel growth has engendered long-standing interest in the identification of molecules or synthetic compounds that block angiogenesis. The search for angiogenic inhibitors has followed three independent paths:

(1) *identification of inhibitors in tissues that lack blood vessels*: Proteins present in cartilage that antagonize angiogenesis[15-18];

(2) *identification of synthetic or natural substances that normally antagonize the effect of stimulators*: Prostaglandin synthetase inhibitors,[19] protamine (antagonist of heparin),[20] fumagillin (AGM1470), a compound that blocks EC migration and proliferation,[21] antibodies that block VEGF/VPF,[22] and antibodies against $\alpha v\beta 3$;[23]

(3) *characterization of inhibitors that are synthesized or processed as such by tumors*: This approach led to the characterization of angiostatin[24] and endostatin.[25]

At this time, the contribution of angiogenesis to the progression of tumors is widely accepted. The search for additional effective inhibitors is underway in both academic and private sectors. Nonetheless, to date, very few inhibitors have been submitted to clinical trials. Some of the currently recognized angiogenic suppressors are poor candidates for systemic treatment because of their collateral effects. Finally, it is conceivable that specific inhibitors of vessel growth could be efficient in certain pathologies, but ineffective in the control of cancer-mediated angiogenesis. Therefore, it is necessary to identify nontoxic, endothelial-specific, and vascular bed-specific effector molecules that can block rampant growth of tumor-induced capillaries, yet ideally not compromise repair-mediated angiogenesis.

It is our premise that potent and tissue-specific inhibitors are those normally existent *in vivo*. Based on the work of many laboratories, including our own, it has become clear that TSP1 has considerable angiostatic/antiangiogenic activity[26–29] and that, in fact, this molecule is an endogenous modulator of physiologic angiogenesis in the human endometrium and mammary gland.[29] For almost 10 years, our laboratory and several others have focused our research on the ability of TSP1 and peptide mimetics to regulate angiogenesis in vivo[30] and to suppress the growth of tumors. Experiments using xenograph assays as well as several in vivo models of angiogenesis have consistently supported TSP1 as a negative modulator of angiogenesis with the ability to suppress tumor growth.[31] Together, these findings argue strongly for studies on TSP1 and TSP1-related gene products that could be effective in controlling vascularization in specific settings.

The region responsible for the antiangiogenic properties of TSP1 has been confined to the second and third type 1.[30,32] In an effort to identify new inhibitors of angiogenesis that might contain the TSP1 antiangiogenic repeats, we have screened a large database of ESTs and identified five previously uncharacterized cDNAs. Full-length sequence revealed that two of those cDNAs are highly similar (52% at the amino acid level) and, in addition to the TSP repeats, contain metalloproteinase and disintegrin motifs.[33] On the basis of their structure, we named them METH-1 and METH-2 (ME for metalloproteinase and TH for thrombospondin). Interestingly, another protein with the same structural features was identified and named pNPI for pro-collagen N propeptidase.[34] All three proteins have a metalloproteinase and disintegrin domain followed by a varied number of TSP/type 1 repeats. The metalloproteinase-disintegrin motif is reminiscent of the ADAM family of growth regulatory genes. Recently, the murine homolog of METH-1 was published and named AD-AMTS.[35] A comparison between murine and human genes showed 84% similarity at the amino acid level.[33] We consider all of these proteins as members of a new family of proteins which we have named metallospondins. We believe that this family has at least four additional members, given the ETS Genebank database. The general structure of metallospondins is presented in FIGURE 1.

The TSP repeats in METH-1 and METH-2 are more similar to the second and third TSP repeats of TSP2, the region known to display antiangiogenic function. A comparison of the sequences is provided in FIGURE 2.

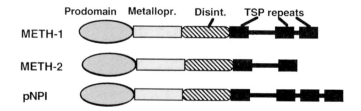

FIGURE 1. Protein structure of metallospondins. The basic structure of METH-1, METH-2, and pNPI includes a prodomain followed by a metalloproteinase domain with a typical zinc-binding motif, disintegrin (cysteine-rich) region, and a variable number of TSP/type 1 domains, 3 in METH-1, 2 in METH-2, and 4 in pNPI.

```
   *  *  *  *              *                          *    *
SPRWSLWSTWAPCSVTCSEGSQLRYRRCVGWNGQCSGKVA-PGTLEWQLQACEDQPCCP   PROPERDIN
DGGWSHWSPWSSCSVTCGDGVITRIRLCNSPSPQMNGKPC--EGEARETKACKKDACPI   TSP-1
DGGWSHWSPWSSCSVTCGVGNITRIRLCNSPVPQMGGKNC--KGSGRETKACQGAPCPI   TSP-2
HGSWGMWGPWGDCSTRCGGGVQYTMRECDNPVPKNGGKYC--EGKRVRYRSCNLEDCP    METH-1
DGGWAPWGPWGECSRTCGGGVQFSHRECKDPEPQNGGRYC--LGRRAKYQSCHTEECP    METH-2
```

FIGURE 2. Type 1/TSP repeats in several proteins. Sequence (single amino acid code) comparison of TSP/type 1 repeats in properdin (first repeat), TSP1 (second repeat), TSP2 (second repeat), METH-1 (first repeat), and METH-2 (first repeat). Common tryptophane (W) and cysteine (C) residues are identified by an *asterisk*.

TSP OR TYPE I REPEATS AND ANGIOGENESIS

The type I repeats of TSP1 have been characterized extensively.[36-38] The sequences have been shown to (1) bind heparin in three regions (KRFK, WSPW, and CSVTCG), (2) activate latent forms of TGF-β via a nonproteolytic pathway by the cooperation of two sequences (K/R-F-K/R and WSPW), (3) bind sulfatide, (4) promote cell adhesion, and (5) inhibit angiogenesis through the CSVTCG sequence. The sequences of CSVTCG and WSPW in METH-1 may well have similar biological functions.

Interestingly, the TSP or type 1 motif is present in several molecules, including TSP-2, complement components C6 to C9,[38] F-spondin,[39] UNC-5 in *Caenorrhabditis elegans*,[40] proteins related to connective tissue growth factor (including CEF-10, CY-61, FISP-12, and NOV),[41-46] and in various parasite proteins such as circumsporozoite and thrombospondin–related anonymous protein (TRAP) in *Plasmodium*.[47-48] The function of the TSP repeats in most of these proteins has not been studied. Nonetheless, removal of the TSP region from the circumsporozoite protein in *P. falciparum* has been shown to impair binding to its receptor on live cells.[49] In properdin, this repeat binds to sulfated glycoconjugates[50-54] and to C3b.[55]

Are all proteins with TSP repeats antiangiogenic? With the exception of studies with TSP1, this question has not been addressed. Because of the identification of METH-1 and METH-2, we have partially addressed the issue by generating recombinant fusion proteins containing TSP repeat sequences from TSP1, properdin, METH-1, and METH-2. FIGURE 3 shows the degree of purity of the recombinant proteins used in angiogenesis assays. All proteins were evaluated for angiogenic activity side-by-side and at the same molar ratio.

Fusion proteins as well as GST alone (negative control) was used on chorioallantoic membrane assays. In this assay, a pellet containing polymerized collagen and angiogenic growth factors (VEGF and FGF-2) was applied to the surface of the CAM to induce a neovascular response in 24 hours. CAM-derived vessels grow against gravity and invade the acellular collagen gel. In the experimental pellets, recombinant proteins were also incorporated to challenge the ability of growth factors to elicit an angiogenic response. When an inhibitor was present, colonization of the collagen gel by vessels was significantly diminished or absent. The degree of angiogenesis was assessed by injection of high molecular weight FITC-dextran into the chicken embryonic circulation. The intensity of fluorescence (equivalent to vascular density) displayed in a 250-μm^2 area was determined using Image 3 software in the

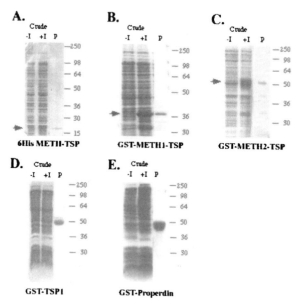

FIGURE 3. Purification of recombinant proteins. SDS-polyacrylamide gel electro-phoresis analysis of total cell lysate and purified *Escherichia coli* recombinant proteins stained with Coommassie blue. Molecular weight of standards is indicated on the *right*. *Lane 1*, total cell lysate prior to IPTG induction; *lane 2*, total cell lysate after IPTG induction; *lane 3*, purified protein. (**A**) 6His-METH1, a histidine-tagged protein containing the first TSP-domain of METH-1; (**B**) GST-METH1, a GST fusion protein containing the first TSP-like domain of METH-1; (**C**) GST-METH-2, a GST fusion protein containing the first TSP-like domain of METH-2; (**D**) GST-TSP1, a GST fusion protein containing the second and third TSP-like type 1 domain of TSP1; and (**E**) GST-properdin, a GST fusion protein containing the first and second TSP-like type 1 domains of properdin.

growth factor-containing pellets and was considered a 100% response. The degree of inhibition of angiogenesis was determined by comparing this value to those dis-played in the experimental pellets. FIGURE 4 shows the degree of vascular response in a 250-μm^2 area after 24 hours of treatment. A dense network of capillaries was detected in the pellets containing growth factors and GST (FIG. 4A). By contrast, GST alone did not promote an angiogenic response (FIG. 4B). A variable degree of inhibition of angiogenesis was seen in the presence of TSP1, METH-1, and METH-2 fusion proteins (FIG. 4C-E). By contrast, the properdin fusion protein did not sup-press the neovascular response mediated by the angiogenic stimulators (FIG. 4F). Results were consistent in seven independent experiments. In addition to the exper-iments performed with the METH-1 and METH-2 type 1 repeats, the entire proteins also displayed angioinhibitory activity.[33]

These results would argue that the presence of TSP repeats alone does not render a protein an angiogenic inhibitor. It appears that differences in the primary structure of these proteins, or perhaps adjacent sequences, participate in the overall antiangio-genic function displayed by these proteins.

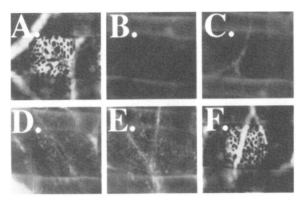

FIGURE 4. Effect of recombinant TSP-repeat fusion proteins on growth factor-mediated angiogenesis. For these experiments 12-day-old white Lenhorn chicken embryos were used. Vitrogen pellets and injection of FITC-dextran was performed as previously described.[30,57] Assays were carried out for 24 hours. Confocal images within the vitrogen pellet are shown in a window of 250 μm². Pellets correspond to: **(A)** VEGF (250 ng/pellet) and FGF-2 (50 ng/pellet) in the presence of GST; note the dense network of capillaries; **(B)** GST alone (negative control) shows no capillary growth; all subsequent pellets contain the same mixture of VEGF and FGF-2 as in **A** in addition to: **(C)** METH-1/GST fusion protein (7 μg/pellet); **(D)** METH-2/GST fusion protein (5 μg/pellet); **(E)** GST-TSP1 (5 μg/pellet); and **(F)** GST-properdin (5 μg/pellet).

Although we have shown that metallospondins have angio-inhibitory activity *in vivo*, the efficacy of these proteins in tumors might be variable. We and others have accumulated sufficient data in animal studies to argue that TSP1 constitutes a likely candidate for antiangiogenic therapy in tumors.[30,31] Whether METH-1 and METH-2 will show the same efficacy within the context of a tumor is still speculative. In angiogenesis assays, both METH-1 and METH-2 intact, full-length proteins appear more potent than either TSP1 or endostatin.[33] Experiments using xenograph assays are currently underway and will determine their efficacy in reducing tumor growth.

CONCLUDING REMARKS

The relationship between tumor progression and induction of a neovascular response has been well documented by several investigators in many independent laboratories. Inhibitors of angiogenesis may prove effective as adjuvant therapy in cancer patients, and several animal studies have demonstrated their efficacy in inhibiting tumor growth or inducing tumor regression.[24,25,31] Furthermore, antiangiogenic treatment of tumor-bearing mice does not induce acquired drug resistance, offering a valuable advantage over conventional cytotoxic therapies that target tumor cell growth.[56] Therefore, the identification and study of angiogenesis inhibitors can provide valuable pharmacologic information to prevent neovascularization in tumors. Here we have introduced a new family of inhibitors, metallospondins. Along with these molecules, novel modulators of endothelial cell function and angiogenic response appear frequently in the literature. Future research efforts should be directed towards further understanding the biology of these inhibitors, their specificity for tumor and other vascular beds, their relative potency, and their mechanism of action.

REFERENCES

1. SANGER, R. 1989. Tumor suppressor genes: The puzzle and the promise. Science **246:** 1406–1412.
2. BISHOP, J.M. 1987. The molecular genetics of cancer. Science **235:** 305–311.
3. HARRIS, H. 1986. The genetic analysis of malignancy. J. Cell Sci. Suppl. **4:** 431–444.
4. WEINBERG, R.A. 1988. Finding the anti-oncogene. Sci. Am. **259:** 34–41.
5. FOLKMAN, J. 1990. What is the evidence that tumors are angiogenic-dependent? J. Natl. Cancer Inst. **82:** 4–6.
6. FOLKMAN, J. 1996. New perspectives in clinical oncology from angiogenesis research. Eur. J. Cancer **32:** 2534–2539.
7. BLOOD, C.H. & B.R. ZETTER. 1990. Tumor interactions with the vasculature: Angiogenesis and tumor metastasis. Biochim. Biophys. Acta **1032:** 89–118.
8. WEIDNER, N. 1992. The relationship of tumor angiogenesis and metastasis with emphasis on invasive breast carcinoma. In Advances in Pathology.: 101–122. Chicago.
9. WEIDNER, N. et al. 1992. Tumor angiogenesis: A new significant and independent prognostic indicator in early-stage breast carcinoma. J. Natl. Cancer Inst. **84:** 1875–1887.
10. WEIDNER, N. et al. 1991. Tumor angiogenesis and metastasis: Correlation in invasive breast carcinoma. N. Engl. J. Med. **324:** 1–8.
11. BOSARI, S. et al. 1992. Microvessel quantitation and prognosis in invasive breast carcinoma. Human Pathol. **23:** 755–761.
12. FOLKMAN, J. et al. 1963. Growth and metastasis of tumor in organ culture. Cancer **16:** 453–467.
13. BARNHILL, R.L. & M.A. LEVY. 1993. Regressing thin cutaneous malignant melanomas (< 1.0 mm) are associated with angiogenesis. Am. J. Pathol. **143:** 99–104.
14. BREM, S.S. et al. 1990. Inhibition of angiogenesis and tumor growth in the brain. Am. J. Pathol. **137:** 1121–1142.
15. LANGER, R. et al. 1976. Isolation of a cartilage factor that inhibits tumor neovascularization. Science **193:** 70–72.
16. LANGER, R.S. et al. 1980. Control of tumor growth in animals by infusion of an angiogenesis inhibitor. Proc. Natl. Acad. Sci. USA **77:** 4431–4335.
17. TAKIGAWA, M. et al. 1985. A factor in conditioned medium of rabbit costal chondrocytes inhibits the proliferation of cultured endothelial cells and angiogenesis induced by B16 melanomas: Its relation with cartilage-derived anti-tumor factor (CATF). Biochem. Int. **14:** 357–363.
18. MOSES, M.A. et al. 1990. Identification of an inhibitor of neovascularization from cartilage. Science **248:** 1408-1410.
19. PETERSON, H.I. 1986. Tumor angiogenesis inhibition by prostaglandin synthetase inhibitors. Anticancer Res. **6:** 251-254.
20. TAYLOR, S. & J. FOLKMAN. 1982. Protamine is an inhibitor of angiogenesis. Nature **297:** 307–312.
21. INGBER, D. et al. 1990. Synthetic analogues of fumagillin that inhibit angiogenesis and suppress tumor growth. Nature **348:** 555–558.
22. FERRARA, N. 1995. The role of vascular endothelial growth factor in pathological angiogenesis. Breast Cancer Res. Treat. **36:** 127–137.
23. BROOKS, P.C. et al. 1995. Anti-integrin $\alpha v \beta 3$ blocks human breast cancer growth and angiogenesis in human skin. J. Clin. Invest. **96:** 1815–1822.
24. O'REILLY, M.S. et al. 1994. Angiostatin: A novel angiogenesis inhibitor that mediates the suppression of metastases by a Lewis lung carcinoma. Cell **79:** 315–328.

25. O'REILLY, M.S. *et al.* 1997. Endostatin: An endogenous inhibitor of angiogenesis and tumor growth. Cell **88:** 277–285.

26. RASTINEJAD, F. *et al.* 1989. Regulation of the activity of a new inhibitor of angiogenesis by a cancer suppressor gene. Cell **56:** 345–355.

27. GOOD, D.J. *et al.* 1990. A tumor suppressor-dependent inhibitor of angiogenesis is immunologically and functionally indistinguishable from a fragment of thrombospondin. Proc. Natl. Acad. Sci. USA **87:** 6624–6628.

28. IRUELA-ARISPE, M.L *et al.* 1991. Thrombospondin exerts an antiangiogenic effect on tube formation by endothelial cells in vitro. Proc. Natl. Acad. Sci. USA **88:** 5026–5030.

29. IRUELA-ARISPE, M.L *et al.* 1996. Thrombospondin-1, an inhibitor of angiogenesis, is regulated by progesterone in human stromal cells. J. Clin. Invest. **97:** 403–412.

30. IRUELA-ARISPE, M.L *et al.* 1999. Inhibition of angiogenesis by thrombospondin-1 is mediated by two independent regions within the type 1 repeats. Circulation. In press.

31. GUO, N.H. *et al.* 1997. Antiproliferative and antitumor activities of D-reverse peptides derived from the second type1 repeats of thrombospondin. Structural requirements for heparin binding and promotion of melanoma cell adhesion and chemotaxis. J. Pept. Res. **50:** 210–221.

32. TOLSMA, S.S. *et al.* 1993. Peptides derived from two separate domains of the matrix protein thrombospondin-1 have anti-angiogenic activity. J. Cell Biol. **122:** 497–511.

33. VAZQUEZ, F. 1999. METH1 and METH2, members of a new family of proteins with angio-inhibitory domains. J. Biol. Chem. In press.

34. COLIGE, A. *et al.* 1997. cDNA cloning and expression of bovine procollagen I N-proteinase: A new member of the superfamily of zinc-metalloproteinases with binding sites for cells and other matrix components. Proc. Natl. Acad. Sci. USA **94:** 2374–2379.

35. KUNO, K. *et al.* 1997. Molecular cloning of a gene encoding a new type of metalloproteinase-disintegrin family protein with thrombospondin motifs as an inflammation associated gene. J. Biol. Chem. **272:** 556–562.

36. GUO, N.H. *et al.* 1992. Heparin- and sulfatide-binding peptides from the type I repeats of human thrombospondin promote melanoma cell adhesion. Proc. Natl. Acad. Sci. USA **89:** 3040–3044.

37. GUO, N.H. *et al.* 1992. Heparin-binding peptides from the type I repeats of thrombospondin. Structural requirements for heparin binding and promotion of melanoma cell adhesion and chemotaxis. J. Biol. Chem. **267:** 19349–19355.

38. SCHULTZ-CHERRY, S. *et al.* 1995. Regulation of transforming growth factor ß activation by discrete sequences of thrombospondin 1. J. Biol. Chem. **270:** 7304–7310.

39. KLAR, A. *et al.* 1992. F-spondin, a gene expressed at high levels in the floor plate encodes a secreted protein that promotes neural cell adhesion and neurite extension. Cell **69:** 95–103.

40. LEUNG-HAGESTEIJN, C. *et al.* 1992. Unc-5, a transmembrane protein with immunoglobulin and thrombospondin type 1 domains, guides cell and pioneer axon migrations in *Caenorhabditis elegans.* Cell **71:** 289–299.

41. SIMMONS, D.L. *et al.* 1989. Identification of a phorbol ester-repressible v-src inducible gene. Proc. Natl. Acad. Sci. USA **86:** 1178–1187.

42. O'BRIEN, T.P. *et al.* 1990. Expression *cyr*61, a growth factor-inducible immediate-early gene. Mol. Cell Biol. **10:** 3569–3576.

43. RYSECK, R.-P. *et al.* 1991. Structure, mapping, and expression of *fisp*-12, a growth factor-inducible gene encoding a secreted cysteine rich protein. Cell Growth Differ. **2:** 225–232.

44. BRADHAM, D.M. *et al.* 1991. Connective tissue growth factor: A cysteine-rich mitogen secreted by vascular endothelial cells is related to the *src*-induced immediate early gene product CEF-10. J. Cell. Biol. **114:** 1285–1294.
45. JOLIOT, V. *et al.* 1992. Proviral rearrangements and overexpression of a new cellular gene (*nov*) in myeloblastosis-associated virus type 1-induced nephroblastomas. Mol. Cell. Biol. **12:** 10-19.
46. BRUNNER, A. *et al.* 1991. Identification of a gene family regulated by transforming growth factor ß. DNA Cell Biol. **10:** 293–305.
47. OZAKI, L.S. *et al.* 1983. Structure of the *Plasmodium knowlesi* gene coding for the circumsporozoite protein. Cell **34:** 815–821.
48. ROBSON, K.J.H. *et al.* 1988. A highly conserved amino acid sequence in thrombospondin, properdin, and in proteins from sporozoites and blood stages of a human malaria parasite. Nature **335:** 79–86.
49. CERAMI, C. *et al.* 1992. The basolateral domain of the hepatocyte plasma membrane bears receptors for the circumsporozoite protein *Plasmodium falciparum* sporozoites. Cell **70:** 1021–1032.
50. HOLT, G.D. *et al.* 1990. Properdin binds to sulfatide (Gal(3-SO4)ß1-1Cer) and has a sequence homology with other proteins that binds sulfated glycoconjugates. J. Biol. Chem. **265:** 2852–2863.
51. PRATER, C.A. *et al.* 1991. The properdin-like repeats of thrombospondin contain a cell attachment site. J. Cell Sci. **112:** 1031–1039.
52. PANCAKE, S.J. *et al.* 1992. Malaria sporozoites and circumsporozoite proteins bind specifically to sulfated glycoconjegates. J. Cell Biol. **117:** 1351–1361.
53. FREVERT, U. *et al.* 1993. Malaria circumsporozoite proteins binds to heparan sulfate proteoglycans associated with the surface membrane of hepatocytes. J. Exp. Med. **177:** 1287–1291.
54. MÜLLER, H.-M. *et al.* 1993. Thrombospondin-related anonymous protein (TRAP) of *Plasmodium falciparum* binds specifically to sulfated glycoconjugates and to HepG2 hepatoma cells suggesting a role for this molecule in sporozoite invasion of hepatocytes. EMBO J. **12:** 2881–2893.
55. HIGGINS, J.M.G. *et al.* 1995. Characterization of mutant forms of recombinant human properdin lacking single thrombsopondin type 1 repeats. J. Immunol. **155:** 5777–5785.
56. BOEHM, T. *et al.* 1997. Antiangiogenic therapy of experimental cancer does not induce acquired drug resistance. Nature **39:** 404–407.
57. IRUELA-ARISPE, M.L. & H. DVORAK. 1997. Angiogenesis: A dynamic balance of stimulator and inhibitors. Thromb. Haematol. **78:** 672–677.

Immunotherapy of Cancer

ELIZABETH M. JAFFEE

Department of Oncology, The Johns Hopkins University School of Medicine, 720 Rutland Avenue/Ross 350, Baltimore, Maryland 21205-2196

ABSTRACT: The goal of cancer treatment is to develop modalities that specifically target tumor cells, thereby avoiding unnecessary side effects to normal tissue. Vaccine strategies that result in the activation of the immune system specifically against proteins expressed by a cancer have the potential to be effective treatment for this purpose. An early vaccine approach that was developed by our group involves the insertion of the granulocyte-macrophage colony stimulating factor (GM-CSF) gene into cancer cells that are then used to immunize patients. These genetically modified tumor cells produce the immune activating protein GM-CSF in the local environment of the tumor cells, specifically activating the patient's T cells to eradicate cancer at metastatic sites. We have performed many studies that demonstrate that this vaccine can cure mice of cancer. We recently demonstrated that this approach can activate an immune response in patients with renal cell carcinoma. We are currently testing a similar approach in patients with pancreatic cancer. Until recently, whole tumor cells were used to produce the vaccine because the proteins expressed by the tumor cells that can be recognized by the immune system were unknown. However, recent advances have allowed the identifiation of many of the proteins expressed by some cancers. In addition, significant attention has been focused on the mechanisms by which antitumor immunity can be modulated. These active areas of research will undoubtably lead to the devleopment of more specific and more potent vaccine strategies in the near future. The first part of this paper focuses on data from two recent clinical trials that evaluated the whole tumor cell approach. The second part of this paper discusses some of the more exciting antigen-specific vaccine approaches that are under development for the treatment of cancer.

INTRODUCTION

Cancer afflicts about 1.2 million Americans each year. About 50% of these cancers are curable with surgery, radiation therapy, and chemotherapy. Despite significant technical advances in these three treatment modalities, each year more than 500,000 Americans will die of cancer. Because most recurrences are at distant sites such as liver, brain, bone, and lung, improved systemic therapies are urgently needed.

ADVANTAGES OF VACCINES THAT INDUCE T-CELL IMMUNE RESPONSES

Immunotherapy has the potential to provide an alternative systemic treatment for most types of cancer. The advantage of immunotherapy over radiation and chemotherapy is that it can act specifically against the tumor without causing normal tissue damage. Vaccines, one form of immunotherapy, can also provide active immunization which allows for amplification of the immune response. In addition, vaccines can generate a memory immune response. Recent advances in our understanding of the mechanisms of immune system activation have revealed that any cellular protein (expressed in virally infected cells or cancer cells) can be recognized by the immune system if those proteins are presented to the immune system in a form that results in activation rather than ignorance or tolerance to that antigen. In addition, T cells rather than B cells are usually responsible for this recognition.

It is important to point out that when we discuss vaccines for cancer we are referring to treatment rather than to prevention, because the antigens expressed by tumor cells (which are the immunogens recognized by the immune system) are not yet known. In contrast, we can use vaccines to prevent infectious diseases because the causative agent and/or its proteins that can serve as the immunogen are already known. Because we do not know what proteins expressed by pancreatic cancers are recognized by the immune system, the best way to design a pancreatic cancer vaccine is to use the whole tumor cell as the antigen source.

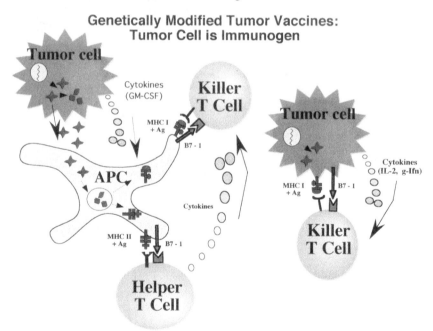

FIGURE 1. Model of two genetically modified whole cell tumor vaccine approaches. In the first model (**left**), tumor cells are genetically modified to express cytokines that attract professional antigen-presenting cells (APCs) to the tumor vaccine site. These APCs then take up the tumor proteins and process them using their own cellular machinery for more effective presentation to both helper and killer T cells. In the second model (**right**), tumor cells are genetically altered to express cytokines that attract killer T cells to the vaccine site, as well as with surface co-stimulatory molecules to enhance T-cell activation, where they are then directly activated by the vaccinating cells.

FIGURE 1 illustrates the two ways in which pancreatic and other tumor cells are currently being genetically modified to more efficiently present their tumor antigens to the immune system, thereby resulting in potent activation of a systemic antitumor immune response. In the first model, tumor cells are genetically modified to express cytokines (proteins normally expressed as paracrine factors by immune cells to orchestrate immune responses) that attract professional antigen-presenting cells (APCs), such as macrophages or dendritic cells, to the site of the tumor cell where these APCs then take up the tumor cell's proteins and process them using their own cellular machinery to more effectively present them to helper and killer T cells. APCs have the ability to activate both helper and killer T cells. Evidence suggests that helper T cells can significantly potentiate killer T-cell activity by secreting cytokines such as interleukin-2 which are potent killer T-cell growth factors. In the second model, tumor cells are genetically modified to express co-stimulatory surface molecules or cytokines that can directly attract and activate killer T cells, often bypassing the helper T-cell arm.

PRE-CLINICAL AND CLINICAL STUDIES OF WHOLE CELL VACCINE APPROACHES

Both of the foregoing approaches have been tested in preclinical models.[1] Dranoff and colleagues were the first to perform a head-to-head comparison of more than 10 known immune activating cytokines using one of the most non-immunogenic murine tumors, B16 F10 melanoma. In this particular study, only one cytokine, granulocyte-macrophage colony stimulating factor (GM-CSF), stood out as the most potent cytokine in curing mice of this very aggressive tumor.[2] GM-CSF is now known to be a potent growth factor for professional APCs including dendritic cells and macrophages. Therefore, this study supports the feasibility of genetically modifying tumor cells to attract professional APCs as intermediates required for helper and killer T-cell activation.

Genetically modified tumor cell vaccines that express various cytokines are already being tested in phase I studies. One study evaluating autologous renal tumor cells that have been genetically modified to express GM-CSF in patients with stage 4 renal cell carcinoma has already been completed.[3] This study demonstrated only local erythema and induration at the vaccine site that was self-limited. No other toxicities were observed. In addition, immune responses in the form of delayed type hypersensitivity (DTH) reactions against autologous tumor cells postvaccination were observed in three of three patients receiving an active vaccine dose of 4×10^7 GM-CSF secreting vaccine cells. Interestingly, one of the three patients demonstrated an associated partial response of pulmonary metastases. Similar DTH responses were observed in other autologous vaccine studies testing different cytokines for activity against other tumors, particularly malignant melanoma.[4]

These early studies testing autologous cytokine-secreting tumor vaccines have demonstrated promising results, encouraging further evaluation of this basic immunotherapy approach. However, these early studies also revealed several problems that limit the feasibility of autologous tumor vaccines. First, it is technically difficult to isolate and expand *in vitro* autologous tumor cells for vaccine production for most histologic tumor types including pancreatic cancers. Second, an autologous vaccine implies that it is individual therapy and therefore not generalizable to all patients with the same cancer. Third, it is very expensive to produce for each individual patient.

To overcome these limitations, we have developed an allogeneic paracrine cytokine vaccine approach. Allogeneic vaccine cells that have been genetically modified to express GM-CSF should be feasible because GM-CSF attracts the intermediate professional APCs for the purpose of activating helper and killer T cells.[5] Therefore, the tumor cell itself does not have to be major histocompatibility complex (MHC) compatible with the host's T cells to activate an immune response. Second, in malignant melanoma, which is the only human tumor for which many tumor antigens have been identified, most antigens recognized by T cells are shared antigens expressed by over 50% of other patients' tumors.[6,7] Thomas et al.[8] recently demonstrated the ability of an allogeneic GM-CSF secreting tumor vaccine to generate potent systemic immunity that was equivalent to the corresponding autologous GM-CSF secreting vaccine cells.[8] In addition, it was shown that this vaccine generated tumor-specific cytotoxic T cells (the critical effector cells for providing systemic immunity) in addition to allogeneic cytotoxic T cells. Therefore, it should be possible to vaccinate patients with a histologically similar set of established tumor lines and still activate systemic antitumor immunity.

We are now testing this approach in patients with stage 1, 2, and 3 pancreatic adenocarcinoma.[9] Patients receive intradermal injections of allogeneic pancreatic vaccine cells that have been genetically modified to express GM-CSF 6 to 8 weeks after undergoing pancreaticoduodenectomy. Four weeks after vaccination patients are evaluated for DTH responses against autologous tumor cells. Patients are then treated with adjuvant radiation and chemotherapy. Four to eight weeks after completion of adjuvant chemotherapy, patients still in remission are given a second vaccination. This study is still ongoing, and the results are preliminary. However, we are observing DTH responses to autologous tumor cells following the first vaccination in some patients.

ANTIGEN-SPECIFIC VACCINE: A LOOK TOWARD THE FUTURE

Even as we test these early vaccine approaches in patients, new and more potent vaccine approaches are being developed in preclinical models. These approaches employ tumor-associated antigens either in the form of proteins or peptides mixed with defined adjuvants administered intradermally or subcutaneously or as genes expressed in viral vectors administered systemically. Antigen-based vaccines get rid of the need for the genetic manipulation of tumor cells. This simplifies the vaccine production process and should result in more generalizable vaccines. In addition, antigen-based vaccines allow for greater control over the amount of antigen formulated in the vaccine, which should translate into improved efficacy. In fact, some of these strategies have been demonstrated in preclinical models to be magnitudes more potent than the whole cell vaccine approach.[10] Recent advances in molcular biology have allowed the direct isolation of tumor-associated antigens that are the targets of cytotoxic T cells. Tumor-associated antigens have now been identified for several

TABLE 1. Categories of identified human tumor antigens

Antigen Category	Human Tumor Antigen
Mutated gene products	Cyclin-dependent kinase 4 (melanoma) Mutated intron B33-B (melanoma) β-catenin (squamous cell carcinoma of head and neck)
Reactivated silent gene products	MAGE gene family (melanoma) BAGE gene family (melanoma) GAGE gene family (melanoma)
Tissue-specific antigens (different antigens)	Tyrosinase (melanoma) Melan-A/MART-1 (melanoma) gp100 (melanoma) gp75 (melanoma)
Idiotypic epitopes	Ig (B cell lymphoma) TCR (T lymphoma)
Viral gene products	EBV (Burkitt's lymphoma) HPV (cervical cancer) HBV (hepatoma)
Oncogene products	bcr/abl rearrangement product (CML) K-ras mutation products (pancreas and colorectal cancers) HER-2/neu overexpression (breast, lung, ovarian cancers)
Mutated tumor suppressor gene products	Mutated p53 gene products (most cancers)

ABBREVIATIONS: Ig, immunoglobulin; TCR, T-cell receptor; EBV, Epstein-Barr virus; HPV, human papilloma virus; HBV, human hepatitis virus; CML, chronic myelogenous leukemia.

cancers including adenocarcinoma of the breast, colon, and pancreas, as well as for malignant melanoma. These antigens can be classified by tissue distribution and function (TABLE 1). Many of these antigens have been found to be shared among other patients' tumors of the same histologic site. These shared antigens are potential candidates for vaccine development. Several of these antigens are currently undergoing phase I testing either mixed with defined antigens or pulsed directly onto autologous dendritic cells (professional APCs) that are isolated from each patient's peripheral blood, expanded and activated *in vitro*, and then given back by adoptive transfer. Future antigen-based vaccine approaches will probably employ newly identified tumor-associated antigens that are delivered in recombinant viral vectors that also contain other immune stimulatory genes and/or genes that target the antigen to particular antigen-processing compartments within a cell to further enhance antitumor immunity. The conduction of well controlled clinical trials will be necessary to identify the most effective approaches for the treatment of advanced cancer. More than likely, it will be necessary to combine vaccine approaches with other cancer treatment modalities to effectively treat larger metastases.

REFERENCES

1. PARDOLL, D.M. 1995. Paracrine cytokine adjuvants in cancer immunotherapy. Annu. Rev. Immunol. **13:** 399–415.

2. DRANOFF, G., E. JAFFEE, A. LAZENBY, P. GOLUMBECK H.I. LEVITSKY, K. BROSE, V. JACKSON, H. HAMADA, D.M. PARDOLL & R.C. MULLIGAN. 1993. Vaccination with irradiated tumor cells engineered to secrete murine granulocyte-macrophage colony-stimulating factor stimulates potent, specific, and long-lasting anti-tumor immunity. Proc. Natl. Acad. Sci. USA **90:** 3539–3543.

3. SIMONS, J.W., E.M. JAFFEE, C. WEBER, H.I. LEVITSKY, W.G. NELSON, L. COHEN, S. CLIFT, C. FINN, K. HAUDA, A. LAZENBY, D.M. PARDOLL, S. PIANTADOSI & A.H. OWENS, R.C. MULLIGAN & F. MARSHALL. 1997. Bioactivity of human GM-CSF gene transduced autologous renal vaccines. Cancer Res. **57:** 1537–1546.

4. CHESON, B.D., P.H. PHILLIPS & M. SZNOL. 1997. National Cancer Institute. Clinical trials. Oncology **11:** 81–90.

5. HUANG, A.Y., P. GOLUMBEK, M. AHMADZADEH, E.M. JAFFEE D.M. PARDOLL & I. LEVITSKY. 1994. Role of bone marrow-derived cells in presenting MHC class I-restricted tumor antigens. Science **264:** 961–965.

6. BOON, T. & P. VAN DER BRUGGEN. 1996. Human tumor antigens recognized by T lymphocytes. J. Exp. Med. **183:** 725–729.

7. ROSENBERG, S.A., Y. KAWAKAMI, P.F. ROBBINS & R. WANG. 1996. Identification of the genes encoding cancer antigens: Implications for cancer immunotherapy. Adv. Cancer Res. **70:** 145–177.

8. THOMAS, M.C., T.F. GRETEN, D.M. PARDOLL & E.M. JAFFEE. 1998. Enhanced tumor protection by granulocyte-macrophage colony-stimulating factor expression at the site of an allogeneic vaccine. Human Gene Ther. **9:** 835–843.

9. JAFFEE, E.M., R. ABRAMS, J. CAMERON, R. DONEHOWER, L. GROCHOW, R. HRUBAN, K.D. LILLEMOE, D.M. PARDOLL, P. SAUTER, C. WEBER & C. YEO. 1998. A phase I clinical trial of lethally irradiated allogeneic pancreatic tumor cells transfected with the Gm-CSF gene for the treatment of pancreatic adenocarcinoma. Human Gene Ther. **9:** 1951–1971.

10. PARDOLL, D.M. 1998. Cancer vaccines. Nature Med. Suppl. **4:** 525–531.

Intracellular Signaling of the TGF-β Superfamily by Smad Proteins

MASAHIRO KAWABATA,[a] TAKESHI IMAMURA, HIROFUMI INOUE, JUN-ICHI HANAI, AYAKO NISHIHARA, AKI HANYU, MASAO TAKASE, YASUHIRO ISHIDOU, YOSHIYUKI UDAGAWA, EIICHI OEDA, DAISUKE GOTO, KEN YAGI, MITSUYASU KATO, AND KOHEI MIYAZONO

Department of Biochemistry, The Cancer Institute, Japanese Foundation for Cancer Research (JFCR), and Research for the Future Program, Japan Society for the Promotion of Science, 1-37-1 Kami-ikebukuro, Toshima-ku, Tokyo 170-8455, Japan

ABSTRACT: TGF-β is a potent inhibitor of cell growth, and accumulating evidence suggests that perturbation of the TGF-β signaling pathway leads to tumorigenesis. Smads are recently identified proteins that mediate intracellular signaling of the TGF-β superfamily. Smads 2 and 3 are phosphorylated by the TGF-β type I receptor. Smad4 was originally identified as a candidate tumor suppressor gene in pancreatic cancers. Smads 2 and 3 form complexes with Smad4 upon TGF-β stimulation. The heteromeric Smad complexes translocate into the nucleus, where they activate expression of target genes. Our recent study demonstrated that Smads exist as monomers in the absence of TGF-β. Smads 2 and 3 form homo- as well as hetero-oligomers with Smad4 upon ligand stimulation. Both homo-oligomers and hetero-oligomers directly bind to DNA, suggesting that the signaling pathway of Smads may be multiplex. Smads 2 and 3 associate with transcriptional coactivators such as p300 in a ligand-dependent manner. p300 enhances transactivation by TGF-β, suggesting that coactivators link Smads to the basal transcriptional machinery. A missense mutation of Smad2 identified in colorectal and lung cancers was introduced to Smad3. The mutant, Smad3(DE), blocked the activation of wild-type Smad2 and Smad3. Thus, the missense mutation not only disrupts the function of the wild-type Smad but also creates a dominant-negative Smad, which could actively contribute to oncogenesis.

INTRODUCTION

Members of the transforming growth factor-β (TGF-β) superfamily, including TGF-βs, activins/inhibins, and bone morphogenetic proteins (BMPs), regulate a wide range of biological phenomena in metazoan organisms.[1] Activins and inhibins were originally identified as factors that regulate secretion of follicle stimulating hormone (FSH) from the pituitary gland and were later shown to regulate fundamental developmental processes such as mesoderm induction. BMPs induce bone and cartilage formation in ectopic tissues. Like activins, BMPs also play pivotal roles in various developmental events including the establishment of the dorsoventral axis, neural induction, and organogenesis of kidneys and eyes. TGF-βs, the prototype of

[a]Phone, Japan-3-3918-0342; fax, Japan-3-3918-0342.
e-mail, mkawabat-ind@umin.u-tokyo. ac.jp

73

the superfamily, are potent growth inhibitors of various lineages of cells including epithelial, endothelial, and hematopoietic. Disruption of the signaling pathway of TGF-β is thus implicated in the initiation of tumors. Indeed, many cancer cells have lost responsiveness to TGF-β. TGF-β also induces production of extracellular matrices, cell migration, angiogenesis, and immunosuppression through which TGF-β may provide the environment that promotes tumor invasion. Therefore, elucidation of the signaling pathway of TGF-β is important in understanding the molecular basis of carcinogenesis.

TGF-β superfamily members bind to two different classes of serine/threonine kinase receptors, termed type I and type II.[1] Receptor activation upon ligand binding is best characterized in TGF-β. TGF-β type II receptor (TβR-II) is a constitutively active kinase that can bind the ligand on its own. Ligand-bound TβR-II then recruits type I receptor (TβR-I/ALK5) and transphosphorylates TβR-I at the "GS domain" rich in glycines and serines. Phosphorylation of the GS domain induces activation of the TβR-I kinase, which in turn phosphorylates cytoplasmic substrates. The downstream events of the receptors have recently begun to be elucidated.[2] Signaling pathway of the TGF-β superfamily is conserved through invertebrates and vertebrates. Genetic studies using *Drosophila* and *Caenorhabditis elegans* have resulted in the identification of the downstream components of the receptors for BMP-like ligands in the organisms. *Mothers against dpp* (*Mad*) in *Drosophila* and *sma*-2, -3, and -4 in *C. elegans* share considerable similarity in the amino acid sequence, suggesting that Mad-related proteins mediate intracellular signaling of the serine/threonine kinase receptors. *DPC4* was isolated as a candidate tumor suppressor gene in pancreatic cancers and shown to be structurally related to *Mad* and *smas*. An increasing number of the vertebrate members belonging to the novel protein family have subsequently been identified and are now denoted Smad.

Eight Smads are known in mammals and are classified into three groups based on their structures and functions (FIG. 1). Receptor-regulated Smads (R-Smads) are directly phosphorylated by type I serine/threonine kinase receptors. Smads 1, 5, and 8 are activated by BMP receptors type IA (BMPR-IA/ALK3) or type IB (BMPR-IB/ALK6), whereas Smads 2 and 3 respond to TβR-I or activin type IB receptors (ActR-IB/ALK4). Recently, ALK2, which was originally identified as activin type IA receptor (ActR-IA), is shown to bind BMP-7/OP-1 and phosphorylate Smads 1 and 5.[3] The second class of the Smad family is common mediator Smads (Co-Smad) that are shared by distinct signaling pathways. Smad4/DPC4 is the only Co-Smad identified in vertebrates. Smads 6 and 7 interfere with signaling by R-Smads and Co-Smads and belong to Anti-Smads. Smads share two conserved regions (FIG. 1). The MH (Mad homology) 1 region resides in the N-terminal half and the MH2 region is located in the C-terminal half. A middle linker region with a variable amino acid sequence lies between the MH1 and MH2 regions. R-Smads and Co-Smads contain the MH1 and MH2 regions. R-Smads, in addition, have the Ser-Ser-X-Ser (SSXS) motif at the C-terminus, which is a direct phosphorylation site by type I receptors. Anti-Smads only share the MH2 region, and the N-terminal half remarkably diverges from the conserved MH1 region.

Upon ligand binding, R-Smads transiently associate with type I receptors and undergo phosphorylation at the SSXS motif. Phosphorylated R-Smads then associate with Co-Smads. The heteromeric complexes translocate into the nucleus where they bind to and activate target genes. The R- and Co-Smad complexes bind to DNA either directly or indirectly through interaction with other DNA binding proteins. The MH1 region directly binds to DNA, whereas the MH2 region has intrinsic transactivation activity. In this report, we present our recent findings on biochemical functions of *Drosophila* Smads, cytoplasmic and nuclear functions of mammalian Smads, and, finally, negative regulation of signaling by Anti-Smads or a mutant Smad.

SIGNALING IN *DROSOPHILA*

Decapentaplegic (Dpp) is a BMP homolog in *Drosophila*. Dpp acts as a morphogen that establishes the dorsoventral polarity in *Drosophila* embryos. Dpp also regulates other developmental events including outgrowth of imaginal disks and gut formation. Punt is a type II receptor for Dpp, whereas Thick veins (Tkv) and Saxophone (Sax) are type I receptors. It has been shown genetically that Mad acts downstream of Tkv. *Daughters against dpp (Dad)* was identified as a Dpp-inducible gene, and genetic studies show that Dad antagonizes Dpp signaling. Medea was recently cloned by several groups.[4,5] The protein structure of Medea is most similar to that of Smad4 among vertebrate Smads, suggesting that Medea is a Co-Smad in *Drosophila*.

We have characterized biochemical functions of the three *Drosophila* Smads (FIG. 1) using COS cells.[5] Mad transiently interacted with activated Tkv and underwent phosphorylation at serine residues. Mad then formed complexes with Medea and translocated into the nucleus. Dad stably interacted with activated Tkv and in-

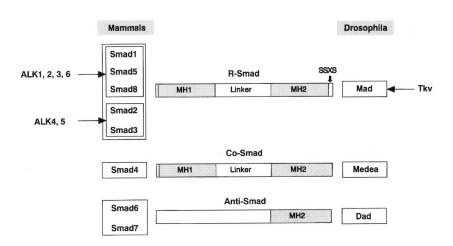

FIGURE 1. Classification and structure of Smads. Smads are grouped into three classes based on structure and function. Mammalian and *Drosophila* Smads are compared. R-Smads are phosphorylated by type I receptors (ALKs) and contain the MH1 and MH2 regions. The C-terminal SSXS motif is the phosphorylation site. Co-Smads lack the SSXS motif. Anti-Smads share only the MH2 region.

terfered with phosphorylation of Mad. Mad existed as a monomer in the absence of receptor stimulation, which will be discussed, and formed homo-oligomers in the presence of Tkv. Dad inhibited homo- and hetero-oligomerization as well as nuclear translocation of Mad. Thus the molecular mechanism of Smad signaling is conserved between *Drosophila* and mammals.

We conducted a two-hybrid screening of a *Drosophila* cDNA library using the cytoplasmic region of Tkv as bait.[6] One of the positive clones was a *Drosophila* inhibitor of apoptosis-1 (DIAP1). DIAP2, which is structurally related to DIAP1, also interacted with Tkv. Overexpression of DIAPs suppresses normally occurring cell death in *Drosophila* eyes, causing rough eye phenotype.[7] Constitutively active Tkv also causes rough eyes.[8] DIAPs may be involved in this process; however, the significance of the DIAP-Tkv interaction *in vivo* awaits further investigation. Neither is it known whether DIAPs play a direct role in Smad signaling at this point.

PHOSPHORYLATION-INDUCED OLIGOMERIZATION OF SMADS

It was shown that ligand-dependent association of R-Smads and Co-Smads is essential for signaling. We studied the interaction between R-Smads upon ligand stimulation. TGF-β induced interaction of Smad2 and Smad3.[9] Smad2 and Smad3 share 91% identity in the amino acid sequence. We therefore examined the possibility of homo-oligomerization of R-Smads.[10] FLAG- and Myc-tagged Smad2 were ex-

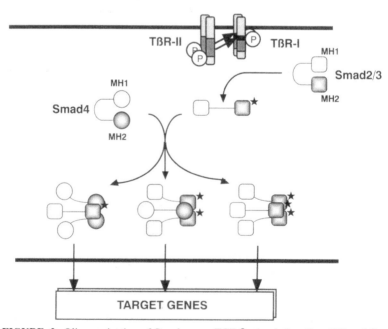

FIGURE 2. Oligomerization of Smads upon TGF-β stimulation. Smad2/3 and Smad4 exist as monomers in the absence of TGF-β. Upon ligand binding, Smad2/3 and Smad4 form trimeric oligomers composed of various numbers of each Smad.

pressed in COS cells in the presence or absence of constitutively active TβR-I. Cells were lysed and subjected to immunoprecipitation with anti-FLAG antibody and immunoblotting with anti-Myc antibody. In the absence of TGF-β stimulation, no oligomers were detected. However, in the presence of activated TβR-I, Smad2 formed homo-oligomers. Smad3 also existed as a monomer in the absence of ligand, and TGF-β induced homo-oligomerization of Smad3. Smad4 is not required for homo-oligomerization, because Smad2 formed oligomers in SW480.7 cells lacking Smad4. Ligand-induced homo-oligomerization was confirmed using gel chromatography. Most of the phosphorylated Smad2 eluted in fractions with sizes of oligomers, whereas unphosphorylated Smad2 eluted as monomers. When Smad2 was coexpressed with Smad4 in the presence of activated TβR-I, the size of the oligomers shifted to smaller fractions, suggesting that Smad2-Smad4 hetero-oligomers form more compact or condensed conformation than do Smad2 homo-oligomers. We also found that Smad2 and Smad4 compete with each other in forming oligomers, indicating that R-Smads and Co-Smads share common binding sites. Detection of homo-oligomers using a chemical cross-linker revealed that Smad2 can form oligomers that contain at least three Smad2 molecules. Crystal structure study of the MH2 domain of Smad4 demonstrated that Smads have a propensity to form trimers. Taken together, the Smad oligomers are likely to be trimers (FIG. 2).

NUCLEAR FUNCTIONS OF SMADS

Smads act as transcriptional activators in the nucleus. We studied the nuclear functions of Smads. It was shown that Smad3-Smad4 hetero-oligomeric complexes bind to DNA.[11] We then investigated whether Smad3 homo-oligomers can bind to DNA. Gel shift assays were performed using a Smad binding sequence from a TGF-β–responsive luciferase reporter, p3TP-Lux, and lysates from COS cells expressing both Smad3 and Smad4 with or without activated TβR-I. TGF-β stimulation induced formation of two distinct DNA binding complexes. Anti-Smad3 antibody supershifted both complexes, and anti-Smad4 antibody supershifted only one of them. The results suggest that one of the complexes contains both Smad3 and Smad4, whereas the other complex consists of Smad3 homo-oligomers. This was confirmed by using Smad4 mutant incapable of oligomerization. The combination of Smad3 and the mutant Smad4 gave only one DNA binding complex. Thus, Smad3 homo-oligomers directly bind to DNA. The physiologic role of the homo-oligomeric DNA binding complex in transcriptional regulation remains to be determined.

Smad2 binds to DNA through interaction with other DNA binding proteins.[12] However, direct DNA binding of Smad2 has not been detected. Although Smad2 is highly similar to Smad3, several differences exist between the two TGF-β–regulated Smads. One of them is an insert in the MH2 region of Smad2, which derives from an extra exon (exon 3) in the Smad2 gene. We constructed a mutant Smad2, Smad2Δex3, which lacks the insert.[13] DNA binding was compared between Smad2 and Smad2Δex3 in gel shift assays. The same probe from p3TP-Lux described above was used. Although Smad2 did not bind to DNA, Smad2Δex3 bound to the probe as efficiently as did Smad3. Thus, the insert in the MH1 region prevents Smad2 from binding to DNA. Smad3 is more potent than Smad2 in activating p3TP-Lux.

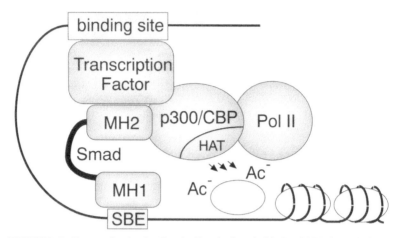

FIGURE 3. Transactivation by Smads. Smads directly bind to DNA through the MH1 region. SBE denotes Smad binding element. Smads also bind to DNA via interaction with other sequence-specific DNA binding transcription factors. The MH2 region recruits co-activators such as p300/CBP. Coactivators interact with proteins of the basal transcription machinery such as RNA polymerase II (Pol II) and loosen chromatin by neutralizing positive charges of histones with histone acetylase (HAT) activity.

Smad2Δex3 induced transactivation as efficiently as did Smad3, suggesting the contribution of direct DNA binding of Smad to activation of the reporter.

An adenoviral oncoprotein, E1A, antagonizes growth inhibition by TGF-β. E1A binds to the retinoblastoma tumor suppressor gene product (pRb), thereby intercepting the growth-regulating pathway of TGF-β. E1A also binds to transcriptional co-activators such as p300 and CBP. p300/CBP associates with a variety of transcription factors. These findings prompted us to investigate the role of p300 in gene regulation by TGF-β.[14] In p3TP-Lux assay, p300 enhanced the activation of the reporter gene by TGF-β, whereas E1A blocked the transactivation. The inhibition by E1A required the p300 binding region in the oncoprotein. In COS cells, Smad3 interacted with p300 in a TGF-β–dependent manner. Smad2 interacted with p300 as well. The binding region in Smad3 was mapped to the MH2 region that has been shown to have an intrinsic transactivation activity. An array of p300 deletion mutants was constructed and tested for the interaction with Smad3. The binding region was mapped to its C-terminal 678 amino acids out of the entire 2414 amino acids. This region inhibited activation of p3TP-Lux by TGF-β in a dominant-negative manner, suggesting that endogenous p300/CBP proteins are required for transactivation of p3TP-Lux by TGF-β. Similar results were reported by several other groups.[15–18] The current model of transcription by Smads is illustrated in FIGURE 3.

ANTAGONIZATION OF SIGNALING BY SMADS

Signaling of the TGF-β superfamily is regulated both positively and negatively by Smad proteins. We identified Smad6 as a novel member of the Smad family from the expressed-sequence tag (EST) database.[19] Smad6 interfered with phosphorylation of Smad1 and Smad2 by BMP and TGF-β, respectively, suggesting that Smad6 inhibits signaling at the receptor level. R-Smads have been shown to directly interact with type I receptors. The interaction is transient and detectable only when phosphorylation is blocked either by using a kinase-defective form of type I receptors or by mutating the SSXS motif. In contrast, Smad6 interacted with both the wild-type and kinase-defective type I receptors. Smad6 is thus recruited to type I receptors upon ligand binding and remains bound to the receptors, thereby inhibiting phosphorylation of R-Smads. Smad7 and *Drosophila* Dad have been shown to inhibit signaling in the identical manner.[5,20,21] Dad was isolated as a gene whose expression is induced by Dpp.[22] Expression of Smad7 is upregulated by TGF-β,[21] whereas Smad6 is induced by BMPs.[23] Thus, Anti-Smads are likely to form autoregulatory negative feedback loop in signaling of the TGF-β superfamily.

Mutations of Smad2 and Smad4 have been found in various cancers. Many of the mutations are mapped to the MH2 region. One such mutation in Smad2 is alteration of the conserved aspartic acid 450 to glutamic acid. The corresponding mutation was introduced into Smad3.[24] The mutant, Smad3(DE), was no longer phosphorylated by TβR-I and stably associated with the receptor. As a result, Smad3(DE) inhibited phosphorylation of Smad2 or Smad3 by TβR-I. In contrast to Anti-Smads, however, Smad3(DE) did not inhibit phosphorylation of Smad1 by BMPR-IB, indicating that the inhibitory action of Smad3(DE) is specific to ligand. The effect of Smad3(DE) on TGF-β–induced growth regulation of HaCaT cells was investigated by establishing cell lines stably expressing various amounts of Smad3(DE). HaCaT cells expressing a low amount of Smad3(DE) was less efficiently inhibited by TGF-β than were the wild-type cells. Cells with a high level of Smad3(DE) expression were completely resistant to TGF-β. The mutation thus disrupts the growth-regulating function of TGF-β in a dominant negative fashion, which could actively contribute to oncogenesis.

SUMMARY

Various laboratories have studied the molecular function of the Smad proteins. Most of the functions are carried out separately by the MH1 or MH2 region. The MH1 and MH2 regions repress activation of each other by forming intramolecular interaction, and phosphorylation of the C-terminus of R-Smads releases this mutual repression. Ligand-induced association of R-Smads with Co-Smads may presumably cause the conformational change that activates Co-Smads. The MH1 region of Smad3 or Smad4 directly binds to DNA. The MH2 region of R-Smads associates with type I receptors and undergoes phosphorylation at the SSXS motif. Both homo- and hetero-oligomerization of Smads are mediated by the MH2 region. The MH2 region also mediates interaction with other nuclear proteins including sequence-specific DNA binding proteins and transcriptional coactivators. The association with coactivators may account for the intrinsic transactivation activity of the MH2 region. Some nuclear proteins, such as c-Jun and Evi-1, interact with the MH1 region.

Smad4 was identified as a candidate tumor suppressor in pancreatic cancers. Recent studies revealed that a subset of juvenile polyposis families carry germline mutations in Smad4.[25] Mutations of Smad2 or Smad4 have also been reported in cancers derived from tissues such as colon, biliary tract, head and neck, and lung. The role of Smads in carcinogenesis was investigated by gene targeting in mice. Smad2 and Smad4 knockout mice died before birth.[26–30] The results revealed the roles of these Smads in early development, but it was not possible to study the outcome of gene targetings in carcinogenesis. Mice with concomitant heterozygous mutation of Smad4 and Apc, a gene responsible for familial adenomatous polyposis, were established.[31] The mice developed more malignant intestinal tumors than the simple Apc heterozygotes, suggesting that the loss of Smad4 contributes to malignant progression of tumors. Smad3 null mice are viable and developed metastatic colorectal cancers.[32] The results provide evidence that disruption of TGF-β signaling is involved in the initiation of colorectal cancer. Elucidation of the functions of Smads will thus allow important insights into the understanding of the molecular basis of carcinogenesis.

REFERENCES

1. DERYNCK, R. & X.-H. FENG. 1997. TGF-β receptor signaling. Biochim. Biophys. Acta **1333:** F105–F150.
2. HELDIN, C.-H., K. MIYAZONO & P. TEN DIJKE. 1997. TGF-β signalling from cell membrane to nucleus through SMAD proteins. Nature **390:** 465–471.
3. MACÍAS-SILVA, M., P.A. HOODLESS, S.J. TANG, M. BUCHWALD & J.L. WRANA. 1998. Specific activation of Smad1 signaling pathways by the BMP7 type I receptor, ALK2. J. Biol. Chem. **273:** 25628–25636.
4. WHITMAN, M. 1998. Smads and early developmental signaling by the TGFβ superfamily. Genes Dev. **12:** 2445–2462.
5. INOUE, H., T. IMAMURA, Y. ISHIDOU, M. TAKASE, Y. UDAGAWA, Y. OKA, K. TSUNEIZUMI, T. TABATA, K. MIYAZONO & M. KAWABATA. 1998. Interplay of signal mediators of decapentaplegic (Dpp): Molecular characterization of Mothers against dpp, Medea, and Daughters against dpp. Mol. Biol. Cell **9:** 2145–2156.
6. OEDA, E., Y. OKA, K. MIYAZONO & M. KAWABATA. 1998. Interaction of Drosophila inhibitors of apoptosis with Thick veins, a type I serine/threonine kinase receptor for Decapentaplegic. J. Biol. Chem. **273:** 9353–9356.
7. HAY, B.A., D.A. WASSARMAN & G.M. RUBIN. 1995. Drosophila homologs of baculovirus inhibitor of apoptosis proteins function to block cell death. Cell **83:** 1253–1262.
8. WIERSDORFF, V., T. LECUIT, S.M. COHEN & M. MLODZIK. 1996. Mad acts downstream of Dpp receptors, revealing a differential requirement for dpp signaling in initiation and propagation of morphogenesis in the Drosophila eye. Development **122:** 2153–2162.
9. NAKAO, A., T. IMAMURA, S. SOUCHELNYTSKYI, M. KAWABATA, A. ISHISAKI, E. OEDA, K. TAMAKI, J. HANAI, C.-H. HELDIN, K. MIYAZONO & P. TEN DIJKE. 1997. TGF receptor mediated signaling through Smad2, Smad3, and Smad4. EMBO J. **16:** 5353–5362.
10. KAWABATA, M., H. INOUE, A. HANYU, T. IMAMURA & K. MIYAZONO. 1998. Smad proteins exist as monomers *in vivo* and undergo homo- and hetero-oligomerization upon activation by serine/threonine kinase receptors. EMBO J. **17:** 4056–4065.
11. YINGLING, J.M., M.B. DATTO, C. WONG, J.P. FREDERICK, N.T. LIBERATI & X.-F. WANG. 1997. Tumor suppressor Smad4 is a transforming growth factor β-inducible DNA binding protein. Mol. Cell. Biol. **17:** 7019–7028.
12. CHEN, X., M.J. RUBOCK & M. WHITMAN. 1996. A transcriptional partner for MAD proteins in TGF-β signalling. Nature **383:** 691–696.

13. YAGI, K., D. GOTO, T. HAMAMOTO, S. TAKENOSHITA, M. KATO & K. MIYAZONO. 1999. Alternatively-spliced variant of Smad2 lacking exon 3: Comparison with wild-type Smad2 and Smad3. J. Biol. Chem. **274:** 703–709.

14. NISHIHARA, A., J. HANAI, N. OKAMOTO, J. YANAGISAWA, S. KATO, K. MIYAZONO & M. KAWABATA. 1998. Role of p300, a transcriptional coactivator, in signaling of TGF-β. Genes Cells **3:** 611–621.

15. JANKNECHT, R., N.J. WELLS & T. HUNTER. 1998. TGF-β-stimulated cooperation of Smad proteins with the coactivators CBP/p300. Genes Dev. **12:** 2144–2152.

16. FENG, X.H., Y. ZHANG, R.Y. WU & R. DERYNCK. 1998. The tumor suppressor Smad4/DPC4 and transcriptional adaptor CBP/p300 are coactivators for Smad3 in TGF-β-induced transcriptional activation. Genes Dev. **12:** 2153–2163.

17. TOPPER, J.N., M.R. DICHIARA, J.D. BROWN, A.J. WILLIAMS, D. FALB, T. COLLINS & M.A. GIMBRONE, JR. 1998. CREB binding protein is a required coactivator for Smad-dependent, transforming growth factor β transcriptional responses in endothelial cells. Proc. Natl. Acad. Sci. USA **95:** 9506–9511.

18. POUPONNOT, C., L. JAYARAMAN & J. MASSAGUÉ. 1998. Physical and functional interaction of SMADs and p300/CBP. J. Biol. Chem. **273:** 22865–22868.

19. IMAMURA, T., M. TAKASE, A. NISHIHARA, E. OEDA, J. HANAI, M. KAWABATA & K. MIYAZONO. 1997. Smad6 inhibits signalling by the TGF-β superfamily. Nature **389:** 622–626.

20. HAYASHI, H., S. ABDOLLAH, Y. QIU, J. CAI, Y.-Y. XU, B.W. GRINNELL, M.A. RICHARDSON, J.N. TOPPER, M.A. GIMBRONE JR., J.L. WRANA & D. FALB. 1997. The MAD-related protein Smad7 associates with the TGFβ receptor and functions as an antagonist of TGFβ signaling. Cell **89:** 1165–1173.

21. NAKAO, A., M. AFRAKHTE, A. MORÉN, T. NAKAYAMA, J.L. CHRISTIAN, R. HEUCHEL, S. ITOH, M. KAWABATA, N.-E. HELDIN, C.-H. HELDIN & P. TEN DIJKE. 1997. Identification of Smad7, a TGFβ-inducible antagonist of TGF-β signalling. Nature **389:** 631–635.

22. TSUNEIZUMI, K., T. NAKAYAMA, Y. KAMOSHIDA, T.B. KORNBERG, J.L. CHRISTIAN & T. TABATA. 1997. *Daughters against dpp* modulates *dpp* organizing activity in *Drosophila* wing development. Nature **389:** 627–631.

23. TAKASE, M., T. IMAMURA, T.K. SAMPATH, K. TAKEDA, H. ICHIJO, K. MIYAZONO & M. KAWABATA. 1998. Induction of Smad6 mRNA by bone morphogenetic proteins. Biochem. Biophys. Res. Commun. **244:** 26–29.

24. GOTO, D., K. YAGI, H. INOUE, I. IWAMOTO, M. KAWABATA, K. MIYAZONO & M. KATO. 1998. A single missense mutant of Smad3 inhibits activation of both Smad2 and Smad3, and has a dominant negative effect on TGF-β signals. FEBS Lett. **430:** 201–204.

25. HOWE, J.R., S. ROTH, J.C. RINGOLD, R.W. SUMMERS, H.J. JARVINEN, P. SISTONEN, I.P. TOMLINSON, R.S. HOULSTON, S. BEVAN, S., F.A. MITROS, E.M. STONE & L.A. AALTONEN. 1998. Mutations in the *SMAD4/DPC4* gene in juvenile polyposis. Science **280:** 1086–1088.

26. SIRARD, C., J.L. DE LA POMPA, A. ELIA, A. ITIE, C. MIRTSOS, A. CHEUNG, S. HAHN, A. WAKEHAM, L. SCHWARTZ, S. KERN, J. ROSSANT & T. MAK. 1998. The tumor suppressor gene *Smad4/Dpc4* is required for gastrulation and later for anterior development of the mouse embryo. Genes Dev. **12:** 107–119.

27. YANG, X., C. LI, X. XU & C. DENG. 1998. The tumor suppressor SMAD4/DPC4 is essential for epiblast proliferation and mesoderm induction in mice. Proc. Natl. Acad. Sci. USA **95:** 3667–3672.

28. WALDRIP, W., E. BIKOFF, P. HOODLESS, J. WRANA & E. ROBERTSON. 1998. Smad2 signaling in extraembryonic tissues determines anterior-posterior polarity of the early mouse embryo. Cell **92:** 797–808.

29. NOMURA, M. & E. LI. 1998. Roles for Smad2 in mesoderm formation, left right patterning, and craniofacial development in mice. Nature **393:** 786–789.
30. WEINSTEIN, M., X. YANG, C. LI, X. XU, J. GOTAY & C.X. DENG. 1998. Failure of egg cylinder elongation and mesoderm induction in mouse embryos lacking the tumor suppressor *smad2*. Proc. Natl. Acad. Sci. USA **95:** 9378–9383.
31. TAKAKU, K., M. OSHIMA, H. MIYOSHI, M. MATSUI, M.F. SELDIN & M.M. TAKETO. 1998. Intestinal tumorigenesis in compound mutant mice of both *Dpc4* (*Smad4*) and *Apc* genes. Cell **92:** 645–656.
32. ZHU, Y., J.A. RICHARDSON, L.F. PARADA. & J.M. GRAFF. 1998. Smad3 mutant mice develop metastatic colorectal cancer. Cell **94:** 703–714.

Bacterial Toxins Inhibiting or Activating Small GTP-Binding Proteins

PATRICE BOQUET[a]

Institut National de la Santé et de la Recherche Médicale (INSERM), Faculté de Médecine, 28 Avenue de Valombrose, 06102 Nice, France

ABSTRACT: Amino acids located on the switch 1 or switch 2 domains of small Gtpases of the Ras and Rho family are targets of several bacterial toxins. Exoenzyme C3 from *Clostridium botulinum* ADP-ribosylates specifically Rho at R43 and prevents the recruitment of Rho on the cell membrane. This blocks the downstream effects of the Rho GTPase. However, exoenzyme C3 is not a toxin, and chimeric proteins fusing C3 with the B moiety of either diphtheria toxin or *Pseudomonas aeruginosa* exotoxin A have been produced to intoxicate cells with low concentration of C3. *C. difficile* toxin B modifies by glucosylation Rho on T37 and Rac and Cdc42 on T35. Glucosylation of Rho, Rac, and Cdc42 blocks the binding of these GTPases on their downstream effectors. *C. sordellii* lethal toxin modifies Ras, Rap, and Rac on T35 by glucosylation. Cytotoxic necrotizing factor 1 (CNF1), from uropathogenic *Escherichia coli* strains, deamidates Q63 of Rho into E63, thereby blocking the intrinsic or GAP-mediated GTPase of Rho. This allows permanent activation of Rho. Thus, Rho GTPases are targets for three different toxin activities. Molecular mechanisms of these toxins are discussed.

INTRODUCTION

Microbes must circumvent, destroy, or totally dissimulate to the host defense mechanisms. To perform these tasks, pathogens have developed astonishingly clever strategies consisting mainly of the use of host-cell systems of regulations. Among the mechanisms elaborated by microbes, production of toxins acting as hormones at a distance or invasion of cells mimicking phagocytosis is particulary powerful. In both of these strategies the cell actin cytoskeleton is clearly a preferred target for toxins and invasive virulence factors.

The Rho subfamily of p21 Ras GTP-binding protein is now the focus of intense study because it is increasingly evident that these GTP-binding proteins are pivotal in the regulation of the actin cytoskeleton.[1] It is therefore not surprising that Rho proteins are also preferred intracellular targets for toxins and virulence factors. We describe and analyze recent advances concerning the mode of action of bacterial toxins and invasion virulence factors on Rho proteins.

The Rho subfamily, which encompasses Rho, Rac, and Cdc42,[1] regulates a wide variety of cellular processes involving actin filaments. For example, Rho regulates cell shape,[2] formation of actin stress fibers,[3–5] cell motility,[6] smooth muscle con-

[a]Phone, 0033493531755; fax, 0033493533509.
e-mail, boquet@unice.fr

traction,[7,8] neurite retraction,[9] and formation of tight junctions.[10,11] Rac regulates formation of lamellipodia,[5] NADPH oxidase-dependent superoxide production.[12] Cdc42 controls the formation of filopodia.[13,14] The downstream targets of Rho proteins, involved in F-actin reorganization, are still not firmly established, but two main activities have emergee to date from the intense research carried out by different groups. Rho is probably mostly involved in smooth muscle contraction by controlling myosin light chain phosphorylation[15] via activation of Rho kinase.[16,17] By bundling actin filaments through myosin activation, Rho induces the formation of actin contractile cables.[18] Rac, on the other hand, acts mainly by polymerizing actin via uncapping of barbed end filaments.[19] Actin filaments are uncapped by removing CapZ from the barbed ends by PIP2 produced through PI 4-5 kinase activation by Rac.

Finally, the role of Rho in the formation of focal points of adhesion implicates a regulating activity on proteins of the ERM family ezrin, moesin, or radixin.[20] However, the precise activity of Rho on ERM proteins is not clear. Does Rho switch on ERM proteins by a mechanism involving PIP2, as described for vinculin?[21] or by phosphorylation through activation of a kinase different from Rok? In any case, one interesting feedback mechanism that might derive from ERM protein activation is the trapping of Rho GDI to the ERM complex with their target membrane proteins such as ezrin bound to CD44.[22] This mechanism would be a simple, efficient process to control activation of Rho, Rac, or Cdc42.

Two types of bacterial exotoxins (referred to here as toxins) interact with the Rho GTP-binding proteins. The first group, by modifying amino acids of the switch 1 Rho domain (effector domain), inhibit the activity of Rho. The second group, by modifying an amino acid of the Rho switch 2 domain (involved in GTPase activity), provokes permanent activation of the GTP-binding protein.

TOXINS INHIBITING RHO

The first group of toxins that inhibit Rho is the family of C3-like ADP-ribosyltransferases which catalyzes ADP-ribosylation of RhoA, B, and C at Asn-41. The second group is the large clostridial cytotoxins that monoglucosylate the Rho subfamily proteins Rho, Rac, and Cdc42 at Thr-37/35.

The C3-like family encompasses several *Clostridium botulinum* C3 isoforms, the *C. limosum* exotoxin and transferases produced by *Bacillus cereus* and *Staphylococcus aureus*.[23] All transferases are single-chained 23-kD exoenzymes with extremely basic isoelectric points (>9). Because they lack a specific binding/translocation domain or component, cell entry is poor and delayed and occurs most likely via fluid phase pinocytosis. The basic isoelectric points of these exoenzymes may allow them to bind nonspecifically to the negatively charged surface of eukaryotic cells. After microinjection or application as fusion toxin, C3 is cytotoxic and causes disorganization of actin filaments due to ADP-ribosylation of RhoA, B, and C proteins at asparagine 41.[24] ADP-ribosylation of Rho at Asn-41 does not impair the binding of GTP of RhoGAP on the GTPase but rather the recruitment of Rho to the membrane.[25] The other Rho subfamily members, Rac and Cdc42, are poor substrates under artificial conditions and do not seem to be relevant *in vivo* targets. C3 has been established as an important tool for studying the functional role of Rho.

The most important members of the family of large clostridial cytotoxins are *C. difficile* toxins A and B. Both are single-chained exotoxins coproduced by pathogenic *C. difficile* strains and show about 60% homology to each other. They have been identified as causative agents of antibiotic-associated pseudomembranous colitis. Whereas TCdA is more enterotoxic, TCdB is about one thousandfold more cytotoxic to cultured cell lines.[26] The cytotoxic effects of both toxins in inducing disaggregation of the microfilament system are mediated by their inherent enzymatic activity. They use the ubiquitously occurring sugar UDP-glucose as a cosubstrate to transfer the glucose moiety to Thr-37 in Rho equivalent to Thr-35 in Rac and Cdc42. Incorporation is maximally one molecule of glucose per molecule of GTPase consistent with a monoglucosylation type of reaction. Glucosylation renders the Rho GTPases inactive, as shown by microinjection of glucosylated Rho, which induces the same effects on the cytoskeleton as does the toxin itself, thus corroborating the notion that toxins A and B are cytotoxic by glucosylating the Rho GTPases.[27,28]

Other members of the family exhibit comparable transferase activity. *C. sordellii* hemorrhagic toxin is identical to toxin A and B,[29] the lethal toxin from the same strain is also a monoglucosyltransferase, but it has different protein substrate specificity; in addition to the Rac protein from the Rho subfamily, Ras proteins (Ras, Rap, and Ral) are modified.[30,31] This is a very exciting aspect, because the protooncogenic function of Ras is blocked by glucosylation. *C. novyi* alphatoxin, however, catalyzes incorporation of *N*-acetylglucosamine into Rho subfamily proteins, a posttranslational modification that is endogenously used in cytoplasmic and nuclear signaling.[32]

The large clostridial cytotoxins are composed of at least three functional domains that reflect the steps of cell entry: the C-terminal part carries the receptor binding domain, the middle part the putative translocation domain, and the *N*-terminal domain harbors the catalytic activity.[33] For TCdB it has clearly been demonstrated that the first fifth of the peptide (aa 1-546 from 2366 aa) is fully catalytic and that neither the putative nucleotide binding site (aa 651-683) nor the conserved cysteines are of any functional relevance for the catalytic activity.[34] The receptor-binding domain shows a repetitive structure that allows binding to at least one membrane receptor, but the repetitive structure argues for recruiting several (possibly identical) receptors per toxin molecule.[33]

TOXINS ACTIVATING RHO

Escherichia coli belong to the normal microflora of the gastrointestinal tract; certain *E. coli* strains, however, are associated with gastroenteritis, urogenital diseases, septicemia, and pleural infections in humans. These pathogenic *E. coli* belong to a restricted number of pathovars defined by the presence of virulence factors determining their host specificity and type of disease produced. CNF1 might be implicated in the pathogenesis of colibacillosis. First, experimental infections of neonatal calves and pigs showed that orally inoculated CNF1-positive *E. coli* cause septicemia enteritis and histologic changes characteristic of toxemic effects in the brain, heart, liver, and kidney. These lesions were similar to those observed after intravenous inoculation of purified CNF1 in the lamb. Second, epidemiologic surveys in

Europe indicate that CNF1-producing strains may represent 10–50% of the *E. coli* strains isolated from extraintestinal infections and 5–30% of the *E. coli* strains isolated from diarrhea.[35]

CNF1, discovered by Caprioli and colleagues[36] as a cell-associated product of *E. coli* strains isolated from young children with diarrhea, causes necrosis of rabbit skin and multinucleation of different types of tissue culture cells. A second type of CNF (CNF2) was found in extracts of certain *E. coli* strains isolated from calves with enteritis.[37]

CNF1 and CNF2 are encoded by a single structural gene with a low GC content (35%).[38,39] This finding suggests a relatively recent acquisition of the *cnf* gene by *E. coli* whose overall GC content is around 50%. Analysis of the deduced amino acid sequences of CNF1 and CNF2 showed that the two toxins are similar (85% identical and 99% conserved residues over 1014 amino acids). Additionally, CNFs are predicted to be relatively hydrophilic proteins with two putative hydrophobic transmembrane domains partially overlapped by two predicted α helices. No classical signal peptide sequence was found in CNFs *N*-terminal 50 residues. A comparison of the predicted amino acid sequence of CNFs with sequences in GenBank revealed that CNFs share regions of homologous amino acids with two other bacterial toxins, *Pasteurella multocida* toxin (PMT)[38,39] and the dermonecrotic toxin of *Bordetella pertussis* (DNT).[39] CNFs, PMT, and DNT form the new family of dermonecrotic toxins.[40]

CNFl can provoke a remarkable reorganization of F-actin structures in cultured cells.[41] This toxin induces intense formation of stress fibers, focal contacts, membrane folding, and retraction fibers. Reorganization of the F-actin cytoskeleton by CNF1 results in the cell's inability to undergo cytokinesis. Cell treatment for over 24 hours with CNF1, at concentrations as low as 10 pg/ml, gives rise to extremely flat large multinucleated cells containing numerous stress fibers.[41]

Treatment of HEp-2 cells with CNFl, for increasing lengths of time (from 4–72 hours), augments the ability of the cells to ingest latex beads.[42] Macropinocytosis is totally blocked when CNFl-treated cells are incubated with the F-actin disrupting drug, cytochalasin B, demonstrating clearly that the process is F-actin dependent.[42] In addition, noninvasive bacteria such as *Listeria innocua* are as invasive as *L. monocytogenes* when incubated with HEp-2 cells pretreated with CNFl.[42]

CNFl induces cells actin reorganization by permanently stimulating the Rho protein. The first hint of this activity was shown as follows: When cytosol from HEp-2 cells previously incubated with CNF1 was ADP-ribosylated with exoenzyme C3, it was observed that the Rho protein had a molecular weight shift to a slightly higher value. This result indicated a possible posttranslational modification of the GTP-binding protein in CNFl-treated cells.[39,43] A CNF1-induced electrophoretic shift of Rho is not due to a block in prenylation (posttranslational modification of the carboxy-terminus ends of small GTP-binding proteins) or to a phosphorylation of Rho.[39] Incubation of HEp-2 cells with CNF1 could also block the cytotoxic activities of two bacterial toxins known to act on the Rho GTP-binding protein, namely, exoenzyme C3 and *C. difficile* toxin B.[44] CNF1 was shown to modify directly *in vitro* Rho without the need for cellular cofactors.[45] Microsequencing of CNF1-modified Rho showed a single modification in the CNF1-treated GTPase compared to the wild type. Rho glutamine 63 was changed into a glutamic acid.[45] Therefore, CNF1

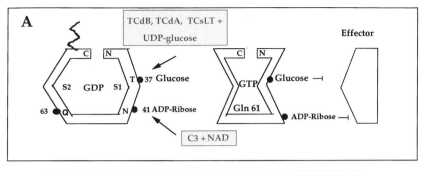

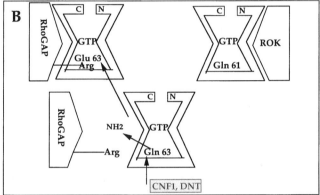

FIGURE 1. Modifications induced by toxins on the Rho small GTPases. Toxins inactivating Rho (**A**) modify the switch 1 (S1) domain, usually when it is exposed to the surface of the GTPase (under the GDP bound form). Modifications of S1 impede the binding of the small GTPase to its effector. Toxins activating Rho (**B**) act on the switch 2 domain (S2). CNF1 and DNT deamidate the Rho glutamine 63 (analogous to Ras glutamine 61) into glutamic acid, which is not suited for the binding of the water molecule required for RhoGAP GTP hydrolysis. Rho stays in the GTP bound form and permanently activates its downstream effector ROK.

exerts specific deamidase activity. Identical activity for CNF1 on Rho was reported using mass spectrometry.[46] Specific deamidation is a hitherto undescribed activity for a bacterial toxin. Indeed, toxin enzymatic activities described at the present time are ADP-ribosylation, depurination, metalloprotease, glucosyltransferase, and adenylate cycling.

CNF1 exerts deamidase catalytic activity on Rho glutamine 63. The equivalent amino acid of Rho glutamine 63 in p21 Ras is glutamine 61. Rho glutamine 63 is an important residue for the intrinsic and RhoGAP-mediated GTPase of Rho.[47] Both CNF1-treated Rho and mutated Rho on glutamine 63 into glutamic acid (RhoQ63E) exhibit a mobility shift upon electrophoresis, identical to that of CNF1-treated Rho. The CNF1-treated Rho and RhoQ63E nucleotide dissociation rate was increased by 2 orders of magnitude, but RhoGAP activity was totally impaired on both CNF1-treated Rho and RhoQ63E. Thus, CNF1 allows Rho to be permanently bound with GTP, enhancing the activity of Rho on Rho effectors. This mechanism is achieved simply by deamidation of Rho glutamine 63. We have localized the Rho deamidase activity onto the CNF1. CNF1 deamidase activity is borne by the 30-kD carboxy-terminus end of the molecule.[40] On the other hand, the cell binding moiety of CNF1 is localized in the amino-terminus of the molecule.[40] CNF1 thus has a toxin architecture comparable to that of *Pseudomonas aeruginosa* exotoxin A.[48] Comparisons of sequence homology between the different dermonecrotic toxins CNF1, CNF2, DNT, and PMT have revealed that CNF1 and CNF2 are highly homologous, sharing both comparable domains for enzymatic and cell binding domains. DNT, however, is a toxin that has a high homology with CNFs for the catalytic domain but differs strongly with CNFs at the level of the cell binding domain. Recently it was shown that DNT, like CNF1, exerts deamidase activity towards Rho.[49] PMT, on the other hand, differs strongly with CNFs and DNT at the level of its putative catalytic domain, but it has a strong homology with the cell binding domains of CNF.[40]

REFERENCES

1. HALL, A. 1998. Rho Gtpases and the actin cytoskeleton. Science **279:** 509–514.
2. RUBIN, E.J. *et al.* 1988. Functional modification of a 21-kilodalton G protein when ADP-ribosylated by exoenzyme C3 of *Clostridium botulinum.* Mol. Cell Biol. **8:** 418–426.
3. CHARDIN, P. *et al.* 1989. The mammalian G protein RhoC is ADPribosylated by *Clostridium botulinum* C3 and affects actin microfilaments in Vero cells. EMBO J. **8:** 1087–1092.
4. PATERSON, H.F. *et al.* 1990. Microinjection of recombinant p21Rho induces rapid changes in cell morphology. J. Cell Biol. **111:** 1001–1007.
5. RIDLEY, A.J. *et al.* 1992. The small GTP-binding protein Rac regulates growth factor-induced membrane ruffling. Cell **70:** 401–410.
6. STASIA, M.J. *et al.* 1991. ADP-ribosylation of a small size GTP-binding protein in bovine neutrophils by the C3 exoenzyme of *Clostridium botulinum* and effect on cell motility. Biochem. Biophys. Res. Commun. **180:** 615–622.
7. KIMURA, K. *et al.* 1996. Regulation of myosin phosphatase by Rho and Rho-associated kinase (Rho-kinase). Science **273:** 245–247.
8. MATSUI, T. *et al.* 1996. Rho-associated kinase, a novel serine/threonine kinase, as a putative target for the small GTP-binding protein Rho. EMBO J. **15:** 2208–2216.
9. JALINK, K. *et al.* 1994. Inhibition of lysophosphatidate-and thrombin-induced neurite retraction and neuronal cell rounding by ADP-ribosylation of the small GTP-binding protein Rho. J. Cell Biol. **126:** 801–810.
10. NUSRAT A. *et al.* 1995. Rho protein regulates tight junctions and perijunctional actin organization in polarized epithelia. Proc. Natl. Acad. Sci. USA **92:** 10629–10633.
11. TAKAHISHI, K. *et al.* 1997. Regulation of cell-cell adhesion by Rac and Rho small G proteins in MDCK cells. J. Cell Biol. **139:** 1047–1059.
12. ABO, A. *et al.* 1991. The small GTP-binding protein, p21 Rac, is involved in the activation of the phagocyte NADPH oxidase. Nature **353:** 668–670.
13. NOBES, C.D. & A. HALL. 1995. Rho, Rac and Cdc42 GTPases regulate the assembly of multi-molecular focal complexes associated with actin stress fibres, lammelipodia and filopodia. Cell **81:** 53–62.
14. KOZMA, R. *et al.* 1996. The GTPase-activating protein n-chimerin cooperates with Rac1 and Cdc42Hs to induce the formation of lammelipodia and filopodia. Mol. Cell Biol. **16:** 5069–5080.
15. KIMURA, K. *et al.* 1996. Regulation of myosin phosphatase by Rho and Rho-associated kinase (Rho-kinase). Science **273:** 245–247.

16. MATSUI, T. et al. 1996. Rho-associated kinase, a novel serine/threonine kinase, as a putative target for the small GTP-binding protein Rho. EMBO J. **15:** 2208–2216.
17. ISHIZAKI, T. et al. 1996. The small GTP-binding protein Rho binds to and activates a 160 kDa ser/thr protein kinase homologous to myotonic dystrophy kinase. EMBO J. **15:** 1885–1893
18. AMANO, M. et al. 1997. Formation of actin stress fibers and focal adhesions enhanced by Rho kinase. Science **275:** 1308–1311.
19. HARTWIG, J.H. et al. 1995. Thrombin receptor ligation and activated Rac uncap actin filament barbed ends through phosphoinositide synthesis in permeabilized human platelets. Cell **82:** 643–653.
20. MACKAY, D.J.G. et al. 1997. Rho-and Rac-dependent assembly of focal adhesion complexes and actin filaments in permeabilized fibroblasts: An essential role for ezrin/radixin/moesin proteins. J. Cell Biol. **138:** 927–938.
21. GILMORE, A.P. & K. BURRIDGE. 1996. Regulation of vinculin binding to talin and actin by phosphatidyl-inositol 4-5 biphosphate. Nature **381:** 531–535.
22. TSUKITA, S. et al. 1997. ERM proteins: Head-to-tail regulation of actin-plasma membrane interaction. Trends Biochem. Sci. **22:** 53–58.
23. BOQUET, P. et al. 1998. Toxins from anaerobic bacteria: Specificity and molecular mechanisms of action. Curr. Opin. Microbiol. **1:** 66–74.
24. SEKINE, A. et al. 1989. Asparagine residue in the Rho gene product is the modification site for botulinum ADP-ribosyltransferase. J. Biol. Chem. **264:** 8602–8605.
25. FUJIHARA, H. et al. 1997. Inhibition of RhoA translocation and calcium sensitization by in vivo ADP-ribosylation with the chimeric DC3B. Mol. Biol. Cell **8:** 2437–2447.
26. SEARS, C.L. & J.B. KAPER. 1996. Enteric bacterial toxins: Mechanisms of action and linkage to intestinal secretion. Microbiol. Rev. **60:** 167–215.
27. JUST, I. et al. 1995. Glucosylation of Rho proteins by Clostridium difficile toxin B. Nature **375:** 500–550.
28. JUST, I. et al. 1995. The enterotoxin from Clostridium difficile (Tox A) monoglucosylates the Rho proteins. J. Biol. Chem. **270:** 13932–13936
29. GENTH, H. et al. 1996. Difference in protein substrates specificity between hemorrhagic toxin and lethal toxin from Clostridium sordellii. Biochem. Biophys. Res. Commun. **229:** 370–374.
30. POPOFF, M.R. et al. 1996. Ras, Rap and Rac small GTP-binding proteins are targets for Clostridium sordellii lethal toxin glucosylation. J. Biol. Chem. **271:** 10217–10224.
31. JUST, I. et al. 1996. Inactivation of Ras by Clostridium sordellii lethal toxin-catalyzed glucosylation. J. Biol. Chem. **271:** 10149–10153.
32. SELZER, J. et al. 1996. Clostridium novyi alpha-toxin-catalyzed incorporation of GlcNAc into Rho subfamily proteins. J. Biol. Chem. **271:** 25173–25177
33. VON EICHEL-STREIBER, C. et al. 1996. Large clostridial cytotoxins-a family of glycosyltransferases modyfying small GTP-binding proteins. Trends Microbiol. **375:** 375–382.
34. HOFMAN, F. et al. 1997. Localization of the glucosyltransferase activity of Clostridium difficile toxin B to the N-terminal part of holotoxin. J. Biol. Chem. **272:** 11074–11078.
35. CAPRIOLI, A. et al. 1983. Partial purification and characterization of an Escherichia coli toxic factor that induces morphological alterations. Infect. Immun. **39:** 1300–1306.
36. DE RYCKE, J. et al. 1990. Evidence for two types of cytotoxic necrotizing factor in human and animal clinical isolates. J. Clin. Microbiol. **28:** 694–699.
37. FALBO, V. et al. 1993. Isolation and nucleotide sequence of the gene encoding cytotoxic necrotizing factor type 1. Infect. Immun. **61:** 4909–4914.

38. OSWALD, E. *et al.* 1990. Cytotoxic necrotizing factor type 2 produced by virulent *Escherichia coli* modifies the small GTP-binding proteins Rho involved in assembly of actin stress fibers. Proc. Natl. Acad. Sci. USA **91:** 3814–3818.
39. LEMICHEZ, E. *et al.* 1997. Molecular localization of the *Escherichia coli* cytotoxic necrotizing factor CNF1 cell-binding and catalytic domains. Mol. Microbiol. **24:** 1061–1070.
40. FIORENTINI, C. *et al.* 1988. Cytoskeletal changes induced in Hep-2 cells by the cytotoxic necrotizing factor of *Escherichia coli*. Toxicon **26:** 1047–1056.
41. FALZANO, L. *et al.* 1993. Induction of phagocytic behaviour in human epithelial cells by *Escherichia coli* cytotoxic necrotizing factor 1. Mol. Microbiol. **9:** 1247–1254.
42. FIORENTINI, C. *et al.* 1994. *E. coli* cytotoxic necrotizing factor 1 increases actin assembly via the p21 Rho GTPase. Zentrabl. Bakteriol. Suppl. **24:** 404–405.
43. FIORENTINI, C. et al. 1994. *Escherichia coli* cytotoxic necrotizing factor 1 increases actin assembly via the p21 Rho protein. P. Zbl. Bakt. Suppl. **24:** 404–405.
44. FIORENTINI, C. *et al.* 1995. *Escherichia coli* cytotoxic necrotizing factor 1: Evidence for induction of actin assembly by constitutive activation of the p21 Rho GTPase. Infect. Immun. **63:** 3936–3944.
45. FLATAU, G. *et al.* 1997. Toxin-induced activation of the G-protein Rho by deamidation of glutamine. Nature **387:** 729–733.
46. SCHMIDT, G. *et al.* 1997. Gln 63 of Rho is deamidated by *Escherichia coli* cytotoxic necrotizing factor 1. Nature **387:** 725–728
47. RITTINGER, K. *et al.* 1997. Structure at 1.65 Angstom of RhoA and its GTPase-activating protein in complex with a transition state analog. Nature **389:** 758–762.
48. ALLURED, V. S. *et al.* 1986. Structure of exotoxin A of *Pseudomonas aeruginosa* at 3.0 Angstrom resolution. Proc. Natl. Acad. Sci. USA **83:** 1320–1324.
49. HORIGUCHI, Y. *et al.* 1997. *Bordetella bronchiseptica* dermonecrotizing toxin induces reorganization of actin stress fibers through deamidation of Gln-63 of the GTP-binding Rho. Proc. Natl. Acad. Sci. USA **94:** 11623–11626.

Farnesyltransferase Inhibitors

Preclinical Development

NANCY E. KOHL[a]

Department of Cancer Research, Merck Research Laboratories, West Point, Pennsylvania 19486, USA

ABSTRACT: The Ras proteins are low molecular weight GTP binding proteins that function in the regulation of the transduction of growth proliferative signals from the membrane to the nucleus. Oncogenically mutated *ras* genes are found in approximately 25% of all human cancers. Localization of the Ras oncoproteins to the inner surface of the plasma membrane is essential for their biological activity. This observation suggested that the enzyme that mediates the membrane localization, farnesyl-protein transferase (FPTase), would be a target for the development of novel anticancer agents. We have developed potent, cell-active inhibitors of FPTase that exhibit antiproliferative activity in cell culture and block the morphologic alterations associated with Ras-induced transformation of mammalian cells in monolayer cultures. *In vivo*, these compounds block the growth of *ras*-transformed fibroblasts in a nude mouse xenograft model and block the growth and, in some cases, cause regression of mammary and salivary tumors in several strains of *ras* transgenic mice in the absence of any detectable side effects. The results of our preclinical studies and those of others suggest that FTIs may have utility against a variety of human cancers, a hypothesis that is curently being tested in the clinic.

INTRODUCTION

The Ras proteins — Harvey (Ha)-, Kirsten (Ki)4A-, Ki4B-, and N-Ras — play an integral role in cell proliferation, acting as a switch in the relay of signals from plasma membrane-bound receptors to the nucleus.[1] Typical of low molecular weight GTP-binding proteins, Ras exists in two forms, an active, GTP-bound form and an inactive, GDP-bound form. Inactivation of Ras is accomplished by GTPase-activating proteins (GAPs) that stimulate the intrinsic GTPase activity of Ras. Mutations in Ras that inhibit GTP hydrolysis result in constitutively active forms of the protein. Such altered forms of Ras, especially Ki4B- and N-Ras, are frequently found in a wide variety of human cancers and are particularly prevalent in human colon, pancreatic, and lung tumors.[2,3]

Ras is synthesized as a biologically inactive, cytosolic precursor that translocates to the plasma membrane and becomes functional following a series of posttranslational modifications (reviewed in ref. 4). The first and obligatory reaction in this series, catalyzed by farnesyl-protein transferase (FPTase), is the transfer of a 15 carbon isoprenoid, farnesyl, from farnesyl diphosphate (FPP) to the cysteine residue 4 ami-

[a]Phone, 215/652-5646; fax, 215/652-7320.
e-mail, nancy_kohl@merck.com

no acids from the C-terminus of the protein. The C-terminal tetrapeptide is referred to as a CA_1A_2X motif, where C is cysteine, A is often an aliphatic amino acid, and X usually serine or methionine. Subsequent to farnesylation, the A_1A_2X residues are proteolytically cleaved and the C-terminal farnesylated cysteine is methylated. In the case of Ha- and N-Ras, a fourth reaction, palmitoylation of one or two cysteines upstream of the CA_1A_2X tetrapeptide, also occurs. The demonstration that farnesylation is essential for the biologic activity of Ras oncoproteins[5–8] has led to the hypothesis that inhibitors of FPTase will be useful in the treatment of human tumors whose uncontrolled growth is dependent on Ras.[9]

FPTase is a heterodimeric enzyme that is expressed in the cytosol of most mammalian cells.[4] FPTase requires both Zn^{2+} and Mg^{2+} for activity: Zn^{2+} is required for binding of the protein substrate and during catalysis appears to be coordinated to the cysteine thiol of the CA_1A_2X substrate.[10] In addition to the Ras proteins, other substrates of FPTase include the nuclear lamins; skeletal muscle phosphorylase kinase; the peroxisomal protein, PxF; the cell regulatory phosphatases PTP1 and PTP2; RhoB; and three proteins of the visual transduction system, transducin, cGMP phosphodiesterase, and rhodopsin kinase.[11,12]

FPTase is a member of a family of prenyltransferases found in mammalian cells. Two additional enzymes, geranylgeranyl-protein transferase (GGPTase) types I and II (also know as Rab GGPTase), catalyze the addition of the 20 carbon isoprenoid, geranylgeranyl, to C-terminal cyteine residues of proteins.[4] GGPTase-I shares many properties with FPTase: it is structurally similar to FPTase and it modifies CA_1A_2X-containing proteins. In contrast to FPTase, GGPTase-I preferentially modifies proteins in which the X residue is either a leucine or phenylalanine. However, the specificity of these two enzymes is not absolute. For example, proteins that are preferentially farnesylated, such as N- and Ki4B-Ras, in which the X residue is a methionine, can be substrates for geranylgeranylation by GGPTase-I,[13–15] particularly when FPTase activity is inhibited.[16–18] GGPTase-II transfers the geranylgeranyl group to both cysteines of proteins that have C-terminal sequences CXC, CC, or CCXX.[4]

DEVELOPMENT OF FPTase INHIBITORS

Several methods have been used to identify inhibitors of FPTase, including random screening of chemical collections and natural products as well as rational design based on the protein and isoprenoid substrates of the reaction. Whereas all of these methods have yielded potent inhibitors of the enzyme, the initial leads were mimetics of the CA_1A_2X tetrapeptide. Early biochemical studies of FPTase demonstrated that CA_1A_2X tetrapeptides can serve as substrates for farnesylation, suggesting that the minimal recognition sequence of the polypeptide substrates of FPTase is the C-terminal tetrapeptide.[19,20] Thus, the CA_1A_2X tetrapeptides inhibit farnesylation by acting as alternative substrates that compete with the polypeptide for farnesylation. These substrate-like tetrapeptides are potent inhibitors of the enzyme, with IC_{50} values similar to the K_m values for the intact proteins. Further biochemical studies demonstrated that substitution of the A_2 residue of the CA_1A_2X with an aromatic group yielded potent, nonsubstrate inhibitors of FPTase.[21,22]

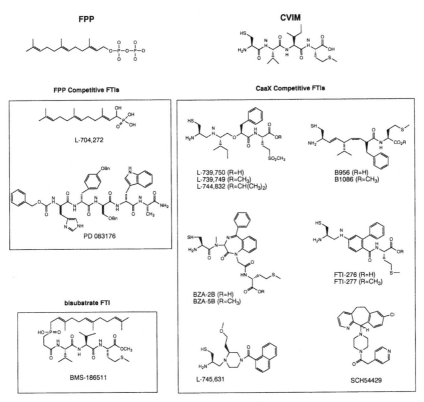

FIGURE 1. Substrate-based FPTase inhibitors.

Since these potent, nonsubstrate CA_1A_2X inhibitors were inactive in whole cell assays, subsequent work focused on improving metabolic stability and cell permeability. Metabolic stability was achieved by incorporating nonhydrolyzable isosteric replacements for the peptide bonds of the CA_1A_2X tetrapeptides (reduced amides,[23–25] olefin[26,27] [as in B956; FIG. 1], or ether linkages[28]) (as in L739-750; FIG. 1). Such modifications have yielded compounds with increased *in vitro* potency against FPTase that are selective for inhibition of FPTase relative to the related enzyme GGPTase-I and are active in whole cells. Because the negatively charged C-terminal carboxylate of the CA_1A_2X peptidomimetics was thought to impede cell penetrability, derivatives were synthesized in which the carboxylate was replaced with an ester or lactone[23,25–28] (see examples in FIG. 1). Such prodrug derivatives are assumed to be converted to the more active free acid once inside the cell. Indeed, while these prodrugs exhibit less potent inhibition of FPTase *in vitro*, they are more potent than the corresponding free acids in whole cell assays and show efficacy in *in vivo* models. Alternatively, cell active, peptide-based FPTase inhibitors have been made by deleting the X residue of the CA_1A_2X[29,30] (for example, L-745,631; FIG. 1). This strategy has yielded potent FPTase inhibitors (IC_{50} in the range of 1–500 nM) that maintain selectivity for inhibition of FPTase relative to GGPTase-I despite deletion of the CA_1A_2X residue responsible for determining the specificity of prenylation. Several of these inhibitors have shown activity in whole cells and in *in vivo* efficacy models.[30]

Extensive structure-activity studies with the CA_1A_2X tetrapeptides demonstrated that a wide range of amino acids are tolerated at the A_1 and A_2 residues. Subsequent replacement of the A_1A_2 region with either an aminobenzoic acid[31] (for example, FTI-276; FIG. 1) or aminobenzodiazepine[32] (for example, BZA-5B; FIG. 1) moiety yielded compounds that inhibit FPTase with nanomolar IC_{50} values and maintain specificity for inhibition of FPTase over GGPTase-I. Importantly, these compounds are active in whole cells in culture and in *in vivo* cancer efficacy models.

Modifications have been made to the cysteine residue of the CA_1A_2X because of its potential for thiol-based toxicity in animals and humans. Cysteine replacements were selected that provide a ligand for an active site zinc ion that was shown to co-ordinate to the thiol group of the CA_1A_2X cysteine residue during catalysis. Replacement of cysteine with histidine or imidazole in a modified CA_1A_2X tetrapeptide yielded potent FPTase inhibitors that were active in whole cells.[33] Screening of a chemical collection has yielded a series of compounds (exemplified by SCH54429 in FIG. 1) that are competitive with CA_1A_2X binding and lack both a thiol and a carboxylic acid residue.[34–37] These compounds possess modest intrinsic FPTase inhibitory activity (IC_{50} = 180 nM for SCH54429), but they are active in whole cell assays and in *in vivo* models.

Compounds that inhibit FPTase through competition with FPP, the isoprenoid substrate in the farnesylation reaction, have also been described. A variety of FPP analogs that lack the pyrophosphate leaving group and are therefore purely competitive inhibitors of FPTase have been synthesized (for example, L-704,272; FIG. 1).[21,38–40] Furthermore, modifications to inhibitors of squalene synthase, another FPP-utilizing enzyme, have yielded potent and selective FPTase inhibitors that are competitive with FPP in the farnesylation reaction.[41,42] Additionally, a number of microbially derived inhibitors that resemble FPP in structure and are competitive with FPP in the farnesylation reaction have been isolated.[43–52] Surprisingly, several peptide-based inhibitors that compete with FPP have also been described[53,54] (for example, PD 083176; FIG. 1). An initial concern with these compounds was the selectivity for inhibition of FPTase relative to inhibition of other FPP-utilizing enzymes. These compounds generally display some selectivity for inhibition of FPTase *in vitro*. Some of the compounds in this class of inhibitors have shown activity in whole cells.[39,41,42,44,45]

Bisubstrate inhibitors designed to mimic the structure of the ternary complex consisting of enzyme, FPP, and CA_1A_2X tetrapeptide have also been synthesized[55–57] (for example, BMS-186511; FIG. 1). Some of these compounds are potent, selective inhibitors of FPTase and are active in whole cells.[56,58]

BIOLOGY OF FPTase INHIBITORS

The vast majority of biological data relating to FPTase inhibitors are derived from the CA_1A_2X -competitive compounds. Biological studies performed in our laboratory have made use of two related peptidomimetics, L-739,749 and L-744,832[28,59]

(FIG. 1). Reduction of the N-terminal peptide bond and replacement of the A_1-A_2 amide bond with an oxyether bond confer metabolic stability to these molecules. L-739,749 and L-744,832 are methyl and isopropyl ester prodrug derivatives, respectively, of L-739,750, a carboxylate-containing inhibitor based on the tetrapeptide CIFM. L-739,750 is a potent and selective inhibitor of FPTase (IC_{50}s of 1.8 nM and 3,000 nM against FPTase and GGPTase-I, respectively). Typical of other cell-active CA_1A_2X peptidomimetics, L-739,749 inhibits the processing of oncogenic Ha-Ras in cultured cells ($IC_{50} = 0.1$–1.0 μM). As expected, L-739,749 is 10-fold more potent than the carboxylate L-739,750 in the processing assay, presumably because of the improved membrane permeance of the ester prodrug.

Numerous biological consequences of inhibiting FPTase in transformed cells have been documented. L-739,749,[60] similar to other cell-active FPTase inhibitors,[32,58,61] can revert the morphology of Ha-*ras*–transformed rodent fibroblasts to that of the untransformed parental cells. Thus, the treated cells flatten, become less refractile, and become contact inhibited. This morphological reversion is accompanied by a rearrangement of the actin cytoskeleton, with actin moving from membrane ruffles and substratum-attachment sites characteristic of *ras*-transformed cells to stress fibers characteristic of normal cells. Typical of the FPTase inhibitors, L-739,749 can reduce the growth rate of Ha-*ras*–transformed cells growing in monolayer culture.[32,58,60] The specificity of this growth inhibition was indicated by the lack of significant effect on the growth rate of the untransformed parental cells or on rodent fibroblasts transformed with v-*raf*, an oncogene downstream of *ras* in the signal transduction pathway that does not require prenylation for biological activity.[60]

One of the most frequently used assays for evaluating the biological consequences of inhibiting FPTase in transformed cells is the soft agar colony formation assay. In this assay, L-739,749 blocked the growth of rodent fibroblasts transformed with oncogenic Ha-*ras* at 2.5–10 μM.[28] At these concentrations, L-739,749 did not inhibit the colony formation of rodent fibroblasts transformed by v-*raf*. This result suggested that the growth inhibitory effect of L-739,749 was not due to nonspecific toxicity.

Several FPTase inhibitors have been shown to inhibit the anchorage-independent growth of human tumor cell lines. L-744,832 inhibited soft agar colony formation of human tumor cell lines derived from various tissues independent of *ras* mutational status.[62] By contrast, a similar analysis using B956[27] revealed a general trend whereby cell lines with activated Ha-*ras* were more sensitive than those with activated N-*ras*. Cell lines with activated Ki-*ras* varied so greatly in sensitivity that some of the lines were comparable in sensitivity to the lines with activated N-*ras* whereas others were no more sensitive than lines that lack an activated *ras* allele. The sensitivity of cell lines harboring an activated Ha-*ras* allele is almost certainly due, at least in part, to inhibition of Ha-Ras processing and thus biological activity in those cells. The mechanism of growth inhibition of cells harboring activated N- or Ki-*ras* or cells lacking an activated *ras* allele is more complicated. Because N- and Ki-*ras* can be geranylgeranylated in cells in which FPTase activity is ablated[17,18] and because a geranylgeranylated form of Ras is transforming when overexpressed in rodent fibroblasts,[63] the singular role of these proteins in growth inhibition by FPTase inhibitors is uncertain. In some cells lacking an activated *ras* allele, sensitivity to the FPTase inhibitor may result from activation of the Ras pathway by alteration of proteins upstream of Ras. The sensitivity of all of these cells is consistent with the involvement of other farnesylated proteins in the biological effect of the FPTase inhibitors. Indeed, RhoB, a protein that is both farnesylated and geranylgeranylated in cells[64] and is solely geranylgeranylated in cells treated with L-739,749,[12] has been implicated in mediating the biological effects of FPTase inhibitors. Thus, rodent fibroblasts transformed with activated Ha-*ras* which also expressed an activated but prenylation-independent form of RhoB were resistant to the biological effects of FPTase inhibitor treatment.[12]

Similar results have been obtained from studies analyzing the *in vivo* efficacy of FPTase inhibitors in a nude mouse xenograft model. L-739,749 effectively inhibited the growth of Ha-, N-, and Ki-*ras*-transformed rodent fibroblasts implanted subcutaneously in nude mice.[28] B956 was similarly shown to inhibit the growth of Ha-*ras*–transformed fibroblasts in a xenograft model in a dose-dependent manner, and this growth inhibition correlated with inhibition of Ha-Ras processing in the tumor.[27] The methyl ester prodrug of B956, compound B1086 (FIG. 1), inhibited the growth in nude mice of human tumor cell lines that express *ras* oncogenes. As observed for B956 in the anchorage-independent growth assay, the sensitivity of a cell line to inhibition of tumor growth depended on which Ras oncoprotein was expressed, with the growth of EJ-1 cells, harboring an activated Ha-*ras*, being completely inhibited while the growth of HCT116 cells, harboring an activated Ki-*ras*, was not significantly altered. However, other compounds, including the nonpeptidic inhibitor SCH55429 (FIG. 1), have shown activity against tumors derived from human tumor cell lines harboring an activated Ki-*ras*.[36,65]

Several strains of oncomice, transgenic mice expressing an oncogenic transgene, have also been used as model systems to test the *in vivo* efficacy of the FPTase inhibitor L-744,832. The MMTV-v-Ha-*ras* oncomice harbor an activated Ha-*ras* gene under the control of the mouse mammary tumor virus (MMTV) promoter/enhancer and spontaneously develop mammary and salivary carcinomas.[66] L-744,832 induced dramatic regression of these tumors in a dose-dependent manner.[59] This tumor regression could be attributed entirely to increased levels of apoptosis.[67] p53 was not required for the L-744,832-induced effects because MMTV-v-Ha-*ras*/p53$^{-/-}$ mice, which lack a functional p53, exhibited tumor regression and increased levels of apoptosis following treatment with L-744,832. Continuous administration of L-744,832 to the MMTV-v-Ha-*ras* mice was required to maintain tumor regression; following cessation of treatment, tumors reappeared.[59] However, most of these tumors regressed upon retreatment. The generation of even a small number of nonresponsive tumors raises the issue of whether or not resistance will be encountered in the clinic.

The tumor regression observed in the treated oncomice would not have been predicted from experiments using cells in culture, where treatment with an FPTase inhibitor results in a cytostatic response rather than a cytotoxic one. This difference between the *in vitro* and *in vivo* situations may be due to the fact that cells must be deprived of attachment to the substratum in order to apoptose upon treatment with an FTI.[68] Thus, tumor cells, which grow anchorage-independently, exhibit apoptosis upon treatment with an FPTase inhibitor, whereas cells grown in monolayer culture cease to proliferate.

The efficacy of L-744,832 also has been evaluated in a strain of MMTV-N-*ras* transgenic mice that develop mammary tumors due to overexpression of wild-type

N-Ras.[69] Although L-744,832 significantly reduced the growth rate of mammary tumors, the effect of the compound was less dramatic than that in the MMTV-v-Ha-*ras* mice. The N-ras protein in the treated tumors remained mainly processed, suggesting that N-Ras may not be the only farnesylated protein mediating the growth inhibitory effect of L-744,832.

In both the nude mouse and oncomouse models, efficacy was achieved in the absence of gross or microscopic toxicity.[28,59] The reason for the sparing of normal tissues, which also depend on Ras for proliferation and in which FPTase should also be inhibited, is not clear. However, similar observations were made in cultured cells. Thus, as just mentioned, FPTase inhibitors block the anchorage-dependent growth of transformed cells at concentrations that minimally affect the growth of untransformed cells. Additionally, the benzodiazepine peptidomimetic BZA-5B interrupts Ras signaling through the mitogen-activated protein kinase cascade in Ha-*ras*–transformed Rat-1 cells but not in untransformed parental cells.[70]

OUTSTANDING ISSUES

Issues related to the preclinical development of the FPTase inhibitors clearly remain to be resolved. Better understanding of the biological target(s) of these compounds might explain some of the current biological anomalies, including why cells lacking an activated *ras* allele can be sensitive to the FPTase inhibitors and why there is little or no effect on normal tissues in mice treated with efficacious doses of the compounds. Equally important are outstanding issues relevant to the clinical use of these compounds. Because sensitivity of a transformed cell to an FPTase inhibitor does not correlate with *ras* mutational status, it is difficult to predict what types of human tumors will respond to treatment with these compounds. Furthermore, the need for continuous dosing of the MMTV-v-Ha-*ras* oncomice to maintain the regressed tumor phenotype suggests that chronic administration of the FPTase inhibitors may be required for optimal efficacy in the clinic. Will such an administration schedule give rise to resistant tumors? Finally, most of the current cancer chemotherapeutics are used in combination in the clinic. Without knowing the biological mechanism of action of the FPTase inhibitors, it is difficult to predict what additional agent might potentiate the clinical effect of these compounds. Whereas many of these questions will be answered by continued investigations in the laboratory, some can only be answered by testing these compounds in humans.

ACKNOWLEDGMENT

I thank Drs. Robert Lobell, Allen Oliff, and Charles Omer for critical reading of the manuscript.

REFERENCES

1. BARBACID, M. 1987. *ras* Genes. Ann. Rev. Biochem. **56:** 779–827.

2. Bos, J.L. 1988. The *ras* gene family and human carcinogenesis. Mutation Res. **195:** 255–271.
3. Bos, J.L. 1989. *ras* oncogenes in human cancer: A review. Cancer Res. **49:** 4682–4689.
4. Zhang, F.L. & P.J. Casey. 1996. Protein prenylation: Molecular mechanisms and functional consequences. Ann. Rev. Biochem. **65:** 241–269.
5. Willumsen, B.M., K. Norris, A.G. Papageorge, N.L. Hubbert & D.R. Lowy. 1984. Harvey murine sarcoma virus p21 *ras* protein: Biological and biochemical significance of the cysteine nearest the carboxy terminus. EMBO J. **3:** 2581–2585.
6. Kato, K., A.D. Cox, M.M. Hisaka, S.M. Graham, J.E. Buss & C.J. Der. 1992. Isoprenoid addition to Ras protein is the critical modification for its membrane association and transforming activity. Proc. Natl. Acad. Sci. USA **89:** 6403–6407.
7. Jackson, J.H., C.G. Cochrane, J.R. Bourne, P.A. Solski, J.E. Buss & C.J. Der. 1990. Farnesol modification of Kirsten-ras exon 4B protein is essential for transformation. Proc. Natl. Acad. Sci. USA **87:** 3042–3046.
8. Hancock, J.F., A.I. Magee, J.E. Childs & C.J. Marshall. 1989. All *ras* proteins are polyisoprenylated but only some are palmitoylated. Cell **57:**1167–1177.
9. Gibbs, J.B. 1991. Ras C-terminal processing enzymes: New drug targets? Cell **65:** 1–4.
10. Reiss, Y., M.S. Brown & J.L. Goldstein. 1992. Divalent cation and prenyl pyrophosphate specificities of the protein farnesyltransferase from rat brain, a zinc metalloenzyme. J. Biol. Chem. **267:** 6403–6408.
11. Gibbs, J.B. & A. Oliff. 1997. The potential of farnesyltransferase inhibitors as cancer chemotherapeutics. Ann. Rev. Pharmacol. Toxicol. **37:** 143–166.
12. Lebowitz, P.F., P.J. Casey, G.C. Prendergast & J.A. Thissen. 1997. Farnesyltransferase inhibitors alter the prenylation and growth-stimulating function of RhoB. J. Biol. Chem. **272:** 15591–15594.
13. Moores, S.L., M.D. Schaber, S.D. Mosser, E. Rands, M.B. O'Hara, V.M. Garsky, M.S. Marshall, D.L. Pompliano & J.B. Gibbs. 1991. Sequence dependence of protein isoprenylation. J. Biol. Chem. **266:** 14603–14610.
14. James, G., J.L. Goldstein & M.S. Brown. 1996. Resistance of K-RasBV12 proteins to farnesyltransferase inhibitors in Rat1 cells. Proc. Natl. Acad. Sci. USA **93:** 4454–4458.
15. Zhang, F.L., P. Kirschmeier, D. Carr, L. James, R.W. Bond, L. Wang, R. Patton, W.T. Windsor, R. Syto, R. Zhang & W.R. Bishop. 1997. Characterization of Ha-Ras, N-Ras, Ki-Ras4A, and Ki-Ras4B as in vitro substrates for farnesyl protein transferase and geranylgeranyl protein transferase type I. J. Biol. Chem. **272:** 10232–10239.
16. Trueblood, C.E., Y. Ohya & J. Rine. 1993. Genetic evidence for in vivo cross-specificity of the CaaX-box proteinprenyltransferases farnesyltransferase and geranylgeranyltransferase-I in *Saccharomyces cerevisiae*. Molec. Cell. Biol. **13:** 4260–4275.
17. Rowell, C.A., J.J. Kowalczyk, M.D. Lewis & A.M. Garcia. 1997. Direct demonstration of geranylgeranylation and farnesylation of Ki-Ras in vivo. J. Biol. Chem. **272:** 14093–14097.
18. Whyte, D.B., P. Kirschmeier, T.N. Hockenberry, I. Nunez-Oliva, L. James, J.J. Catino, W.R. Bishoip & J.-K. Pai. 1997. K- and N-Ras are geranylgeranylated in cells treated with farnesyl protein transferase inhibitors. J. Biol. Chem. **272:** 14459–14464.
19. Reiss, Y., J.L. Goldstein, M.C. Seabra, P.J. Casey & M.S. Brown. 1990. Inhibition of purified p21[ras] farnesyl:protein transferase by Cys-AAX tetrapeptides. Cell **62:** 81–88.
20. Schaber, M.D., M.B. O'Hara, V.M. Garsky, S.D. Mosser, J.D. Bergstrom, S.L. Moores, M.S. Marshall, P.A. Friedman, R.A.F. Dixon & J.B. Gibbs. 1990. Polyisoprenylation of Ras *in vitro* by a farnesyl-protein transferase. J. Biol. Chem. **265:** 14701–14704.

21. POMPLIANO, D.L., E. RANDS, M.D. SCHABER, S.D. MOSSER, N.J. ANTHONY & J.B. GIBBS. 1992. Steady-state kinetic mechanism of ras farnesyl:protein transferase. Biochemistry 31: 3800–3807.
22. GOLDSTEIN, J.L., M.S. BROWN, S.J. STRADLEY, Y. REISS & L.M. GIERASCH. 1991. Nonfarnesylated tetrapeptide inhibitors of protein farnesyltransferase. J. Biol. Chem. 266: 15575–15578.
23. KOHL, N.E., S.D. MOSSER, S.J. DESOLMS, E.A. GIULIANI, D.L. POMPLIANO, S.L. GRAHAM, R.L. SMITH, E.M. SCOLNICK, A. OLIFF & J.B. GIBBS. 1993. Selective inhibition of ras-dependent transformation by a farnesyltransferase inhibitor. Science 260: 1934–1937.
24. GARCIA, A.M., C. ROWELL, K. ACKERMANN, J.J. KOWALCZYK & M.D. LEWIS. 1993. Peptidomimetic inhibitors of ras farnesylation and function in whole cells. J. Biol. Chem. 268: 18415–18418.
25. GRAHAM, S.L., S.J. DESOLMS, E.A. GIULIANI, N.E. KOHL, S.D. MOSSER, A.I. OLIFF, D.L. POMPLIANO, E. RANDS, M.J. BRESLIN, A.A. DEANA, V.M. GARSKY, T.H. SCHOLZ, J.B. GIBBS & R.L. SMITH. 1994. Pseudopeptide inhibitors of Ras farnesyl-protein transferase. J. Med. Chem. 37: 725–732.
26. WAI, J.S., D.L. BAMBERGER, T.E. FISHER, S.L. GRAHAM, R.L. SMITH, J.B. GIBBS, S.D. MOSSER, A.I. OLIFF, D.L. POMPLIANO, E. RANDS & N.E. KOHL. 1994. Synthesis and biological activity of Ras farnesyl protein transferase inhibitors. Tetrapeptide analogs with amino methyl and carbon linkages. Bioorg. & Med. Chem. 2: 939–947.
27. NAGASU, T., K. YOSHIMATSU, C. ROWELL, M.D. LEWIS & A.M. GARCIA. 1995. Inhibition of human tumor xenograft growth by treatment with the farnesyl transferase inhibitor B956. Cancer Res. 55: 5310–5314.
28. KOHL, N.E., F.R. WILSON, S.D. MOSSER, E.A. GIULIANI, S.J. DESOLMS, M.W. CONNER, N.J. ANTHONY, W.J. HOLTZ, R.P. GOMEZ, T.-J. LEE, R.L. SMITH, S.L. GRAHAM, G.D. HARTMEN, J.B. GIBBS & A. OLIFF. 1994. Farnesyltransferase inhibitors block the growth of ras-dependent tumors in nude mice. Proc. Natl. Acad. Sci. USA 91: 9141–9145.
29. DESOLMS, S.J., A.A. DEANA, E.A. GIULIANI, S.L. GRAHAM, N.E. KOHL, S.D. MOSSER, A.I. OLIFF, D.L. POMPLIANO, E. RANDS, T.H. SCHOLZ, J.M. WIGGINS, J.B. GIBBS & R.L. SMITH. 1995. Pseudodipeptide inhibitors of protein farnesyltransferase. J. Med. Chem. 38: 3967–3971.
30. WILLIAMS, T.M., T.M. CICCARONE, S.C. MACTOUGH, R.L. BOCK, M.W. CONNER, J.P. DAVIDE, K. HAMILTON, K.S. KOBLAN, N.E. KOHL, A.M. KRAL, S.D. MOSSER, C.A. OMER, D.L. POMPLIANO, E. RANDS, M.D. SCHABER, D. SHAH, F.R. WILSON, J.B. GIBBS, S.L. GRAHAM, G.D. HARTMAN, A.I. OLIFF & R.L. SMITH. 1996. 2-Substituted piperazines as constrained amino acids. Application to the synthesis of potent, non carboxylic acid inhibitors of farnesyltransferase. J. Med. Chem. 39: 1345–1348.
31. SEBTI, S.M. & A.D. HAMILTON. 1996. Rational design of Ras prenyltransferase inhibitors as potential anticancer drugs. Biochem. Soc. Trans. 24: 692–699.
32. JAMES, G.L., J.L. GOLDSTEIN, M.S. BROWN, T.E. RAWSON, T.C. SOMERS, R.S. MCDOWELL, C.W. CROWLEY, B.K. LUCAS, A.D. LEVINSON & J.J.C. MARSTERS. 1993. Benzodiazepine peptidomimetics: potent inhibitors of Ras farnesylation in animal cells. Science 260: 1937–1942.
33. HUNT, J.T., V.G. LEE, K. LEFTHERIS, B. SEIZINGER, J. CARBONI, J. MABUS, C. RICCA, N. YAN & V. MANNE. 1996. Potent, cell active, non-thiol tetrapeptide inhibitors of farnesyltransferase. J. Med. Chem. 39: 353–358.
34. BISHOP, W.R., R. BOND, J. PETRIN, L. WANG, R. PATTON, R. DOLL, G. NJOROGE, J. CATINO, J. SCHWARTZ, W. WINDSOR, R. SYTO, J. SCHWARTZ, D. CARR, L. JAMES &

P. KIRSCHMEIER. 1995. Novel tricyclic inhibitors of farnesyl protein transferase. J. Biol. Chem. **270:** 30611–30618.

35. NJOROGE, F.G., B. VIBULBHAN, C.S. ALVAREZ, W.R. BISHOP, J. PETRIN, R.J. DOLL, V. GIRIJAVALLABHAN & A.K. GANGULY. 1996. Novel tricyclic animoacetyl and sulfonamide inhibitors of Ras farnesyl protein transferase. Bioorg Med. Chem. Lett. **6:** 2977–2982.

36. MALLAMS, A.K., F.G. NJOROGE, R.J. DOLL, M.E. SNOW, J.J. KAMINSKI, R.R. ROSSMAN, B. VIBULBHAN, W.R. BISHOP, P. KIRSCHMEIER, M. LIU, M.S. BRYANT, C. ALVAREZ, D. CARR, L. JAMES, I. KING, Z. LI, C.-C. LIN, C. NARDO, J. PETRIN, S.W. REMISZEWSKI, A.G. TAVERAS, S. WANG, J. WONG, J. CATINO, V. GIRIJAVALLABHAN & A.K. GANGULY. 1997. Antitumor 8-chlorobenzocycloheptapyridines: A new class of selective, nonpeptidic, nonsulfhydryl inhibitors of Ras farnesylation. Bioorg. Med. Chem. **5:** 93–99.

37. NJOROGE, F.G., R.J. DOLL, B. VIBULBHAN, C.S. ALVAREZ, W.R. BISHOP, J. PETRIN, P. KIRSCHMEIER, N.I. CARRUTHERS, J.K. WONG, M.M. ALBANESE, J.J. PIWINSKI, J. CATINO, V. GIRIJAVALLABHAN & A.K. GANGULY. 1997. Discovery of novel nonpeptide tricyclic inhibitors of Ras farnesyl protein transferase. Bioorg. Med. Chem. **5:** 101–113.

38. PATEL, D.V., R.J. SCHMIDT, S.A. BILLER, E.M. GORDON, S.S. ROBINSON & V. MANNE. 1995. Farnesyl diphosphate-based inhibitors of Ras farnesyl protein transferase. J. Med. Chem. **38:** 2906–2921.

39. MANNE, V., C.S. RICCA, J.G. BROWN, A.V. TUOMARI, N. YAN, D. PATEL, R. SCHMIDT, M.J. LYNCH, C.P. CIOSEK, JR., J.M. CARBONI, S. ROBINSON, E.M. GORDON, M. BARBACID, B.R. SEIZINGER & S.A. BILLER. 1995. Ras farnesylation as a target for novel antitumor agents: potent and selective farnesyl diphosphate analog inhibitors of farnesyltransferase. Drug Dev. Res. **34:** 121–137.

40. OVERHAND, M., E. PIETERMAN, L.H. COHEN, A.R.P.M. VALENTIJN, G.A. VAN DER MAREL & J.H. VAN BOOM. 1997. Synthesis of triphosphonate analogues of farnesyl pyrophosphate. Inhibitors of squalene synthase and protein:farnesyl transferase. Bioorg. & Med. Chem. Lett. **7:** 2435–2440.

41. AOYAMA, T., T. SATOH, M. YONEMOTO, J. SHIBATA, K. NONOSHITA, S. ARAI, K. KAWAKAMI, Y. IWASAWA, H. SANO, K. TANAKA, Y. MONDEN, T. KODERA, H. ARAKAWA, I. SUZUKI-TAKAHASHI, T. KAMEI & K. TOMIMOTO. 1998. A new class of highly potent farnesyl diphosphate-competitive inhibitors of farnesyltransferase. J. Med. Chem. **41:** 143–147.

42. YONEMOTO, M., T. SATOH, H. ARAKAWA, I. SUZUKI-TAKAHASHI, Y. MONDEN, T. KODERA, K. TANAKA, T. AOYAMA, Y. IWASAWA, T. KAMEI, S. NISHIMURA & K. TOMIMOTO. 1998. J-104,871, a novel farnesyltransferase inhibitor, blocks Ras farnesylation in vivo in a farnesyl pyrophosphate-competitive manner. Molec. Pharmacol. **54:** 1–7.

43. DUFRESNE, C., K.E. WILSON, S.B. SINGH, D.L. ZINK, J.D. BERGSTROM, D. REW, J.D. POLISHOOK, M. MEINZ, L. HUANG, K.C. SILVERMAN & R.B. LINGHAM. 1993. Zaragozic acids D and D2: Potent inhibitors of squalene synthase and of ras farnesylprotein transferase. J. Natural Prod. **56:** 1923–1929.

44. GIBBS, J.B., D.L. POMPLIANO, S.D. MOSSER, E. RANDS, R.B. LINGHAM, S.B. SINGH, E.M. SCOLNICK, N.E. KOHL & A. OLIFF. 1993. Selective inhibition of farnesyl-protein transferase blocks ras processing in vivo. J. Biol. Chem. **268:** 7617–7620.

45. HARA, M., K. AKASAKA, S. AKINAGA, M. OKABE, H. NAKANO, R. GOMEZ, D. WOOD, M. UH & F. TAMANOI. 1993. Identification of Ras farnesyltransferase inhibitors by microbial screening. Proc. Natl. Acad. Sci. USA **90:** 2281–2285.

46. LINGHAM, R.B., K.C. SILVERMAN, G.F. BILLS, C. CASCALES, M. SANCHEZ, R. G. JENKINS, S. E. GARTNER, I. MARTIN, M. T. DIEZ, F. PELAEZ, S. MOCHALES, Y.-L. KONG,

R. W. BURG, M. S. MEINZ, L. HUANG, M. NALLIN-OMSTEAD, S. D. MOSSER, M. D. SCHABER, C. A. OMER, D.L. POMPLIANO, J. B. GIBBS & S.B. SINGH. 1993. Chaetomella acutiseta produces chaetomellic acids A and B which are reversible inhibitors of farnesyl-protein transferase. Applied Microbiol. & Biotechnol. **40:** 370-374.

47. SINGH, S.B., D.L. ZINK, J.M. LIESCH, M.A. GOETZ, R.G. JENKINS, M. NALLIN-OMSTEAD, K.C. SILVERMAN, G.F. BILLS, R.T. MOSLEY, J.B. GIBBS, G. ALBERS-SCHONBERG & R.B. LINGHAM. 1993. Isolation and structure of chaetomellic acids A and B from Chaetomella acutiseta: farnesyl pyrophosphate mimic inhibitors of Ras farnesyl-protein transferase. Tetrahedron **49:** 5917–5926.

48. SINGH, S.B., J.M. LIESCH, R.B. LINGHAM, M.A. GOETZ & J.B. GIBBS. 1994. Actinoplanic acid A: A macrocyclic polycarboxylic acid which is a potent inhibitor of Ras farnesyl-protein transferase. J. Am. Chem. Soc. **116:** 11606–11607.

49. SINGH, S.B., J.M. LIESCH, R.B. LINGHAM, K.C. SILVERMAN, J.M. SIGMUND & M.A. GOETZ. 1995. Structure, chemistry, and biology of actinoplanic acids: Potent inhibitors of Ras farnesyl-protein transferase. J. Organ. Chem. **60:** 7896–7901.

50. VAN DER PYL, D., P. CANS, J.J. DEBERNARD, F. HERMAN, Y. LELIEVRE, L. TAHRAOUI, M. VUILHORGNE & J. LEBOUL. 1995. RPR113228, a novel farnesyl-protein transferase inhibitor produced by *Chrysosporium lobatum.* J. Antibiotics 736–737.

51. JAYASURIYA, H., G.F. BILLS, C. CASCALES, D.L. ZINK, M.A. GOETZ, R.G. JENKINS, K.C. SILVERMAN, R.B. LINGHAM & S.B. SINGH. 1996. Oreganic acid: A potent novel inhibitor of Ras farnesyl-protein transferase from an endophytic fungus. Bioorg. Med. Chem. Lett. **6:** 2081–2084.

52. SILVERMAN, K.C., H. JAYASURIYA, C. CASCALES, D. VILELLA, G.F. BILLS, R.G. JENKINS, S.B. SINGH & R.B. LINGHAM. 1997. Oreganic acid, a potent inhibitor of Ras farnesyl-protein transferase. Biochem. Biophys. Res. Commun. **232:** 478–481.

53. WALLACE, A., K.S. KOBLAN, K. HAMILTON, D.J. MARQUIS-OMER, P.J. MILLER, S.D. MOSSER, C.A. OMER, M.D. SCHABER, R. CORTESE, A. OLIFF, J.B. GIBBS & A. PESSI. 1996. Selection of potent inhibitors of farnesyl-protein transferase from a synthetic tetrapeptide combinatorial library. J. Biol. Chem. **271:** 31306–31311.

54. LEONARD, D.M., K.R. SHULER, C.J. POULTER, S.R. EATON, T.K. SAWYER, J.C. HODGES, T.-Z. SU, J.D. SCHOLTEN, R.C. GOWAN, J.S. SEBOLT-LEOPOLD & A.M. DOHERTY. 1997. Structure-activity relationships of cysteine-lacking pentapeptide derivatives that inhibit ras farnesyltransferase. J. Med. Chem. **40:** 192–200.

55. BHIDE, R.S., D.V. PATEL, M.M. PATEL, S.P. ROBINSON, L.W. HUNIHAN & E.M. GORDON. 1994. Rational design of potent carboxylic acid based bisubstrate inhibitors of ras farnesyl protein transferase. Bioorg. & Med. Chem. Letts. **4:** 2107–2112.

56. PATEL, D.V., E.M. GORDON, R.J. SCHMIDT, H.N. WELLER, M.G. YOUNG, R. ZAHLER, M. BARBACID, J.M. CARBONI, J.L. GULLO-BROWN, L. HUNIHAN, C. RICCA, S. ROBINSON, B.R. SEIZINGER, A.V. TUOMARI & V. MANNE. 1995. Phosphinyl Acid-based Bisubstrate Analog Inhibitors Of Ras Farnesyl Protein Transferase. J. Med. Chem. **38:** 435–442.

57. PATEL, D.V., M.G. YOUNG, S.P. ROBINSON, L. HUNIHAN, B.J. DEAN & E.M. GORDON. 1996. Hydroxamic acid-based bisubstrate analog inhibitors of Ras farnesyl protein transferase. J. Med. Chem. **39:** 4197–4210.

58. MANNE, V., N. YAN, J.M. CARBONI, A.V. TUOMARI, C.S. RICCA, J.G. BROWN, M.L. ANDAHAZY, R.J. SCHMIDT, D. PATEL, R. ZAHLER, R. WEINMANN, C.J. DER, A.D. COX, J.T. HUNT, E.M. GORDON, M. BARBACID & B.R. SEIZINGER. 1995. Bisubstrate inhibitors of farnesyltransferase: a novel class of specific inhibitors of ras transformed cells. Oncogene **10:** 1763–1779.

59. KOHL, N.E., C.A. OMER, M.W. CONNER, N.J. ANTHONY, J.P. DAVIDE, S.J. DESOLMS, E.A. GIULIANI, R.P. GOMEZ, S.L. GRAHAM, K. HAMILTON, L.K. HANDT, G.D. HARTMEN, K.S. KOBLAN, A.M. KRAL, P.J. MILLER, S.D. MOSSER, T.J. O'NEILL, E.

RANDS, M.D. SCHABER, J.B. GIBBS & A. OLIFF. 1995. Inhibition of farnesyltransferase induces regression of mammary and salivary carcinomas in ras transgenic
mice. Nature Med. **1:** 792–797.

60. PRENDERGAST, G.C., J.P. DAVIDE, S.J. DESOLMS, E.A. GIULIANI, S.L. GRAHAM, J.B.
GIBBS, A. OLIFF & N.E. KOHL. 1994. Farnesyltransferase inhibition causes morphological reversion of ras-transformed cells by a complex mechanism that
involves regulation of the actin cytoskeleton. Mol. Cell. Biol. **14:** 4193–4202.

61. COX, A.D., A.M. GARCIA, J.K. WESTWICK, J.J. KOWALCZYK, M.D. LEWIS, D.A.
BRENNER & C.J. DER. 1994. The CAAX peptidomimetic compound B581 specifi-
cally blocks farnesylated, but not geranylgeranylated or myristylated, oncogenic
Ras signaling and transformation. J. Biol. Chem. **269:** 19203–19206.

62. SEPP-LORENZINO, L., Z. MA, E. RANDS, N.E. KOHL, J.B. GIBBS, A. OLIFF & N.
ROSEN. 1995. A peptidomimetic inhibitor of farnesyl:protein transferase blocks the
anchorage-dependent and -independent growth of human tumor cell lines. Cancer
Res. **55:** 5302–5309.

63. COX, A.D., M.M. HISAKA, J.E. BUSS & C.J. DER. 1992. Specific isoprenoid modification is required for function of normal, but not oncogenic, ras protein. Mol. Cell.
Biol. **12:** 2606–2615.

64. ADAMSON, P., C.J. MARSHALL, A. HALL & P.A. TILBROOK. 1992. Post-translational
modifications of p21rho proteins. J. Biol. Chem. **267:** 20033–20038.

65. SUN, J., Y. QIAN, A.D. HAMILTON & S.M. SEBTI. 1995. Ras CAAX peptidomimetic
FTI 276 selectively blocks tumor growth in nude mice of a human lung carcinoma
with K-ras mutation and p53 deletion. Cancer Res. **55:** 4243–4247.

66. SINN, E., W. MULLER, P. PATTENGALE, I. TEPLER, R. WALLACE & P. LEDER. 1987.
Coexpression of MMTV/v-Ha-ras and MMTV/c-myc genes in transgenic mice:
Synergistic action of oncogenes in vivo. Cell **49:** 465–475.

67. BARRINGTON, R.E., M.A. SUBLER, E. RANDS, C.A. OMER, P.J. MILLER, J.E. HUNDLEY,
S.K. KOESTER, D.A. TROYER, D.J. BEARSS, M.W. CONNER, J.B. GIBBS, K. HAMIL-
TON, K.S. KOBLAN, S.D. MOSSER, T.J. O'NEILL, M.D. SCHABER, E.T. SENDERAK,
J.J. WINDLE, A. OLIFF & N.E. KOHL. 1998. A farnesyltransferase inhibitor induces
tumor regression in transgenic mice harboring multiple oncogenic mutations by
mediating alterations in both cell cycle control and apoptosis. *Mol. Cell. Biol.* **18:**
85–92.

68. LEBOWITZ, P.F., D. SAKAMUR & G.C. PRENDERGAST. 1997. Farnesyl transferase
inhibitors induce apoptosis of ras-transformed cells denied substratum attachment.
Cancer Res. **57:** 708–713.

69. MANGUES, R., T. CORRAL, N.E. KOHL, W.F. SYMMANS, S. LU, M. MALUMBRES, J.B.
GIBBS, A. OLIFF & A. PELLICER. 1998. Antitumor effect of a farnesyl transferase
inhibitor in mammary and lymphoid tumors overexpressing N-ras in transgenic
mice. Cancer Res. **58:** 1253–1259.

70. JAMES, G.L., M.S. BROWN, M.H. COBB & J.L. GOLDSTEIN. 1994. Benzodiazepine
peptidomimetic BZA-5B interrupts the MAP kinase activation pathway in H-Ras-
transformed Rat-1 cells, but not in untransformed cells. J. Biol. Chem. **269:**
27705–27714.

Selective Inhibition of *ras*-Transformed Cell Growth by a Novel Fatty Acid-Based Chloromethyl Ketone Designed to Target Ras Endoprotease

YULONG CHEN[a]

Department of Medicinal Chemistry, College of Pharmacy, University of Minnesota, Minneapolis, Minnesota 55455, USA

ABSTRACT: A novel fatty acid-based chloromethyl ketone, UM96001, which was designed to be a Ras C-terminal sequence-specific endoprotease inhibitor, at low micromolar concentrations (1 ~ 5.0 μM), potently inhibits *ras*-transformed rat kidney cell growth, whereas the growth of untransformed normal rat kidney cells is not affected under the same conditions. UM96001 almost completely blocks the anchorage-independent clonogenic growth of *ras*-transformed rat and human cancer cells at low micromolar concentrations. Inhibition of *ras*-transformed rat and human cancer cell growth by UM96001 may occur via the mechanism of selective induction of apoptosis of the cells. Furthermore, TPCK and BFCCMK, the known selective inhibitors of Ras C-terminal sequence-specific endoprotease, also yield similar inhibition results. These results provide the first experimental evidence that the endoproteolysis of Ras oncoproteins may be important for Ras-mediated cell growth and apoptosis. Therefore, the Ras C-terminal sequence-specific endoprotease may be a potential anticancer target.

INTRODUCTION

An important family of prenylated proteins, Ras superfamily, has been extensively studied for the last decade. Ras oncogenes have been identified in about 30% of all human cancers and particularly found in 90% of human pancreatic cancers, 50% of colorectal tumors, and 30% of lung cancers.[1] After prenylation, Ras proteins undergo endoproteolysis to remove the AAX amino acid sequence from the Ras C-terminus CAAX (C, cysteine; A, aliphatic amino acid; X, undetermined amino acid), followed by methylation of the newly formed prenylated cysteine C-terminus. The posttranslational modifications of Ras proteins are necessary for many Ras functions.[2–6] The design and synthesis of Ras farnesyltransferase (FTase) inhibitors as anticancer drugs have been an intense research topic in recent years,[7–9] because FTase inhibitors not only inhibit the growth of *ras*-transformed cells,[10–14] but also induce tumor regression in animals without significant toxicity.[15]

[a]Address for correspondence: Department of Pharmacology, Medical School, University of Minnesota, Minneapolis, MN 55455. Phone, 612/626-6539; fax, 612/625-8408.
e-mail, chenx112@tc.umn.edu

By contrast, few studies have been carried out to understand the role of endopro-teolysis of Ras proteins in cell growth and apoptosis. The importance of endopro-teolysis for the localization of Ras proteins to the plasma membrane was demonstrated in an elegant membrane-binding experiment.[16] However, the real physiologic consequence of proteolytic removal of Ras C-terminal three amino acids in mammalian cells is not clear.[17] This author hypothesized that proteolysis of en-dogenous Ras C-terminus is necessary for Ras-mediated tumor growth *in vivo*. Therefore, inactivating Ras endoprotease activity *in vivo* will block Ras-mediated cancer cell growth. In a previous report, I demonstrated that the irreversible inhibi-tors of Ras endoprotease indeed block the growth of *ras*-transformed rodent cells and human cancer cells with K-*ras* mutations, whereas the growth of untransformed NIH/3T3 cells is not affected under the same conditions.[18] The molecular mecha-nism of growth inhibition might occur via induction of *ras*-transformed cells to un-dergo apoptosis.[18] In this report, the author further demonstrates that the growth of normal rat kidney cells (NRK-49F) is not affected under similar conditions, whereas the growth of K-*ras* transformed normal rat kidney cells (KNRK, transformed by Kirsten murine sarcoma virus) is potently inhibited by the novel fatty acid-based chloromethyl ketone UM96001, which was originally designed to be a potent Ras endoprotease inhibitor.[18]

RESULTS AND DISCUSSION

On the basis of the available data from our and other studies of the Ras endopro-tease,[19–23] I proposed a hypothetical active site of Ras endoprotease, which consists of four key components: a hydrophobic lipid-binding pocket, a CAAX-binding pocket, a putative salt bridge formed with the C-terminus of the Ras protein, and a putative active site cysteine (FIG. 1). The design of the novel fatty acid-based chlo-

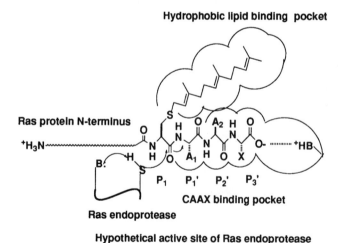

FIGURE 1. Proposed hypothetical active site of Ras endoprotease

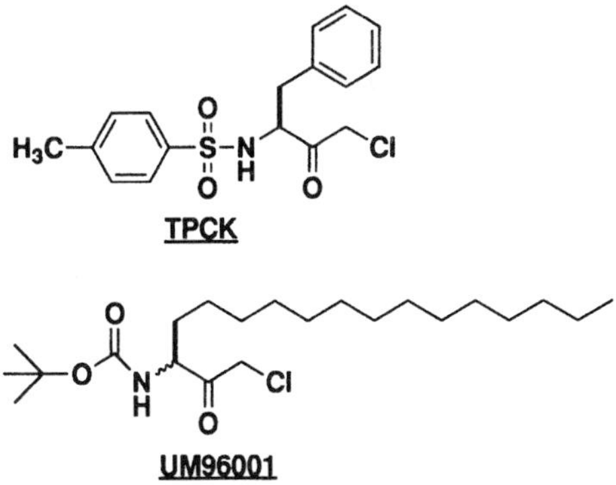

FIGURE 2. Structures of *ras*-transformed cell growth blockers.

romethyl ketone UM96001 (Fig. 2) as a potential Ras endoprotease inhibitor was primarily developed from my earlier finding that hydrophobic chloromethyl ketone TPCK is a specific, potent, and irreversible Ras endoprotease inhibitor[19] and was based on the hypothetical active site of this enzyme (Fig. 1). It was rationalized that inclusion of the substrate-mimicked farnesyl thioether moiety into a chloromethyl ketone molecule would provide better binding and inhibitory potency than would TPCK. The kinetic studies support this rationale. The inhibition mode of these inhibitors is active-site directed, irreversible, and concentration- and time-dependent. The bimolecular rate constants k_{inh}/K_i values for TPCK and N-Boc-S-farnesyl cysteine chloromethyl ketone (BFCCMK) are (77 ± 6) $M^{-1} \cdot min^{-1}$ and $(11.6 \pm 0.6) \times 10^2$ $M^{-1} \cdot min^{-1}$, respectively.[19,20] From the standpoint of hydrophobicity and simple molecular modeling studies, the dodecyl group can substitute for the farnesyl group. Hence, a chloromethyl ketone inhibitor of Ras endoprotease with a similar potency of BFCCMK may be obtained by the substitution of the dodecyl moiety for the farnesyl moiety. Furthermore, because of the chemical lability of the thioether unit of the farnesylcysteine derivatives, replacement of the thioether unit with a methylene unit provides a more stable and cell-permeable compound, UM96001 (Fig. 2).[18] The designing idea of replacement of the farnesyl moiety with fatty acid side chains in our irreversible inhibitors was recently corroborated in studies of substrate specificity by other researchers. A published report[24] demonstrated that replacement of the farnesyl moiety with the pentadecyl group yielded a similar binding affinity of the tetrapeptide substrate for the Ras endoprotease.

Compound UM96001 was tested on KNRK cells. Non-*ras*–transformed NIH/3T3 and NRK-49F cells served as control cell lines. Inhibition of growth of the *ras*-transformed cells and cancer cells with *ras* mutations by all tested inhibitors is time- and concentration-dependent.[18] FIGURE 3 shows the dose-dependent selective inhibition of *ras*-transformed KNRK cell growth versus untransformed NRK-49F by UM96001. The novel fatty acid-based chloromethyl ketone UM96001 almost completely blocks the growth of KNRK cells (~100% inhibition) (Fig. 3), but not that of untransformed NRK-49F cells. TLCK, which did not inhibit the enzyme at this concentration,[19,20] did not inhibit *ras*-transformed cell growth at 5 μM.[18] The positive

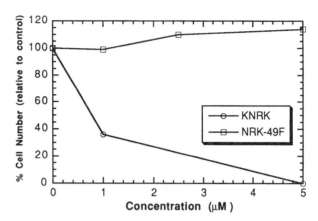

FIGURE 3. Selective inhibition of K-*ras*-transformed normal rat kidney cell growth by UM96001. *Open circles:* Dose-response of KNRK cell growth; each datum point is from triplicate measurements of a typical experiment. *Open squares:* Dose-response of NRK-49F cell growth; each datum point is from an average of two independent experiments. Cell numbers were counted in a hemocytometer using the trypan blue exclusion method. Experimental details were the same as those published.[18]

control TPCK inhibited the growth of KNRK cells to the extent of 42% at 5 μM.[18] This result is consistent with that of the *in vitro* enzymatic activity assay.[19,20] Together, these results demonstrate that the blocking of *ras*-transformed cell growth is selective.

Single suspension cells from KNRK and HEC-1A (a human endometrial cancer cell line containing point mutations in codon 12 of K-*ras*[25]) were cultured in a semi-solid medium, soft agar. Compound UM96001 completely blocked the anchorage-independent clonogenic formations of KNRK cells at 5 μM of concentration (~100%). At 5 μM of concentration of UM96001, the colony formations of HEC-1A cells in soft agar were inhibited by 30%. A higher concentration (20 μM) of UM96001 completely abolished the clonogenic growth of HEC-1A cells in soft agar (~100%). These results are consistent with those of anchorage-dependent cell growth assays.

After treatment with 5 μM of UM96001 for 48 hours, apoptosis in UM96001-treated KNRK cells was observed. The morphologic hallmarks of cell apoptosis, chromatin condensation and then nuclear fragmentation, were clearly demonstrated by fluorescence microscopy.[18] Preliminary studies on morphologic changes in drug-treated and untreated cells suggest that UM96001 is a potent apoptotic inducer of *ras*-transformed KNRK cells.

Ras proteins play a dual role in apoptosis in fibroblasts: they promote or suppress apoptosis.[26] Farnesylation of Ras oncoproteins is important for the survival of *ras*-transformed fibroblasts detached from substratum.[27] Inhibition of farnesylation also decreased the tumor size in animals via apoptosis of tumor cells.[28] Endoproteolysis of Ras oncoproteins, to our knowledge, had never been studied for its role in apoptosis of cells until I first reported that inhibition of *ras*-transformed cell growth by irreversible Ras endoprotease inhibitors might be caused by induction of apoptosis.[18] Cancer cells with *ras* mutations seem more sensitive to Ras endoprotease inhibitors than do untransformed cells.[18] Farnesylation and endoproteolysis of Ras proteins appear to be critical for apoptosis of *ras*-transformed cells.[18,27,28]

UM96001 blocked the growth of *ras*-transformed KNRK cells, but not the growth of untransformed NIH/3T3[18] and normal rat kidney cells at the same concentrations (1 ~ 5 μM) (FIG. 3). At low micromolar concentrations, UM96001 blocked anchorage-independent growth of both *ras*-transformed normal rat kidney cells and human cancer cells.[18] At higher concentrations, chloromethyl ketones had some effect on the growth of untransformed NIH/3T3 cells[18] mainly because of the alkylating nature of these compounds. Therefore, UM96001 itself may not be an ideal anticancer drug candidate. However, it serves as a good lead for further development of the second generation of anti-Ras agents for Ras-mediated cancer growth. Moreover, the inhibition profile in cells by TPCK and BFCCMK is similar to that in partially purified Ras endoprotease.[19,20] These results are consistent with our working hypothesis that inactivation of Ras endoprotease activity blocks the growth of *ras*-transformed cancer cells. In other words, endogenous proteolysis of Ras *in vivo* may be required for Ras to mediate the malignant growth of *ras*-transformed cells. For normal cells, proteolysis of Ras proteins might not be essential for survival of the cells. Interestingly, our results in mammalian cells reflect those from yeast and *Xenopus*. In yeast, a gene, *RCE1*, was identified as being responsible for the endoproteolysis of both Ras protein and **a**-factor.[29] Disruption of *RCE1* resulted in defects in Ras localization and signaling, but *RCE1* is not essential for the survival of normal yeast cells.[29] In *Xenopus*, proteolysis and methylation are also required for the membrane binding and function of Ras.[30]

In summary, a novel fatty acid-based chloromethyl ketone, UM96001, has been designed and synthesized. New observations indicate that UM96001 produces potent inhibition of the growth of *ras*-transformed rat kidney cells and human cancer cells with *ras* mutations, in comparison with the untransformed cells, and induces apoptosis of *ras*-transformed cells. Results from this laboratory strongly suggest that UM96001 is definitely worthy of further investigation as an anticancer lead agent and that the Ras endoprotease may be a potential anticancer target.

ACKNOWLEDGMENTS

This work was supported in part by a start-up fund from the University of Minnesota Academic Health Center and by grant IRG-58-001-40-IRG-03 from the American Cancer Society. The main data in this paper were published recently in *Cancer Letters*. The author thanks Drs. Carston R. Wagner and Patrick E. Hanna for generously sharing their laboratory facilities with me.

REFERENCES

1. BOS, J.L. 1989. Cancer Res. **49:** 4682–4689.
2. LOWY, D.R. & B.M. WILLUMSEN. 1993. Annu. Rev. Biochem. **62:** 851–891.
3. CLARKE, S. 1992. Annu. Rev. Biochem. **61:** 355–386.
4. CASEY, P.J. 1995. Science **268:** 221–225.

5. HALL, A. 1998. Science **279:** 509–514. Heimbrook, D. C. & A. Oliff. 1998. Curr. Opin. Cell Biol. **10:** 284–288.
6. DOWNWARD, J. 1998. Curr. Opin. Gene. Dev. **8:** 49–54.
7. KOBLAN, K.S. *et al.* 1996. Biochem. Soc. Trans. **24:** 688–692.
8. KELLOFF, G.J. *et al.* 1997. Cancer Epidemiol. Biomarkers & Prev. **6:** 267–282.
9. COX, A.D. & C.J. DER. 1997. Biochim. Biophy. Acta **1333:** F51–F71.
10. KOHL, N.E. *et al.* 1993. Science **260:** 1934–1937.
11. JAMES. G.L. *et al.* 1993. Science **260:** 1937–1942.
12. GARCIA, A.M., C. ROWELL, K. ACKERMANN, J.J. KOWALCZYK & M.D. LEWIS. 1993. J. Biol. Chem. **268:** 18415–18418.
13. QIAN, Y. *et al.* 1994. J. Biol. Chem. **269:** 12410–12413.
14. MANNE, V. *et al.* 1995. Oncogene **10:** 1763–1779.
15. KOHL, N.E. *et al.* 1995. Nat. Med. **1:** 792–797.
16. HANCOCK, J.F., K. CADWALLADER & C. MARSHALL. EMBO J. **10:** 641–646.
17. KATO, K. *et al.* 1992. Proc. Natl. Acad. Sci. USA **89:** 6403–6407.
18. CHEN, Y. 1998. Cancer Lett. **131:** 191–200.
19. CHEN, Y. 1995. ASBMB/DBC-ACS Joint Meeting in San Francisco, Late Breaking Abstract LB 46 [Addendum]. FASEB J. **9**(6).
20. CHEN, Y., Y.-T. MA & R.R. RANDO. 1996. Biochemistry **35:** 3227–3237.
21. ASHBY, M.N., D.S. KING & J. RINE. 1992. Proc. Natl. Acad. Sci. USA **89:** 4613–4617.
22. MA, Y.-T., A. CHAUDHURI & R.R. RANDO. 1992. Biochemistry **31:** 11775–11776.
23. JANG, G.-F., K. YOKOYAMA & M.H. GELB. 1993. Biochemistry **32:** 9500–9507.
24. JANG, G-F. & M. H. GELB. 1998. Biochemistry **37:** 4473–4481.
25. ENOMOTO, T. *et al.* 1990. Cancer Res. **50:** 6139–6145.
26. KAUFFMANN-ZEH, A. *et al.* 1997. Nature **385:** 544–548.
27. LEBOWITZ, P.F., D. SAKAMURO & G.C. PRENDERGAST. 1997. Cancer Res. **57:** 708–713.
28. BARRINGTON, R.E. *et al.* 1998. Mol. Cell. Biol. **18:** 85–92.
29. BOYARTCHUK, V.L., M.N. ASHBY & J. RINE. 1997. Science **275:** 1796–1800.
30. GELB, M.H. Science **275:** 1750–1751.

Azatyrosine

Mechanism of Action for Conversion of Transformed Phenotype to Normal

YOSHIAKI MONDEN,[a] FUMIE HAMANO-TAKAKU,[a]
NOBUKO SHINDO-OKADA,[b] AND SUSUMU NISHIMURA[a,c]

[a]Banyu Tsukuba Research Institute in collaboration with Merck Research Laboratories,
Okubo 3, Tsukuba, Ibaraki 300-2611, Japan
[b]Biology Division, National Cancer Center Research Institute, Tsukiji 5-1-1, Chuo-ku,
Tokyo 104-0045, Japan

ABSTRACT: Azatyrosine [L-β-(5-hydroxy-2-pyridyl)-alanine] has the unique property of converting *ras*- or c-*erbB*-2 transformed phenotype to normal. The administration of azatyrosine also inhibits tumor formation in transgenic mice harboring the normal human c-Ha-*ras* which is mutated during treatment with various chemical carcinogens.To elucidate the molecular mechanism, we investigated how azatyrosine functions and what are its major targets. Azatyrosine functions downstream of *ras*; azatyrosine does not alter either the level of GTP-bound Ras or the total amount of Ras. Instead, azatyrosine inhibits the activation of c-Raf-1 kinase by oncogenic c-ErbB-2, resulting in inactivation of AP1. It is interesting that azatyrosine also restores the expression of the *rhob* gene, the product of which regulates the formation of actin stress fibers. Azatyrosine is incorporated into cellular proteins to replace tyrosine. Several experiments indicate that replacement of tyrosine is likely to be a cause for its conversion of transformed phenotype to normal. To prove this hypothesis, we are attempting to develop a mutant of tyrosyl-tRNA synthetase that, unlike wild type, can aminoacylate azatyrosine more efficiently than can tyrosine.

INTRODUCTION

In 1989, we reported that the antibiotic azatyrosine, isolated from *Streptomyces chibanensis* (L-β-(5-hydroxyl-2-pyridyl)-alanine; FIG. 1) induces reversion of activated c-Ha-*ras*–transformed NIH3T3 cells to the apparently normal phenotype.[1] Azatyrosine also caused reversion of transformed NIH3T3 cells transfected by activated c-Ki-*ras*, N-*ras*, c-*raf*, or c-*erbB*-2.[1] It also caused reversion of human cancer cell lines, such as pancreatic adenocarcinoma PSN-1 cells, which are known to have a c-Ki-*ras* point mutation, amplification of c-*myc* and a *p53* mutation,[2] and colon cancer HCT-116 cells having activated c-Ki-*ras*.[3] However, azatyrosine was unable to convert the transformed phenotype of NIH3T3 cells transfected with *hst*, *ret*, or *src*, indicating that the target(s) of azatyrosine is in the *ras* signaling pathway.[1]

When NIH3T3 cells transformed by activated c-Ha-*ras* were incubated with azatyrosine for more than 6 days in a culture medium, permanent conversion cells

[c]Phone, +81-298-77-2003; fax, +81-298-77-2034.
e-mail, nismrasm@banyu.co.jp

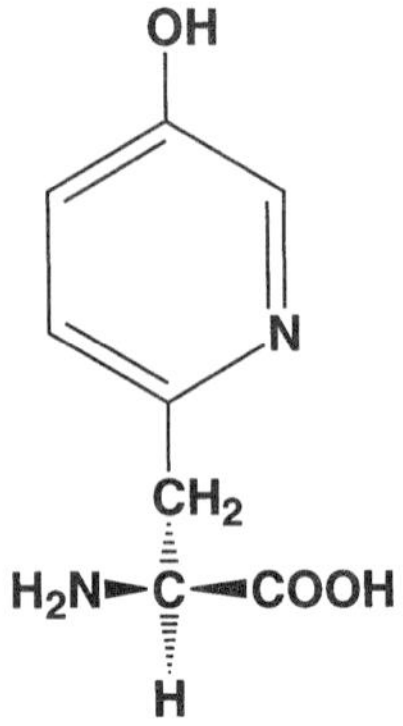

FIGURE 1. Structure of azatyrosine.

were obtained. Such reverent cells maintained a normal phenotype in the absence of azatyrosine during prolonged culture. By adopting differential hybridization with ^{32}P-labeled cDNAs from the original ras-transformed NIH3T3 cells and the reverent cells, a λgt10 cDNA library was screened.[4] The gene specifically expressed in the reverent cells thus isolated was the ras recision gene (rrg), which was previously isolated as a tumor suppressor gene by Contente et al.[5] and subsequently identified as the gene for lysyl oxidase.[6] Other genes such as collagen type III, rhoB, intracisternal A particle (IAP) genome, and Ca-31 (the gene for a Ca binding protein) were also expressed.[4] Those genes (rrg and rhoB) as well as the gene for fibronectin began to be expressed within several days when ras-transformed NIH3T3 cells were incubated with azatyrosine. These results suggested that azatyrosine blocked signal transduction in the ras signaling pathway, thereby activating several cellular genes in ras-transformed cells, and that these activated genes acted cooperatively to counteract ras function and fix the normal phenotype.

Azatyrosine inhibited neurite outgrowth (NOG) of PC12 cells induced by expression of either ras or raf oncogene[7] and inhibited NOG induced by microinjected oncogenic Ras protein, but not NGF-induced NOG. These results also suggested that the target of azatyrosine is in abnormal signal transduction of Ras pathway.

The other intriguing function of azatyrosine is its inhibitory activity of tumor formation in vivo.[8] We used transgenic mice harboring the normal human c-Ha-ras gene.[9] These transgenic mice were very susceptible to induction of tumors. The tumors produced in these transgenic mice by the administration of chemical carcinogens almost all contained a somatically mutated c-Ha-ras gene.[10] Application of azatyrosine to the skin of transgenic mice after initiation with 7,12-dimethylbenz[a]anthracene (DMBA) greatly reduced the incidence, number of papillomas per mouse (as shown in FIG. 2), as well as their size. The administration of azatyrosine ip after initiation with methylnitrosourea also completely prevented the formation of forestomach papillomas.[8] These results clearly indicate that azatyrosine inhibits the chemical carcinogenesis involved in ras activation in vivo.

In the following sections, recent work on azatyrosine using c-erbB-2 transformed cells is described. The aim of these studies is to elucidate the mechanism of action of azatyrosine in more detail, attempting to identify the signal-transduction process triggered by activated c-ErbB-2 and inhibited by azatyrosine.

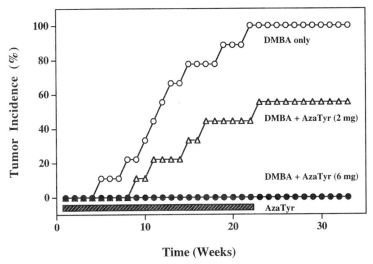

FIGURE 2. Inhibition of skin papilloma formation induced by a single dose of DMBA by azatyrosine. The skin was painted with 200 mg of DMBA (5 mg/kg body weight). Beginning 2 days after treatment, azatyrosine dissolved in 50% ethanol was applied to the skin at indicated doses every 3 days. The control group received only the same amount of 50% ethanol after DMBA treatment.

REVERSION OF THE MORPHOLOGIC PHENOTYPE OF THE C-*ERBB*-2–TRANSFORMED CELL

We used A4 cells, a variant of NIH3T3 cells, transformed with oncogenic c-erbB-2.[11] On day 2 after azatyrosine was added to the culture medium, the growth of A4 cells was inhibited in a dose-dependent manner, as shown in FIGURE 3. Treatment with azatyrosine 1 mg/ml completely inhibited cell growth, but growth inhibition at 500 µg/ml was marginal. Morphologic analysis showed that azatyrosine at more than 500 µg/ml induced all of the cells to revert to normal morphology within 2 days after treatment. Thus, azatyrosine showed the ability to revert the transformed phenotype of c-erbB-2–transformed cells, as in the case of ras-transformed cells. It should be mentioned that the morphologic change of c-erbB-2–transformed cells to normal phenotype is not permanent, because the reverted cells could acquire transformed phenotype when the cells are cultured in the absence of azatyrosine, contrary to ras-transformed NIH3T3 cells.[1,12]

STIMULATION OF EXPRESSION OF *RHO* GENES IN C-*ERB*B-2–TRANSFORMED CELLS BY AZATYROSINE

We previously reported that expression of the *rhoB* gene is induced in c-Ha-ras–transformed NIH3T3 cells upon incubation with azatyrosine.[4] In this study, expression of a member of the *rho* family of genes was examined with c-erbB-2–trans-

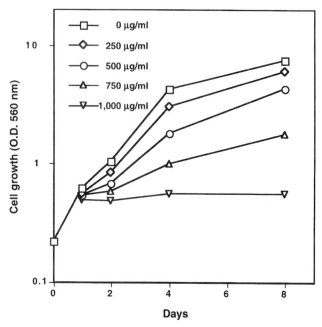

FIGURE 3. Effects of azatyrosine on the growth of A4 cells. A4 cells were cultured in the presence or the absence of azatyrosine at the concentrations indicated.

formed cells (A4 cells) in the presence or absence of azatyrosine as well as normal NIH3T3 cells.[13] The level of expression of the *rho* family of genes in A4 cells such as *rhoA, rhoB*, and *rhoC* was low compared with that in NIH3T3 cells. The amount of *rho*B and *rho*C mRNAs in A4 cells was less than 10% of that in NIH3T3 cells. The expression of *rho*A in A4 cells was also reduced to 20% of that in NIH3T3 cells. On the other hand, when A4 cells were treated with azatyrosine, expression of the *rho* genes was restored. The level of expression of the *rhoA* gene in A4 cells treated for 1 day with azatyrosine at 800 µg/ml was the same as that in NIH3T3 cells, whereas the expression of *rhoB* and *rhoC* in A4 cells treated with azatyrosine was approximately 50% of that in NIH3T3 cells. These results indicate that azatyrosine restores the expression of rho family genes in A4 cells.

INDUCTION OF ACTIN STRESS FIBER FORMATION IN
C-*ERBB*-2–TRANSFORMED CELLS BY AZATYROSINE

Cellular transformation is characterized by alteration of cell morphology, enhancement of cell proliferation, and acquisition of the capacity for anchorage independent growth. These features of transformed cells, in particular morphologic changes, are considered to be related to disassembly of the cytoskeleton.[14,15] In addition, cell morphology is regulated by Rho proteins via the assembly of actin stress fibers.[16–20]

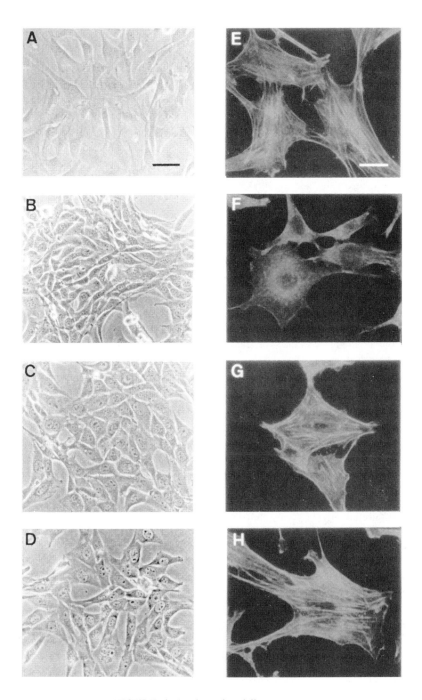

FIGURE 4. *See legend on following page.*

Since expression of *rho* family genes in *c-erbB*-2–transformed cells was enhanced by azatyrosine, the formation of actin stress fibers was also examined in these cells incubated with azatyrosine.[21] As shown in FIGURE 4, actin stress fibers were clearly observed in NIH3T3 cells, whereas they disappeared in A4 cells concomitant with morphologic changes. By contrast, azatyrosine induced actin stress fiber formation in A4 cells together with reversion of the cells to flatter cells. Our results indicated that the mechanism by which azatyrosine restores *c-erbB*-2–transformed cells to a normal morphology is associated with induction of actin stress fibers and they also implied that the restoration of expression of *rho* genes is connected with the formation of actin stress fibers. Moreover, the *c-erbB*-2–transformed cells that overexpressed the *rhoB* gene were flatter than the parental *c-erbB*-2–transformed cells, and the formation of actin stress fibers was observed in these flatter cells.[21]

EFFECTS OF AZATYROSINE ON SIGNAL TRANSDUCTION INDUCED BY ACTIVATED C-*ERBB*-2

Activation of c-ErbB-2 kinase transmits cellular signaling from the cellular membrane to the nucleus via several factors. The resultant activation of transcriptional factors stimulates expression of particular genes that are relevant to proliferation of cells.[22,23] To elucidate the mechanism of action of azatyrosine in cellular transformation, an attempt was made to identify the signal transduction step(s) affected by azatyrosine.[12]

First, we investigated the effect of azatyrosine on activation of Ras induced by oncogenic c-ErbB-2. In A4 cells, the amount of Ras-bound GTP was approximately twice that of normal NIH3T3 cells. Treatment of A4 cells with azatyrosine did not alter either the amount of GTP-bound Ras or the total amount of Ras, indicating that activation of Ras still occurred to the same extent in the azatyrosine-treated A4 cells.

The c-*raf*-1 protooncogene encodes a cytoplasmic serine/threonine protein kinases that is operated downstream of Ras.[24–28] Activation of c-*Raf*-1 is induced by growth factors and membrane-bound products of oncogenes and is accompanied by its hyperphosphorylation.[29,30] Therefore, we next examined the effect of azatyrosine on the phosphorylation of c-Raf-1. c-Raf-1 was more phosphorylated in A4 cells than in normal NIH3T3 cells, indicating that c-ErbB-2 activates c-Raf-1 protein as previously reported. A4 cells treated with azatyrosine 500 μg/ml showed a 50% reduction in phosphorylation of c-Raf-1 with no effect on the amount of c-Raf-1 protein. These results indicate that azatyrosine inhibits the activation of c-Raf-1 kinase triggered by oncogenic c-ErbB-2. Activated c-ErbB-2 protein and activated c-Raf-1

FIGURE 4. Effects of azatyrosine on the morphology of A4 cells and on the formation of actin stress fibers in A4 cells. NIH 3T3 cells were cultured in the absence of azatyrosine (**A** and **E**). A4 cells were cultured in the absence of azatyrosine (**B** and **F**), in the presence of azatyrosine at 400 μg/ml (**C** and **G**), and in the presence of azatyrosine at 800 μg/ml (**D** and **H**). Cells were photographed 3 days after the start of treatment with azatyrosine (**A, B, C,** and **D**). Bar, 50 μm. After a 3-day incubation, cells were fixed, stained with rhodamine-phalloidin, and observed under a fluorescence microscope (**E, F, G,** and **H**). Bar, 20 μm.

protein are known to activate transcription factor AP1.[22,23] Activation of AP1 plays a crucial role in cell transformation.[31,32] To examine the effect of azatyrosine on stimulation of AP1 activity, NIH3T3 cells were cotransfected with reporter plasmid pTREtkCAT and oncogenic c-*ErbB*-2 expression plasmid pCOB2A7 in the presence or absence of azatyrosine.[12] The pTREtkCAT plasmid contains TRE in the region upstream of the promoter of thymidine kinase and CAT genes. When the cells were treated with azatyrosine 800 μg/ml, stimulation of AP1 activity measured by CAT assay was significantly inhibited, whereas the background level of CAT activity from the transfectant with only pTREtkCAT was not affected at all. Therefore, it was concluded that azatyrosine inhibits the activation of AP1 by oncogenic c-ErbB-2. The activity of AP1 is regulated by induction of transcription and posttranslational modification of Fos and Jun.[33–37] Inasmuch as activated c-*erbB*-2 increases the extent of phosphorylation of c-Jun,[38] we investigated the effect of azatyrosine on phosphorylation and expression of c-Jun.[12] In A4 cells, the level of phosphorylated c-Jun was increased compared with that in normal NIH3T3 cells. Treatment of A4 cells with azatyrosine reduced the level of phosphorylation up to 50% without affecting the expression level of c-Jun. This result suggested that azatyrosine inhibited AP1 activity via inhibition of phosphorylation of c-Jun.

Recent studies showed that active, GTP-bound Ras associates directly with c-Raf-1 kinase, resulting in activation of c-Raf-1.[27–29] However, azatyrosine can also convert transformed phenotype caused by the oncogenic *raf* mutant,[1] which lacks the N-terminal Ras-binding domain.[27–29] Therefore, it is more likely that azatyrosine inhibits c-Raf-1 activity through a mechanism other than simply blocking the Ras-Raf interaction.

INCORPORATION OF AZATYROSINE INTO PROTEINS

Because of the structural similarity of azatyrosine and tyrosine, it is likely that azatyrosine is incorporated into cellular proteins to replace tyrosine. To prove this possibility, we cultured A4 cells in the presence of [³H]azatyrosine and examined its incorporation into proteins. As shown in FIGURE 5, [³H]azatyrosine was in fact incorporated into proteins.[39] To investigate whether azatyrosine replaces tyrosine in protein, A4 cells were cultured with [³H]tyrosine or [³H]azatyrosine in the presence of different amounts of unlabeled azatyrosine or tyrosine. Unlabeled tyrosine inhibited incorporation of [³H]azatyrosine into proteins in a dose-dependent manner. In addition, unlabeled azatyrosine inhibited incorporation of [³H]tyrosine. These results indicated that azatyrosine and tyrosine compete in the incorporation into proteins. SDS-polyacrylamide gel electrophoresis has revealed that many distinct proteins were labeled with [³H]azatyrosine, suggesting that incorporation of azatyrosine into proteins is not restricted to particular proteins(s), but more or less randomly into many protein molecules. However, the efficiency of incorporation of azatyrosine may be different depending on the type of proteins, because the radioactive pattern of the gel labeled with [³H]azatyrosine is different from that labeled with [³H]tyrosine.

To determine if incorporation of azatyrosine is relevant to its ability to convert transformed phenotype to normal, we added excess amounts of tyrosine to the cul-

A   B

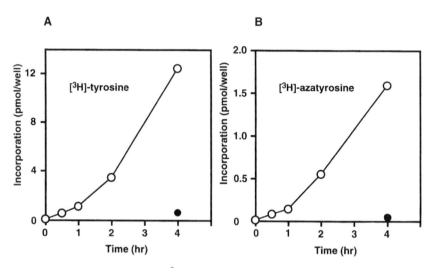

FIGURE 5. Incorporation of [³H]azatyrosine into A4 cells. A4 cells were cultured with [³H]tyrosine (**A**) or [³H]azatyrosine (**B**) for the times indicated (*open circles*). Cycloheximide, as an inhibitor of protein synthesis, was added before [³H]tyrosine or [³H]azatyrosine (*filled circles*). Radioactivity of the TCA-insoluble fractions of cell lysates was measured.

ture medium and examined the ability of azatyrosine in phenotype conversion of A4 cells. When A4 cells were cultured in the original medium containing 72 μg/ml of tyrosine, 500 μg/ml of azatyrosine could convert the transformed phenotype of A4 cells to normal. By contrast, when A4 cells were cultured with 500 μg/ml of azatyrosine in the presence of 1 mg/ml of tyrosine, A4 cells retained their transformed morphology.[39] Thus, high concentrations of tyrosine interfered with the ability of azatyrosine to convert transformed phenotype to normal, similar to its inhibition of incorporation of azatyrosine into proteins.

INEFFICIENT PHOSPHORYLATION OF AZATYROSINE RESIDUE IN PEPTIDE

Tyrosine residues in cellular proteins are known to be phosphorylated by various kinases. Phosphorylation of tyrosine residues in proteins plays an important role in activation in the Ras signal transduction pathway.[40,41] Thus, it is hypothesized that azatyrosine is incorporated into a crucial protein(s) in which tyrosine phosphorylation is important in signal transduction and azatyrosine inhibits phosphorylation, thereby maintaining normal phenotype. Therefore, as a model experiment, the fragment of EGFR that contains azatyrosine instead of tyrosine was chemically synthesized, and its phosphorylation by EGFR kinase was examined. As shown in FIGURE 6, the extent of phosphorylation of azatyrosine residue in the peptide is approximately 20% compared with phosphorylation of tyrosine residue in the corresponding peptide, indicating that azatyrosine is an inferior acceptor for phosphorylation.

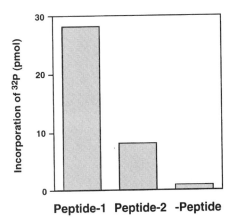

Peptide-1 : RRKGSTAENAEYLRVA

Peptide-2 : RRKGSTAENAE^{AZA}YLRVA

FIGURE 6. Incorporation of ^{32}P into synthetic peptide containing azatyrosine by EGFR kinase. Peptides correspond to the autophosphorylation site of the EGFR carboxyl terminal tail. Peptides (40 nmol) were incubated with EGFR kinase obtained by STRAT-AGENE and γ-^{32}P-ATP, and radioactivity of the TCA-insoluble fractions was randomly measured.

AN ATTEMPT TO MUTATE TYROSYL-tRNA SYNTHETASE FOR EFFICIENT INCORPORATION OF AZATYROSINE

The effective concentration of azatyrosine required to convert the transformed phenotype to normal is high, likely because of the inefficient aminoacylation of azatyrosine by tyrosyl-tRNA synthetase. If we can make a mutant of tyrosyl-tRNA synthetase that can aminoacylate azatyrosine more efficiently than can tyrosine, and if transfection of such mutated tyrosyl-tRNA synthetase gene into A4 cells resulted in a reduction of the concentration of azatyrosine needed for the morphologic change, it should be the final proof of our hypothesis that incorporation of azatyrosine into protein causes phenotype conversion.

For this purpose, an attempt was made to create a mutant of *Escherichia coli* aminoacyl-tRNA synthetase that can accept more efficiently azatyrosine than normal tyrosine. *E. coli* tyrosyl-tRNA gene was randomly mutagenized by employing the modified polymerase chain reaction. The library plasmids that contain mutated tyrosyl-tRNA synthetase were introduced into *E. coli*. The transformed *E. coli* was screened by monitoring incorporation of azatyrosine to obtain mutated tyrosyl-tRNA synthetase (FIG. 7). One mutant thus isolated could in fact incorporate azatyrosine 15-fold more than it could tyrosine. Tyrosyl-tRNA synthetase isolated from the mutant showed the same *in vitro* activity. Transfection of this mutated *E. coli* tyrosyl-tRNA synthetase together with *E. coli* tRNA^{Tyr} gene into A4 cells is now underway. The advantage of using *E. coli* tyrosyl-tRNA synthetase instead of a mammalian one is that both *E. coli* and mammalian synthetases can only recognize tRNA^{Tyr} from the same species. Therefore, in future studies, when the mutated *E. coli* tyrosyl-tRNA synthetase gene and amber suppressor *E. coli* tRNA^{Tyr} gene are transfected into mammalian cells, together with the gene that contains the amber nonsense codon in

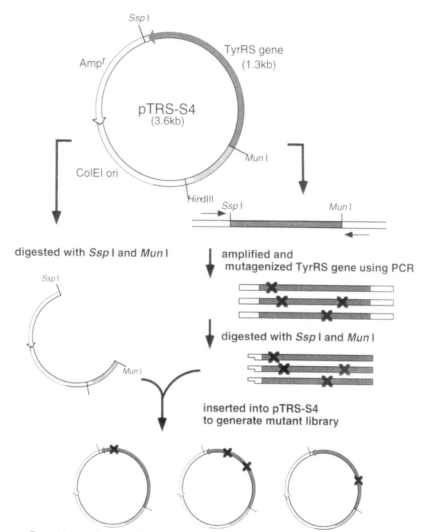

FIGURE 7. Scheme for illustrating the method of random mutagenesis of the tyrosyl-tRNA synthetase (TyrRS) gene using a modified PCR. The *E. coli* TyrRS gene was amplified and mutagenized by a modified PCR according to the method described by Leung *et al.*[42] In this method, to reduce the fidelity of DNA synthesis by Taq polymerase, 0.5 mM of Mn^{2+} was added in the reaction. The PCR products were digested with *Ssp*I and *Mun*I and inserted into TyrRS expression vectors pTRS-S4, instead of the wild-type TyrRS gene.

a particular position, we can make a protein containing azatyrosine in a specific position(s). Such an alloprotein(s) should be useful both for elucidation of basic problems on cancer as well as from a biotechnological point of view.

REFERENCES

1. SHINDO-OKADA, N., O. MAKABE, H. NAGAHARA & S. NISHIMURA. 1989. Permanent conversion of mouse and human cells transformed by activated *ras* or *raf* genes to apparently normal cells by treatment with the antibiotic azatyrosine. Mol. Carcinogen **2**: 159–67.
2. YAMADA, H., H. SAKAMOTO, M. TAIRA, S. NISHIMURA, T. SHIMOSATA, M. TERADA & T. SUGIMURA. 1996. Amplification of both c-Ki-*ras* with a point mutation and c-*myc* in a primary pancreatic cancer and its metastatic tumors in lymph nodes. Jpn. J. Cancer Res. (Gann) **77**: 370–375.
3. SHIRASAWA, S., M. FURUSE, N. YOKOYAMA & T. SASAZUKI. 1993. Altered growth of human colon cancer cell lines disrupted at activated Ki-*ras*. Science **260**: 85–88.
4. KRZYZOSIAK,W.J., N. SHINDO-OKADA, H. TESHIMA, K. NAKAJIMA & S. NISHIMURA. 1992. Isolation of genes specifically expressed in flat revertant cells derived from activated *ras*-transformed NIH3T3 cells by treatment with azatyrosine. Proc. Natl. Acad. Sci. USA **89**: 4879–4883.
5. CONTENTE, S., K. KENYON, D. RIMOLDI & R.M. FRIEDMA. 1991. Expression of gene *rrg* is associateed with reversion of NIH3T3 transformed by LTR-c-H-*ras*. Science **249**: 796–798.
6. KENYON, K., S. CONTENTE, P.C. TRACKMAN, J. TANG, H.M. KAGAN & R.M. FRIEDMAN. 1991. Lysyl oxidase and *rrg* messenger RNA. Science **253**: 802.
7. FUJITA-YOSHIGAKI, J., S. YOKOYAMA, N. SHINDO-OKADA & S. NISHIMURA. 1992. Azatyrosine inhibits neurite outgrowth of PC12 cells induced by oncogenic Ras. Ongocene **7**: 2019–2024.
8. IZAWA, M., S. TAKAYAMA, N. SHINDO-OKADA, S. DOI, M. KITAMURA, M. KATSUKI & S. NISHIMURA. 1992. Inhibition of chemical carcinogenesis *in vivo* by azatyrosine. Cancer Res. **52**: 1628–1630.
9. SAITOH, A., M. KIMURA, R. TAKAHASHI, M. YOKOYAMA, T. NOMURA, M. IZAWA, T. SEKIYA, S. NISHIMURA & M. KATSUKI. 1990. Most tumors in transgenic mice with human c-Ha-*ras* gene contained somatically activated transgenes. Oncogene **5**: 1195–1200.
10. ANDO, K., A. SAITO, O. HINO, R.-L. TAKAHASHI, M. KIMURA & M. KATSUKI. 1992. Chemically induced forestomach papillomas in transgenic mice carry mutant human c-Ha-*ras* transgenes. Cancer Res. **52**: 978–982.
11. SHAN, J., S. MATSUDA, M. IHCINO & T. YAMAMOTO. 1992. Detetion of the ligand activity of the c-*erb*B-2 protein in calf serum. Jpn. J. Cancer Res. **83**: 15–19.
12. MONDEN, Y., T. NAKAMURA, K. KOJIRI, N. SHINDO-OKADA & S. NISHIMURA. 1996. Azatyrosine inhibits the activation of c-Raf-a, c-Jun and AP1 but not the activation of Ras during signal transduction triggered by oncogenic c-ErbB-2. Oncol. Rep. **3**: 33–40.
13. MONDEN, Y., T. NAKAMURA, K. KOJIRI, N. SHINDO-OKADA & S. NISHIMURA. 1996. Stimulation of the expression of *rho*B contributes to the ability of azatyrosine to convert C-*erb*B-2 transformed cells to a normal morphology. Oncol. Rep. **3**: 49–55.
14. WEBER, K., E. LAZARIDES, R.D. GOLDMEN, A. VOGEL & R. POLLACK. 1974. Localization and distribution of actin fibers in normal, transformed and revertant cells. Cold Springs Harbor Symp. Quant. Biol. **39**: 363–369.
15. POLLACK, R., M. OSBORN & K. WEBER. 1975. Patterns of organization of actin and myosin in normal and transformed cultured cells. Proc. Natl. Acad. Sci. USA **72**: 994–998.
16. RUBIN, E.J., D.M. GILL, P. BOQUET & M.R. POPOFF. 1988. Functional modification of 21 kilodalton G protein when ADP-ribosylated by exoenzyme C3 of *Clostridium botulinum*. Mol. Cell Biol. **8**: 418–426.
17. CHARDIN, P., P. BOQUET, P. MADAULE & M.R. POPOFF. 1989. The mammalian G protein *rho*C is ADP-ribosylated by *Clostridium botulinum* exoenzyme C3 and affects actin microfilaments in Vero cells. EMBO J. **8**: 1087–1092.

18. PATERSON, H.F., A.J. SELF, M.D. GARRETT, L. JUST, K. AKTORIES & A. HALL. 1990. Microinjection of recombinant p21^{rho} induces rapid changes in cell morphology. J. Cell. Biol. **111:** 1001–1007.

19. RIDLEY, A.J. & A. HALL. 1992. The small GTP-binding protein *rho* regulates the assembly of focal adesions and actin stress fibers in response to growth factors. Cell **70:** 389–399.

20. MIURA, Y., A. KIKUCHI, T. MUSHA, S. KURODA, H. YAKU, T. SASAKI & Y. TAKAI. 1993. Regulation of morphology by *rho* p21 and its inhibitory GDP/GTP exchange protein (*rho* GDI) in Swiss 3T3 cells. J. Biol. Chem. **268:** 510–515.

21. MONDEN, Y., T. NAKAMURA, K. KOJIRI, K. SHINDO-OKADA & S. NISHIMURA. 1996. Stimulation of the expression of *rho*B contributes to the ability of azatyrosine to convert c-*erb*B-transformed cells to a normal morphology. Oncol. Rep. **3:** 49–55.

22. SISTONEN, L., E. HOELTTA, H. LEHVASLAIHO, L. LEHTOLA & K. ALITALO. 1989. Activation of the *neu* tyrosine kinase induces the *fos/jun* transcription factor complex, the glucose transporter, and ornithine decarboxylase. J. Cell. Biol. **109:** 1911–1919.

23. FUJIMOTO, A., S. KAI, T. AKIYAMA, K. TOYOSHIMA, K. KAIBUCHI, Y. TAKAI & T. YAMAMOTO. 1991. Transactivation of the TPA-responsive element by the oncogenic c-*erb*B-2 protein is partly mediated by protein kinase C. Biochem. Biophys. Res. Commun. **178:** 724–732.

24. KOLCH, W., G. HEIDECHER, P. LLOYD & U.R. RAPP. 1991. Raf-1 protein kinase is required for growth of induced NIH3T3 cells. Nature **349:** 426–428.

25. DICKSON, B., F. SPRENGER, D. MORRISON & E. HATEN. 1992. Raf functions downstream of Ras-11 in the sevenless signal transduction pathway. Nature **360:** 600–603.

26. MOODIE, S.A., B.M. WILLUMSEN, M.J. WEBER & A. WOLFMAN. 1993. Complexes of Ras: GTP with Raf-1 and mitogen-activated protein kinase kinase. Science **260:** 1658–1661.

27. WARNE, P.H., P.R. VICIANA & J. DOWNWARD. 1993. Direct interaction of Ras and the amino-terminal region of Raf-1 *in vitro*. Nature **364:** 352–355.

28. ZHANG X., J. SETTLEMAN, J.M. KYRIAKIS, E. TAKEUCHI-SUZUKI, S.T. ELLEDGE, M.S. MARSHALL, J.P. BRUDER, U.R. RAPP & J. AVRICH. 1993. Normal and oncogene p21 ras proteins bind to the amino-terminal regulatory domain of c-Raf-1. Nature **364:** 308–313.

29. MORRISON, D.K., D.R. KAPLAN, U.R. RAPP & T.M. ROBERT. 1988. Signal transduction from membrane to cytoplasm. Growth factors and membrane-bound oncogene products increase Raf-1 phosphorylation and associated protein kinase activity. Proc. Natl. Acad. Sci. USA **85:** 8855–8859.

30. HEIDECKER, G., W. KOELCH, D.K. MORRISON & U.R. RAPP. 1992. The role of Raf-1 phosphorylation in signal transduction. Adv. Cancer Res. **58:** 53–73.

31. WASYLYK, C., J.L. IMLER & B. WASYLYK. 1988. Transforming but not immortalizing oncogenes activate the transcription factor PEA1. EMBO J. **7:** 2475–2488.

32. SCHOENTHAL, A., P. HERRLICH, H.J. RAHMSDORF & H. PONTA. 1988. Requirement for *fos* gene expression in the transcriptional activation of collagenase by other oncogenes and phorbol esters. Cell **54:** 325–334.

33. BINETRUY, B., T. SMEAL & M. KARIN. 1991. Ha-Ras augments c-Jun activity and stimulates phosphorylation of its activation domain. Nature **351:** 122–127.

34. BOYLE, W.J., T. SMEAL, L.H. KEFIZE, P. ANGEL, J.R. WOODGETT, M. KARIN & T. HUNTER. 1991. Activation of protein kinase C decreases phosphorylation of c-Jun at sites that negatively regulate its DNA-binding activity. Cell **64:** 573–584.

35. PULVERER, B.J., J.M. KYRIAKIS, J. AVRICH, E. NIKOLAKAKI & J.R. WOODGETT. 1991. Phosphorylation of c-*jun* mediated by MAP kinases. Nature **353:** 670–674.

36. SMEAL, T., B. BINETRUY, D.A. MERCOLA, M. BIRRER & M.KARIN. 1991. Oncogenic and transcriptional cooperation with Ha-Ras requires phosphorylation of c-Jun on serine 63 and 73. Nature **354:** 494–496.

37. SMEAL, T., B. TINETRUY, D. MERCOLA, B.A. GROVER, G. HEIDECKER, U.R. RAPP & M. KARIN. 1992. Oncoprotein-mediated singling cascade stimulates c-Jun activity by phosphorylation of serines 63 and 73. Mol. Cell Biol. **12:** 3507–3513.

38. FUJIMOTO, A., S. KAI, T. AKIYAMA, K. TOYOSHIMA, K. KAIBUCHI, Y. TAKAI & T. YAMAMOTO. 1991. Transactivation of the TPA-responsive element by the oncogene c-*erb*B-2 protein is partly mediated by protein kinase C. Biochem. Biophys. Res. Commun. **178:** 724–732.

39. MONDEN, Y., T. NAKAMURA, K. KOJIRI, N. SHINDO-OKADA & S. NISHIMURA. 1996. Azatyrosine is incorporated into proteins instead of tyrosine residues, with the resultant conversion of transformed cells to cells with a normal phenotype. Oncol. Rep. **3:** 625–629.

40. ULLRICH, A. & J. SCHLESSINGER. 1990. Signal transduction by receptors with tyrosine kinase activity. Cell **61:** 203–212.

41. FANTL, W.J., D.E. JOHNSON & L.T. WILLIAMS. 1993. Signalling by receptor tyrosine kinases. Annu. Rev. Biochem. **62:** 458–481.

42. LEUNG, D.W., E. CHEN & D.V. GOEDDEL. 1989. A method for random mutagenesis of a defined DNA segment using a modified polymerase chain reaction. Technique **1:** 11–15.

SCH 51344, An Inhibitor of RAS/RAC-Mediated Cell Morphology Pathway

C. CHANDRA KUMAR,[a,d] KAZUMASA OHASHI,[b] KYOKO NAGATA,[b] AMY WALSH,[c] DAFNA BAR-SAGI,[c] AND KENSAKU MIZUNO[b]

[a]Department of Tumor Biology, Schering-Plough Research Institute, 2015 Galloping Hill Road, Kenilworth, New Jersey 07033, USA

[b]Department of Biology, Faculty of Science, Kyushu University, Fukuoka 812-8581, Japan

[c]Department of Molecular Genetics and Microbiology, State University of New York at Stony Brook, Stony Brook, New York 11794, USA

ABSTRACT: RAS interacts with multiple targets in the cell and controls at least two signaling pathways, one regulating extracellular signal-regulated kinase (ERK) activation and the other controlling membrane ruffling formation. These two pathways appear to act synergistically to cause transformation. Human smooth muscle α-actin promoter is repressed in RAS-transformed cells and derepressed in revertant cell lines, suggesting that it is a sensitive marker to follow phenotypic changes in fibroblast cells. SCH 51344 is a pyrazoloquinoline derivative identified on the basis of its ability to derepress α-actin promoter in RAS-transformed cells. Previous studies have shown that SCH 51344 is a potent inhibitor of RAS transformation. However, SCH 51344 had very little effect on the activities of proteins in the ERK pathway, suggesting that it inhibits RAS transformation by a novel mechanism. Recently, we have demonstrated that SCH 51344 specifically blocks membrane ruffling induced by activated forms of H-RAS, K-RAS, N-RAS, and RAC. Treatment of fibroblast cells with this compound had very little effect on RAS-mediated activation of ERK and JUN kinase activities. SCH 51344 was effective in inhibiting the anchorage-independent growth of Rat-2 fibroblast cells transformed by the three forms of oncogenic RAS and RAC V12. These results indicate that SCH 51344 inhibits a critical component of the membrane ruffling pathway downstream from RAC and suggest that targeting this pathway may be an effective approach to inhibiting transformation by RAS and other oncogenes.

INTRODUCTION

Ras is a key regulator of cell growth in all eukaryotic cells. Ras proteins are plasma membrane-bound GTP-binding proteins that function as nucleotide-dependent molecular switches.[1,2] In the GDP-bound state they are inactive, but upon binding with GTP they undergo an activating conformational change.[3] Ras in its GTP-bound state couples the signals of activated growth factors to downstream effectors. Recent genetic and biochemical studies indicate that Ras exerts its biological effects by interacting with multiple effectors in the cell, which include Raf, phosphatidyl inositol

[d]Phone, 908-740-7328; fax: 908-740-3918.
e-mail, Chandra.kumar@spcorp.com

RAS interacts with multiple targets in the cell and activates diverse signaling cascades

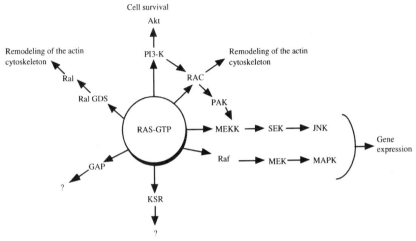

FIGURE 1. Ras mediates its cellular effects presumably through interaction with multiple downstream effectors and activation of diverse signaling cascades. Our current understanding of the downstream targets of each of the Ras effectors is shown. PI3K, phosphotidylinositol-3 kinase; MEKK, MEK kinase; SEK, SAPK/JNK kinase; KSR, kinase suppressor of Ras.

(P I)-3 kinase, p120 GTPase activating protein (GAP), and Ral-GDS, a guanine nucleotide dissociation factor, AF-6/Canoe, RIN1, and so forth (FIG. 1).[4] Through its ability to interact with multiple effectors, Ras activates many signaling pathways that control diverse processes such as regulation of gene expression, remodeling of the actin cytoskeleton, cell survival, and programmed cell death and differentiation.[4,5]

The question then arises of what is the contribution of different signaling pathways to Ras-induced malignant transformation? One elegant approach to understanding the contributions of different signaling pathways to Ras-mediated transformation is the use of Ras effector domain mutants that are defective in binding to specific targets.[6] Presumably these effector domain mutants allow the binding of a subset of normal effectors. Studies using effector domain mutants have shown that at least two functions of Ras are critical for transformation in mammalian cells, one regulating gene expression and the other controlling actin cytoskeletal organization.[7,8] The first signaling pathway, referred to as an extracellular signal-regulated kinase (ERK) pathway, involves a series of cytoplasmic serine/threonine kinases that eventually lead to phosphorylation of specific transcription factors and activation of immediate early genes.[9] The second pathway, referred to as the cell morphology pathway or membrane ruffling pathway, is mediated by Rac, a member of the Rho family of proteins.[10,11] Studies with effector-domain mutants have revealed bifurcation of the signaling pathways downstream of Ras, leading to remodeling of the cy-

Requirement of two signaling pathways for Ras-mediated transformation
(Bar-Sagi/Wigler)

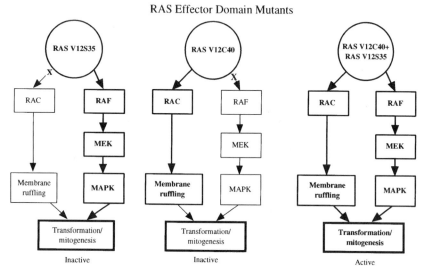

RAS Effector Domain Mutants

FIGURE 2. Selective activation of Ras-dependent signaling cascade by effector binding loop mutants. Effector binding loop mutants of both Ras and Rac have enabled us to determine that Ras-induced mitogenesis requires activation of both MAP kinase and Rac-mediated membrane ruffling pathways.

toskeleton and regulation of gene expression.[7] The effector domain mutant RasV12S35, with an alteration of threonine to serine at position 35, binds Raf and can activate the MAP kinase cascade. However, it fails to stimulate the membrane ruffling pathway. RasV12C40, an activated mutant of Ras with an alteration of tyrosine to cysteine at position 40 in the effector domain, does not interact with Raf and is thus unable to activate the MAP kinase cascade.[7] However, this mutant can cause membrane ruffling in a Rac-dependent manner. Neither RasV12S35 nor RasV12C40 can initiate DNA synthesis and cause transformation of fibroblast cells, suggesting that activation of neither the MAP kinase cascade nor the Rac-mediated membrane ruffling pathway is sufficient to cause mitogenesis or transformation (FIG. 2). When these mutants were expressed together, transformation and mitogenesis were achieved, suggesting that both pathways are required for Ras-induced transformation.[7,8]

In tumor cells, RAS becomes oncogenically activated as a result of point mutations that interfere with the protein's intrinsic GTPase activity, thereby causing RAS to become constitutively bound to GTP.[1,2] An estimated 30% of all human tumors contain an activating mutation in Ras. The frequency of Ras mutations varies with the tumor type, the highest frequencies being seen in lung, colon, thyroid, and pancreatic carcinomas.[12] This frequency of Ras mutations is likely an underestimation, because chronic upregulation of the Ras pathway can also occur in the absence of mutations in Ras itself. Aberrant signaling pathways that lie downstream of Ras are a recurring theme in the initiation and/or progression of human malignancies.

Several approaches have been taken to identify drugs that inhibit the transforming activity of the RAS protein either directly or indirectly. A promising approach in targeting Ras for cancer treatment involves the use of farnesyl transferase inhibitors (FTIs).[13] FTIs block Ras function by preventing its posttranslational modification by the farnesyl isoprenoid. However, the function of RAS and its downstream kinase cascade is central to many cellular processes. Although current evidence supports the potential use of FTIs in cancer treatment, the ultimate utility of FTIs against human cancers must await evaluation in the clinic.[14] Because Ras protein function is believed to be central to so many cellular processes, blocking its function by FTIs may inhibit all of its functions and thus limit the usefulness of FTIs. Therefore, another approach to targeting Ras protein function involves the development of inhibitors that prevent activated Ras from relaying its downstream signaling by interfering at different points in its signaling cascades. The diversity of Ras target proteins and the necessity for activation of at least two effector pathways for malignant transformation open new directions for the design of additional therapeutic interventions that may negate Ras transformation without abolishing all Ras functions.

AN α-ACTIN PROMOTER-BASED REPORTER GENE ASSAY SYSTEM TO IDENTIFY INHIBITORS OF RAS TRANSFORMATION

We have developed a general approach to identify drugs that can inhibit Ras transformation by acting either directly on Ras or indirectly on other effectors of Ras. The rationale for the development of this assay system was based on observations that human smooth muscle forms of myosin light chain-2 (MLC-2) and α-actin mRNA and protein levels are repressed in RAS-transformed fibroblast cells.[15–17] Revertants of RAS-transformed cells showed normal levels of MLC-2 gene expression, suggesting that the expression of these cytoskeletal markers is modulated by

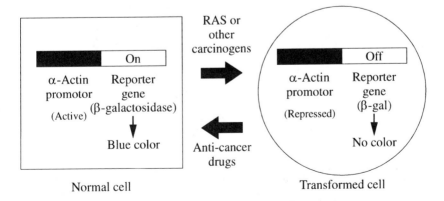

FIGURE 3. Schematic representation of the strategy for setting up a system for screening drugs based on derepression of reporter-gene activity. See text for details.

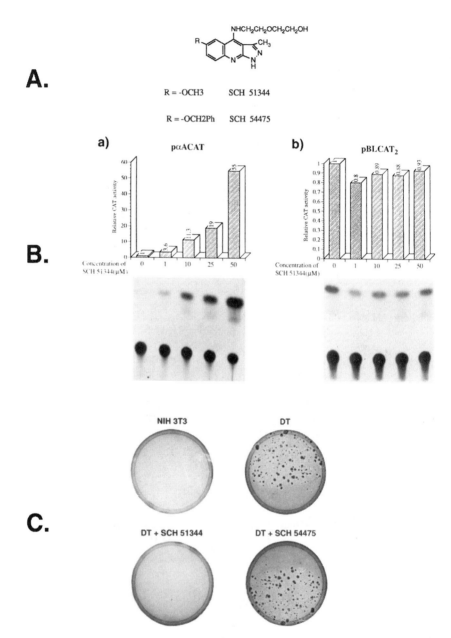

FIGURE 4. (A) Structures of SCH 51344 and SCH 54475, a benzyloxy analog of SCH 51344. (B) Rat-2 (HO6) cells were transfected with 20 μg of pαACAT or 5 μg of pBLCAT2 for 6 hours before washing twice with phosphate-buffered saline and adding fresh medium containing either DMSO or different concentrations of SCH 51344. CAT activities were determined 60 hours later after adjusting for equal amounts of protein. The fold increase in CAT activity compared to control is shown above the bars. (C) Inhibition of the growth of Ras-transformed DT cells in soft-agar by SCH 51344.

RAS transformation. Using plasmids containing 59-upstream sequences of the human smooth muscle α-actin gene fused to different reporter genes, we showed that changes in α-actin mRNA and protein levels are due to changes at the transcriptional level.[16] A schematic illustration of the α-actin promoter-based reporter gene assay system is shown in FIGURE. 3. Initially, stable fibroblast cell lines expressing β-galactosidase (β-gal) under the control of the human α-actin promoter were derived. Transformation of these stable cells by RAS resulted in repressed reporter gene activity. These Ras-transformed cell lines were used to identify agents that can revert Ras transformation by their ability to derepress α-actin promoter driven reporter gene activity.[15] To validate this assay system, revertants of Ras-transformed cells were isolated to demonstrate derepression of reporter gene activity. A major advantage of this system is that cytotoxic agents such as nonspecific inhibitors of DNA, RNA, and protein synthesis will not be scored as false positives, because derepression of reporter gene activity requires the cells to actively synthesize mRNA and protein.

SCH 51344

Using this cell-based reporter gene assay system, we identified a novel class of molecules known as pyrazoloquinolines among the library of compounds at the Schering-Plough Research Institute.[18] A representative compound in this series, SCH 51344 (6-methoxy-4-[2-[(2-hydroxyethoxyl)-ethyl]amino]-3-methyl-1M-pyrazolo [3,4]quinoline) (FIG. 4), was used to (1) evaluate its effectiveness in blocking Ras transformation and (2) determine the mechanism by which these compounds inhibit RAS transformation. The following observations supported the conclusion that SCH 51344 inhibits Ras transformation: (1) treatment of RAS-transformed Rat-2 cells with increasing concentrations of SCH 51344 led to a significant increase (3- to 50-fold) in α-actin promoter-driven CAT activity, whereas it had very little effect on thymidine kinase promoter-driven CAT activity (FIG. 4B); (2) treatment of RAS-transformed cells with SCH 51344 restored organized actin filament bundles; (3) SCH 51344 was effective in inhibiting the anchorage-independent growth of K-RAS transformed NIH 3T3 cells (DT) and human colon and pancreatic tumor-derived cell lines such as Panc-1, SW-480, and DLD-1; and (4) SCH 51344 was also effective in blocking RASV12-induced maturation of *Xenopus* oocytes.[18]

One interesting feature about SCH 51344 is the apparent lack of toxic effect on normal cells. Treatment of PC 12 cells with SCH 51344 for 3 days did not inhibit nerve growth factor-induced neurite outgrowth, suggesting that SCH 51344 has very little effect on normal signaling pathways mediated by RAS. In addition, pretreatment of Rat-2 fibroblast cells with SCH 51344 did not abolish serum-induced activation of *c-fos* promoter activity (unpublished observations), indicating that SCH 51344 selectively suppresses RAS transformation without affecting normal cell functions.

SCH 51344 TREATMENT HAS NO EFFECT ON RAS-INDUCED ERK1/ERK2 AND JNK ACTIVATION

To understand the mechanism by which SCH 51344 inhibits RAS transformation, we tested the compound on various signaling pathways activated by Ras. Treatment of normal fibroblast cells with SCH 51344 did not block the EGF or serum-induced activation of MEK, MAPK, and p90RSK activities.[18,19] Next, we determined if the drug had any effect on activation of ERK or c-Jun kinase (JNK) in response to expression of the three isoforms of oncogenic RAS proteins. Transient expression of the activated forms of H-RAS, K-RAS, and N-RAS in normal fibroblast cells resulted in significant activation of ERK-2 and JNK activity, and treatment with SCH 51344 did not block this stimulation.[19,20] These results suggested that inhibition of RAS-mediated activation of ERK and JNK pathways is not obligatory in blocking the transforming function of RAS and that SCH 51344 acts on a signaling pathway distinct from these signaling pathways.[18]

INHIBITION OF CELL MORPHOLOGY PATHWAY BY SCH 51344

The next logical step was to analyze if SCH 51344 inhibited the cell morphology pathway activated by RAS. In these studies, REF-52 cells were pretreated with diluent or SCH 51344 for 24 hours prior to microinjection with a plasmid encoding T7-tagged H-RAS V12. Induction of membrane ruffling was analyzed by phase contrast microscopy. Pretreatment of the cells with SCH 51344 completely inhibited RAS-induced membrane ruffling (FIG. 4, top panel). Immunofluorescence staining of the injected cells confirmed that drug treatment had no apparent effect on the expression and subcellular distribution of the H-RAS V12 protein.[20] Pretreatment of the cells with 25 mM SCH 51344 for 5 hours prior to microinjection was sufficient to inhibit

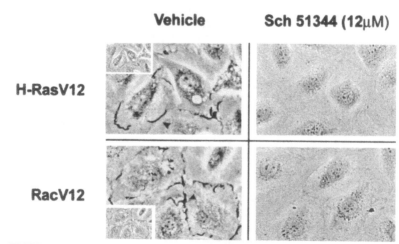

FIGURE 5. Inhibition of H-RASV12– and RACV12–induced membrane ruffling by SCH 51344. REF 52 cells were treated with 12.5 mM SCH 51344 or DMSO (1:2000) for 24 hours prior to microinjection with H-Ras V12 and Rac V12 (50 ng/ml) expression plasmids. Ruffling activity was scored by the appearance of transient phase bands actively traversing the upper surface of the cell. Ruffling images were captured at 32× magnification 4 hours after microinjection. Ruffles were enhanced by the autotrace function of Corel Draw computer software. **Insets** show the unprocessed images. Cells were also fixed and immunostained with anti-T7 antibody (1:300) to monitor the expression of RAS and RACV12 proteins.

the membrane ruffling induced by H-RAS V12. In addition, the inhibitory effect was reversible, because membrane ruffles could readily be seen within 45 minutes of removal of the drug. The rapid reversibility of the inhibitory effects of the drug rules out the possibility that these effects reflect a general toxic effect of the drug. SCH 51344 was effective in inhibiting the membrane ruffling induced by activated forms of H-RAS, K-RAS, and N-RAS. The compound was also effective in blocking Rac-induced membrane ruffling, indicating that the drug interferes with the ability of RAS to induce membrane ruffling at a point downstream from RAC. These results clearly showed that stimulation of the membrane ruffling pathway is critical in the transforming activity of RAS, and SCH 51344 represents a pharmacologic agent that targets this pathway specifically at a point downstream from RAC.

    The pathway by which RAS and RAC stimulate the membrane ruffling pathway is not clearly established. Recently, some RAC1-interacting proteins were isolated using the yeast two-hybrid system.[21,22] POR1 binds directly to RAC1 in a GTP-dependent fashion, and truncated versions of POR1 inhibit the induction of membrane ruffling by an activated mutant of RAC1, suggesting a potential role for POR1 in the RAC-mediated cell morphology pathway. Recent studies showed that Rac activates LIMKinase-1 (LIMK-1), which in turn phosphorylates and inactivates cofilin, an essential protein that is required for turnover of actin filaments.[23-25] It was

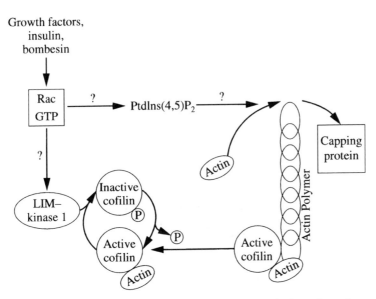

FIGURE 6. Proposed model for Rac-induced changes in actin dynamics to form membrane ruffles. Activation of Rac by either growth factors or RasV12 leads to activation of LIMkinase-1 which in turn phosphorylates cofilin. This may inhibit localized disassembly of actin filaments and release cofilin from the actin monomers. Rac also stimulates the production of phosphatidylinositol-4,5-biphosphate (PIP_2) by PIP_5 kinase, which is believed to cause filament uncapping. Removal of a capping protein from the end of an actin filament could then allow the polymerization of actin to resume. The intermediates that activate LIMK-1 and PIP_5 kinase are unknown.

observed that Rac-dependent formation of lamellipodia is blocked by dominant negative forms of LIMK-1, and dominant negative Rac leads to decreased phoshorylation of cofilin, whereas activated Rac modestly increases phosphorylation.[24,25] The current model for the Rac-induced formation of membrane ruffles is shown in FIGURE 6. Rac activates LIM kinase-1, which in turn phosphorylates cofilin. This may inhibit localized disassembly of actin filaments and help to release cofilin from the actin monomers.[23] To induce the formation of membrane ruffles, Rac must also induce the polymerization of actin. One possible mechanism involves Rac-induced increases in the levels of phosphatidylinositol 4,5-biphosphate (PIP2), which is thought to cause filament uncapping. Removal of the capping protein from the end of an actin filament could then allow the polymerization of actin to resume.[23,26]

Next, we tested the effect of SCH 51344 on RacV12-induced activation of LIMK-1. For these studies, COS-7 cells were transfected with the expression plasmids of LIMK-1 and RacV12 and incubated with SCH 51344 or diluent. Following 30 hours of incubation, LIMK-1 was immunoprecipitated and assayed for kinase activity using His6-cofilin as the substrate. As shown in FIGURE 7, RacV12 expression caused slight but significant (1.6-fold) activation of LIMK-1, and SCH 51344 treatment prevented this activation. The compound did not have any effect on LIMK-1 enzymatic activity *in vitro*, suggesting that SCH 51344 inhibits a downstream effector of Rac, which in turn stimulates LIMK-1 (results not shown). We are currently using radiolabeled compound to identify the target protein that is inhibited by SCH 51344, which may provide a novel, therapeutically useful target for RAS-mediated malignancies.

REFERENCES

1. BARBACID, M. 1990. *Ras* oncogenes: Their role in neoplasia. Eur. J. Clin. Invest. **20:** 225–235.
2. BOS, J.L. 1989. Ras oncogenes in human cancer: A review. Cancer Res. **49:** 4682–4689.
3. McCORMICK, F. 1994. Activators and effectors of ras p21 proteins. Curr. Opin. Genet. Dev. **4:** 71–76.
4. VOJTEK, A.J. & C.J. DER. 1998. Increasing complexity of the Ras signaling pathway. J. Biol. Chem. **273:** 19925–19928.
5. SHARON, L., R. CAMPBELL, K.L. KHOSRAVI-FAR, G.J. ROSSMAN, G.J. CLARK & C.J. DER. 1998. Increasing complexity of Ras signaling. Oncogene **17:** 1395–1413.
6. WHITE, M.A., C. NICOLETTE., A. MINDEN, A. POLVERINI, L. VAN AELST, M. KARIN & M.H. WIGLER. 1995. Multiple *ras* functions can contribute to mammalian cell transformation. Cell **80:** 533–541.
7. JONESON, T., M. WHITE, M. WIGLER & D. BAR-SAGI. 1996. Stimulation of membrane ruffling and MAP kinase activation by distinct effectors of RAS. Science **271:** 810–812.
8. JONESON, T. & D. BAR-SAGI. 1997. Ras effectors and their role in mitogenesis and oncogenesis. J. Mol. Med. **259:** 7–13.
9. EGAN, S.E. & R.A. WEINBERG. 1993. The pathway to signal achievement. Nature **365:** 781–783.
10. SYMONS, M. 1996. Rho family of GTPases: The cytoskeleton and beyond. Trends Biochem. Sci. **21:** 178–181.
11. HALL, A. 1998. Rho GTPases and the actin cytoskeleton. Science **279:** 509–514.
12. CLARK, G.J. & C.J. DER. 1993. GTPases in Biology. :259–288. Springer-Verlag. Berlin.

13. GIBBS, J.B. 1991. Ras C-terminal processing enzymes—new drug targets? Cell **65**: 1–4.

14. KOHL, N.E., F.R. WILSON, S.D. MOSSER, E. GUILIANI, J. DESOLMS, S. DESOLMS, M.W. CONNER, N.J. ANTHONY, W.J. HOLTZ, R.P. GOMEZ, T.J. LEE, R.L. SMITH, S.L. GRAHAM, G.D. HARTMAN, J.B. GIBBS & A. OLIFF. 1994. Protein farnesyl transferase inhibitors block the growth of *ras*-dependent tumors in nude mice. Proc. Natl. Acad. Sci. **USA 91**: 9141–9145.

15. KUMAR, C.C. & C. CHANG. 1992. Human smooth muscle myosin light chain-2 gene expression is repressed in ras transformed fibroblast cells. Cell Growth Differ. **3**: 1–10.

16. Kumar, C.C., P. Bushel., S. Mohan-Peterson & F. Ramirez. 1992. Regulation of smooth muscle α-actin promoter in *ras*-transformed cells: Usefulness for setting up reporter gene based assay system for drug screening, Cancer Res. **52**: 6877–6884.

17. LEAVITT, J., P. GUNNING, L. KEDES & R. JARIWALA. 1985. Smooth muscle α-actin is a sensitive marker for the transformed phenotype. Nature **316**: 840–842.

18. KUMAR, C.C., C. PROROCK-ROGERS, J. KELLY, Z. DONG, J.J. LIN, L ARMSTRONG, H.F. KUNG, M.J. WEBER & A. AFONSO. 1995. SCH 51344 inhibits *ras* transformation by a novel mechanism. Cancer Res. **55**: 5106–5117.

19. KUMAR, C.C. 1998. SCH 51344: An inhibitor of Ras/Rac-mediated membrane ruffling pathway. *In* G Proteins, Cytoskeleton and Cancer. H. Maruta & K. Kohama, Eds.: 303–315. R.G. Landes Company. Georgetown, TX.

20. WALSH, B.A., N. DHANASEKHARAN, D. BAR-SAGI & C.C. KUMAR. 1997. SCH 51344–induced reversal of Ras-transformation is accompanied by the specific inhibition of the Ras and Rac-dependent cell morphology pathway. Oncogene **15**: 2553–2560.

21. VAN AELST, L., T. JONESON & D. BAR-SAGI. 1996. Identification of a novel Rac1-interacting protein involved in membrane ruffling. EMBO J. **15**: 3778–3786.

22. VAN AELST, L. & C. D'SOUZA-SCHOREY. 1997. Rho GTPases and signaling networks. Genes Dev. **11**: 2295–2322.

23. ROSENBLATT, J. & T.J. MITCHISON. 1998. Actin, cofilin and cognititon. Nature **393**: 739–740.

24. ARBER, S., F.A. BARBAYANNIS, H. HANSER, C. SCHNEIDER, C.A. STANYON, O. BERNARD & P. CARON. 1998. Regulation of actin dynamics through phosphorylation of cofilin by LIM-kinase. Nature **393**: 805–809.

25. YANG, N., O. HIGUCHI, K. OHASHI, K. NAGATA, A. WADA, K. KANGAWA, E. NISHIDA & K. MIZUNO. 1998. Cofilin phosphorylation by LIM-kinase 1 and its role in Rac-mediated actin organization. Nature **393**: 809–812.

26. HARTWIG, J. H., G.M. BOKOCH, C.L. CARPENTER, L.A. JANMEY, A. TAYLOR, A. TOKER & T.P. STOSSEL. 1995. Thrombin receptor ligation and activated Rac uncap actin filament barbed ends through phosphoinoside synthesis in permeabilized human platelets. Cell **82**: 643–653.

Activation of Apoptosis and Its Inhibition

DOUGLAS K. MILLER[a]

Department of Immunology and Rheumatology, Merck Research Laboratories, Rahway, New Jersey 07065, USA

ABSTRACT: The induction of apoptosis, or controlled cell death, by various stimuli has been shown to activate a cascade of endoproteases, called caspases, that cleave numerous cellular proteins necessary for cellular homeostasis. This review discusses this family of proteases together with a variety of mammalian and viral regulatory proteins that act to control this activation.

INTRODUCTION

Apoptotic cell death has been characterized by a progressive series of morphologic cellular changes ranging from membrane blebbing and cell shrinkage to nuclear condensation and fragmentation.[1,2] Accompanying biochemical changes include the appearance on cell surfaces of phosphatidyl serine and proteins that induce phagocytosis of the cells,[3,4] proteolytic cleavage of a host of intracellular proteins,[5] and specific DNA cleavage into nucleosomal fragments.[6] Induced by a host of stimuli such as chemotherapeutic agents, radiation, activated oxygen, and growth factor withdrawal, the execution of apoptosis has been associated with members of the caspases, a family of cysteinyl endoproteases that cleave after Asp.[7] These proteases, when activated, cleave a variety of cytoplasmic and nuclear proteins that contribute to the initiation and progression of cell death.

DISCOVERY AND CHARACTERISTICS OF CASPASES

The conceptual framework for the various steps in the apoptotic process and the specific importance of the caspase family were provided by the laboratory of R. Horvitz where they showed in *Candida elegans* that the protein, Ced-3, was essential for the execution of apoptosis[8] (FIG. 1). Ced-3 was identified as a member of what came to be known as the caspase family, and mutations of Ced-3 that prevented its catalytic activity prevented apoptosis.[9]

The first and prototypic member of the caspase family, caspase-1 (FIG. 2), was identified as a cytoplasmic protease that activated the proinflammatory cytokine interleukin-1β and hence was called interleukin-1β converting enzyme (ICE).[10,11] The purified active enzyme was composed of two subunits, p20 and p10, which were both sequentially processed from a precursor domain within an inactive 45 kD pre-

[a]Address all correspondence to: Dr. Douglas K. Miller, Department of Inflammation Research, Merck Research Laboratories, PO Box 2000, R80N-A32, Rahway, New Jersey 07065. Phone, 908/594-6838; fax, 908/594-3111.
e-mail, douglas_miller@merck.com

cursor protein that was preformed and present in relatively large quantities in the cytosol. The active enzyme, however, was a tetramer composed of two p20 and two p10 subunits with two active sites.[12,13] The active enzyme recognized minimally a tetrapeptide with a P_1 Asp, which was buried deep within the p20 subunit of the enzyme. The p20 subunit contained the active site Cys and His necessary for catalytic activity, whereas the p10 subunit contained the residues specifying the P_2-P_4 binding site.[10] The P_4 residue was second in importance only to the P_1 Asp as necessary to the determination of whether a peptide sequence could be recognized.[14,15]

The realization that the proapoptotic Ced-3 was similar to caspase-1 stimulated a search for other mammalian caspase family members. These caspases fall into two broad phylogenetic categories based on their sequence alignment: those that are related to caspase-1 and those that are related to Ced-3 (FIG. 2). Sequence analysis shows that what distinguishes each subfamily is the presence or absence of loop extensions principally beyond the conserved beta sheets or alpha helices found within the core structure. Particularly important is the presence of an extended loop within the p10 subunit of Ced-3 subfamily members that more rigidly surrounds and defines the pocket recognizing the signature P_4 residue.[16] All of those members identified within the Ced-3 subfamily are known to be involved in apoptotic functions, whereas evidence for an apoptotic role for caspase-1 and the other members in that subfamily is less clear. More likely, the members of this subfamily are probably involved in proteolytic activation, such as those previously observed for IL-1β or interleukin-18.[17-20]

The discovery of the various caspase family members has been amply reviewed over the last several years.[21-23] To this list has been added two less well-defined caspases, caspase-13 (ERICE, evolutionarily related interleukin-1β converting enzyme[24]) and recently caspase-14,[25,26] both of which belong to the caspase-1 subfamily.

MECHANISMS OF INDUCTION OF CELL DEATH

In *C. elegans*, while Ced-3 was shown to be essential to produce the cleavages necessary to induce apoptosis, cytoplasmic protein Ced-4 was identified as an adapter protein that activated this protease.[27,28] The mitochondrial protein Ced-9, in turn, controlled the activation of Ced-4,[29,30] whereas the cytoplasmic protein Egl-1[31,32] modulated the activity of Ced-9. As shown in FIGURE 1, these *C. elegans* proteins have been shown to have mammalian counterparts in the most general of the two well recognized induction pathways for apoptosis, the pathway involving stimuli that lead to mitochondrial damage. Mitochondrial permeability is affected by a host of proapoptotic factors including the activation of p53, growth factor withdrawal, irradiation, activated oxygen, and cytotoxic drugs.[33] Like Ced-3, caspase-9 is an essential protease[34] whose activity is modulated by the Ced-4-like adaptor protein Apaf-1 (apoptosis-activating factor 1).[35,36] Apaf-1 is activated by cytochrome c, a mitochondrial protein released during proapoptotic mitochondrial damage.[37] In addition to a cytochrome c-binding WD motif, Apaf-1 contains a nucleotide binding domain and a globular caspase recruitment domain (CARD[38]) that is essential for interaction with a corresponding CARD region in caspase-9 to form a ternary complex.[39,40] The complex of Apaf-1, cytochrome c, and caspase-9 has been termed the

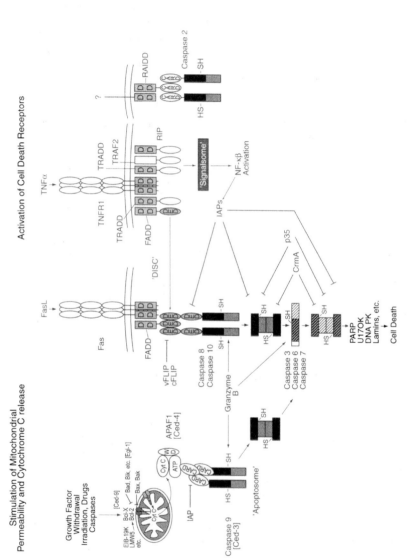

FIGURE 1. See legend on facing page.

"Apoptosome."[41] Members of the Bcl-2 family, including Bcl-x residing in the inner mitochondrial membrane, are highly homologous to Ced-9, and they control mitochondrial function, modulating release of cytochrome c.[42–44] Cytoplasmic proapoptotic Bcl-2 family members such as Bad or Bik, like Egl-1, can inhibit the activity of the antiapoptotic Bcl-2 family members. An added mammalian layer of complexity is provided by membrane-bound proapoptotic Bcl-2 family members such as Bax or Bak.[45]

A parallel pathway of death induction in mammals is the activation of one of at least five different cell death receptors, all members of the TNF receptor superfamily, which are activated by TNF family member ligands.[46] Shown in FIGURE 1 are the two prototypical receptors, Fas and the type I TNF receptor (TNFR1), which are respectively stimulated by the Fas ligand and TNFα. These are trimeric Type I receptors activated by trimeric ligands. In the cytoplasmic domain of all of the death receptors there is an 80 amino acid region, termed the death domain (DD),[47] which is a globular domain that promotes protein complexing between comparable proteins that contain it.[48] When ligated, these death receptors activate two closely related caspases, caspase-8 and caspase-10, via secondary adaptor proteins such as FADD (Fas-associated death domain).[49] FADD contains both a death domain to bind to the receptors as well as a second globular 80 amino acid long protein sequence, termed the death effector domain (DED), which is essential for binding to a similar region in caspase-8 and caspase-10.[50] This receptor, adaptor protein, and caspase complex has been termed the "death-inducing signaling complex" (DISC).[51] A third potential receptor-signaling complex utilizes caspase-2 and the adaptor protein RAIDD. RAIDD contains both a CARD domain that binds to the corresponding CARD domain of caspase-2 as well as a DD that can bind to an as yet unidentified receptor.[52,53] Like caspase-8, caspase-2 is activated very early in the apoptotic cascade.[54]

Like caspase-9 and caspase-2, caspase-8 and caspase-10 are characterized by being caspases that in their inactive precursor state have a large prodomain N-terminal

---

FIGURE 1. Mechanisms of induction of apoptotic cell death. Apoptosis is induced by two generalized pathways by factors inducing mitochondrial permeability and cytochrome c release and by activation of cell death receptors. Mitochondrial permeability is controlled by the Bcl-2 family of channel regulators which are either antiapoptotic (Bcl-2/Bcl-x) or proapoptotic (Bax/Bak) or (Bad/Bik). Released cytochrome c enables the adaptor protein APAF1 to bind and activate caspase-9 (the apoptosome). Active caspase-9 (shown as a caspase tetramer with active site Cys on the longer subunit) activates effector caspase-3, caspase-7, and ultimately caspase-6. These active caspases perform the majority of apoptotic cleavages. Death receptors Fas and TNFR1 activate caspase-8 or caspase-10 via complexing by the adaptor protein FADD (the death-inducing signaling complex, DISC). Active caspase-8/10 can then activate independently the effector caspases or can directly act on mitochondria and Bcl-2 homologs to induce mitochondrial permeability and hence increase caspase-9 activation. An identified receptor activates caspase-2 via its adaptor protein RAIDD. Various viral or cellular inhibitors modulate the activation including the adaptor protein inhibitors of apoptosis (IAP), Flice-like (caspase-8) inhibitor proteins (FLIPs), and Bcl-2 family homologs (E1B-19K and LMW5 proteins). CrmA and p35 are viral proteins that directly inhibit caspase activity. TNFR1 receptor complex utilizes the adaptor proteins TRADD and TRAF2 to activate transcription factor NF-κB. This pathway uses a separate protein complex of kinases and adaptor proteins (the signalsome) and upregulates antiapoptotic inhibitor proteins such as IAPs and Bcl-2 homologs.

to their catalytic p20 and p10 regions. The CARD or DED domain found within this precursor region enables them to be complexed to adaptor proteins for activation. Following that activation, their major role is to initiate a caspase cascade by cleaving a series of secondary effector caspases that contain only a vestigial prodomain devoid of any complex-forming domains. These downstream, or effector, caspases, such as caspase-3, caspase-6, and caspase-7, are the caspases that perform the majority of protein cleavages associated with apoptosis. Hence, in mammals, instead of a single round of caspase activation as is apparently the case in *C. elegans*, the pattern is to have two stages, a first stage of initiator caspases activated by a variety of stimuli and a second stage of executioner caspases activated as a final common pathway. Activation of both caspase stages can be induced by a serine protease, called granzyme B, that is found in the granules of killer T cells and introduced into target cells following their fusion. Granzyme B, like the caspases, cleaves proteins after Asp residues.[55,56]

Activation of TNFR1 and other TNF receptor family members also stimulates NF-κB activation in addition to apoptosis. Mediated by a family of adaptor proteins such as TRAF2 (see ref. 57), an 800-kD complex of kinases and adaptor proteins (termed the "signalsome"[58]) induces the phosphorylation of the IκBα inhibitor of NF-κB (see refs. 59 and 60 for recent reviews). The resultant phosphorylated IκBα is degraded by proteosomes, and the liberated NF–κB translocates to the nucleus where it transcribes a variety of antiapoptotic proteins such as cellular inhibitors of

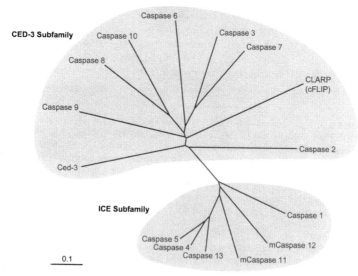

FIGURE 2. Caspase family phylogenetic tree. The sequences of 13 of the known caspase members (all human save for mouse caspase-11 and caspase-12) were aligned and plotted using CLUSTAL W.[284] The genbank references include caspase-1 (M87507), caspase-2 (U25804), caspase-3 (U26943), caspase-4 (U28014), caspase-5 (U28015), caspase-6 (U20536), caspase-7 (U39613), caspase-8 (U58143), caspase-9 (U56390), caspase-10 (U60519), mcaspase-11 (Y13089), mcaspase-12 (Y13090), and caspase-13 (AF078533).

apoptosis proteins (IAps[61]; see below). Inhibition of NF–κB activation produces a corresponding increase in apoptosis, indicating that the balance of cell viability versus cell death is maintained by the degree of NF–κB activation.[61–64]

ACTIVATION OF CASPASES

All caspases are present as precursors that must be cleaved to enable separation of the p20 and p10 catalytic fragments from the adaptor protein CARD or DED domain. The precursors have low intrinsic activity towards peptide substrates and essentially no activity towards their protein substrates.[65,66] Processing of the precursor caspase enables reorganization of the p20 and p10 subunits in the final active quaternary structure and increased enzymatic activity.[12,65] Exactly when and how that reorganization occurs vary from one caspase to another; for caspase-1 and caspase-9 activation, for example, cleavage has to occur first at the p20 C-terminal domain,[65,67] whereas for caspase-8, cleavage has to occur first at the junction of the prodomain and p20 N-terminus.[68,69] Because the sites of cleavage occur after Asp, activation occurs either autocatalytically or in a concerted fashion by other caspases or by the serine protease granzyme B. Hence, mutations of the Asp residues at the sites of cleavage as well as of the active site Cys prevent activation of the caspases.[66,68–70] Chimeric precursor caspases assembled with the p10 subunit prior to that of the p20, mimicking a spatial organization found in the mature active form of the enzyme, are spontaneously activated intramolecularly.[71] This indicates that a major reason for caspase precursor inactivity is a structural one in which the catalytic domains are assembled apart from one another in such a fashion that only cleavage of the precursor enables active enzyme assembly (see also ref. 65).

The CARD, DED, and DD domains found in the activator caspases and their associated adaptor proteins are all globular domains with six internal amphipathic alpha helices that produce charged surface domains.[72] These domains bind to each other by attraction and assembly of corresponding acidic and basic patches such as those found in RAIDD and caspase-2 and in Apaf-1 and caspase-9.[73] For the long precursor domain caspases, the critical process enabling autocatalysis is the assembly of multimeric members of the caspases through complexing of their precursor domains. Removal of that precursor domain prevents both complex formation and subsequent activation, such as that found with caspase-1.[74] The precursor domains themselves, however, are not inhibitory towards caspase activity. This activation complex can be artificially induced by the generation of chimeric caspase molecules in which the precursor domain is replaced by receptors or the FK506 binding protein. The resultant molecules are brought together by complexing the receptors or adding cross-linked FK506.[51,68,69,75] This clustering-induced proximity enables caspase dimers to cleave each other[69,76,77] and then reassemble the p20 and p10 fragments in the active tetramer in such a way that the p20 from one precursor comes together with the p10 subunit from the other precursor.[12]

The short precursor domain caspases (-3, -6, and -7) are not autocatalytically activated unless they are attached in a chimera to a domain that can enable them to form multimers.[78] Instead, these caspases are cleaved by upstream caspases in a cascade fashion. Both caspase-8 and caspase-9 have been shown to cleave all the foregoing three caspases following their autoactivation; cleavage of caspase-3 and caspase-7 occurs first, and then caspase-3 activates caspase-6.[67,79–84] The first cleavage site to enable catalytic activation for all the caspases occurs at the C-terminus of the p20 fragment (FIG. 3), enabling release of the smaller p10 fragment followed by cleavage of the precursor domain region.[21,65,85] For most of the caspases the P_4 residue at this site of cleavage is a hydrophobic residue (FIG. 3), and this reflects the specificity of the activating protease. Substrate specificity of the active long precursor proapoptotic caspases (-2, -8, -9, and -10) that are autocatalytic is homologous to the sequence at their activation site. For the short precursor caspases, the cleavage sequence is a reflection not of their own activity, but rather that of the activating caspase; hence, for caspase-3 the activation sequence is similar to the IETD activity of caspase-8, caspase-9, or caspase-10 rather than that of the DEVD sequence found in caspase-3 itself. Following its initial activation, subsequent cleavages such as that removing the caspase-3 short precursor peptide, are characteristic of caspase-3 activity and are inhibited by a caspase-3 inhibitor DEVD-aldehyde, but not an IETD-aldehyde which inhibits the upstream caspases.[85]

Because of the sequence similarity at the site of activation of the caspases, granzyme B with its IEPD activity[86,87] was found to process essentially all of the caspases (see ref. 21), particularly caspase-3, caspase-7, and caspase-10.[56,88,89] This enables granzyme B to efficiently activate both activator and effector caspases. Furthermore, granzyme B separately cleaves such caspase-sensitive targets as DNA-protein kinase and NuMA as well as other unique proteins not normally cleaved by caspases.[90] That the primary effects of granzyme B work through caspase activation and subsequent activity has been confirmed where a pancaspase inhibitor, z-VAD-fmk, blocks granzyme B-induced apoptosis.[91]

SUBSTRATES OF CASPASES

Many proteins have been found to be cleaved by caspases following apoptotic signaling, and cleavage of these substrates resulting in functionally active or inactive proteins provides the biochemical basis behind the phenotypic effects seen with apoptosis. Those targets include proteins associated with normal nuclear repair and homeostasis, structural proteins for cytoplasmic and nuclear membranes, and a variety of signaling proteins—kinases, transcription factors, and cytoplasmic proteins involved in a variety of cellular functions. Those proteins for which the site of cleavage is known are listed in TABLE 1, and those cleavage sites reflect the substrate specificities of the caspase activities (FIG. 3). The catalytic activities of those caspases that have been studied in detail tend to fall into three distinct groups based on careful examination of the substrate specificity of the active members using a combinatorial peptide substrate library[15,92]: caspase-1, caspase-4, and caspase-5 prefer a large aromatic or hydrophobic group such as Trp; caspase-6, caspase-8, caspase-9, and caspase-10 prefer an aliphatic hydrophobic group such as Leu or Val; wheras caspase-2, caspase-3, and caspase-7 prefer an Asp (FIG. 3). The largest number of substrates are those that contain an Asp in the P_4 position (TABLE 1), and these are cleaved principally by caspase-3 and caspase-7. For example, cleavage of the nuclear repair enzyme polyADP ribose polymerase (PARP) by caspase-3 is one of the ear-

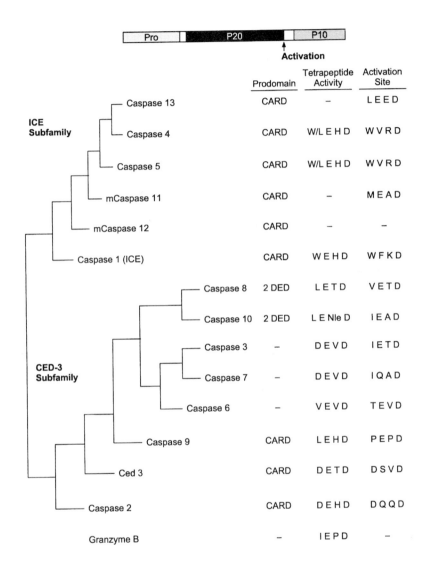

FIGURE 3. Caspase family structure, activation sites, and tetrapeptide substrate activity. Caspases are found as inactive precursor molecules that contain an N-terminal prodomain of different length together with two other fragments, a ~20 kD-sized fragment that contains the catalytic Cys and His, and a ~10 kD-sized fragment that determines the P_4 specificity of the enzyme. The prodomain is either extremely short (caspases-3, -7, and -6) or contains either a single CARD or two DED domains that complex with adaptor proteins. Activation occurs by cleavage after an Asp residue at the C-terminus of the p20 fragment through either autocatalytic or upstream initiator caspase activity. The optimum activities of the caspases and of granzyme B were determined with peptide combinatorial libraries (see refs. 15 and 21–23 for details).

TABLE 1. Targets of apoptotic caspases[a]

Group	Enzyme	Cleavage Site	References
Nuclear repair/ nucleic acid cleavage	PARP	DEVD-G	93
	DNA-PK$_{cs}$	DEVD-N	250
	U1-70 kDa	DGPD-G	250
	hnRNA C	DXXD-X	251
	DSEB/RF-C140	DEVD-G, DLVD-S	252,253
	DFF45/ICAD	DETD-S, DAVD-T	96
	Topoisomerase I	DDVD-Y	254
Structural proteins	NuMA	DSLD-L	255,256
	α-Fodrin	DSLD-S	103
	gelsolin	DQTD-G	257
	G-Actin	ELPD-G	258
	Lamin B1	VEID-N	100
	Gas 2	SRVD-G	259
Signaling proteins	PKCδ	DMQD-N	260,261
	PKCθ	DEVD-K	262
	FAK	DQTD-X, VSWD-X	101
	PAK2	DEVD-G	263
	PRK2	DITD-C	264
	MEKK1	DTVD-G	265
	Mst1	DEMD-S	266,267
	Mst2	DELD-S	267
	P21$^{cip1/Waf1}$	DHVD-L	268,269
	P27^{Kip1}	DPSD-S	268
	RasGAP	DTVD-G	270
	SREBP1/2	DEPD-S	271
	MDM2	DVPD-G	272
	P50 (NF-κB)	DVSD-S	273
	Rb	DEAD-G	274
	D4-GDP dis factor	DELD-S	275
	p35	DQMD-G	186
	PP2A	DEQD-S	276
	cPLA$_2$	DELD-S	277
	Nedd4	DQPD-X	278
	Huntingtin	DSLD-X	279
	Presenilin-1	AQRD-S	280
	HPAK65	SHVD-G	281
	PITSLRE kinase	YVPD-S	282
	BID	LQTD-G	104,105
	Stat1	MELD-G	283

[a]Tetrapeptide recognition sites for caspase cleavage of the indicated substrates are indicated.

liest and most sensitive indicators of apoptosis.[93–95] Likewise, the distinctive nuclear changes associated with caspase activation include the cleavage by caspase-3 at the inhibitor of the caspase-activated deoxynuclease (ICAD), also called DNA fragmentation factor 45 (DFF45). Inactivation of this inhibitor frees a cytosolic apoptosis-specific nuclease to cleave DNA into the nucleosome-sized fragments characteristic of apoptosis.[6,96–98] Many of the substrates cleaved by these two closely related caspases can be cleaved by either one; for example, in the genetic absence of caspase-3, caspase-7 activity can cleave PARP, Rb, PAK2, DNA-PK$_{cs}$, and gelsolin.[99] Caspase-6 activity was first associated with the cleavage of lamins, the meshwork of intermediate filaments at the nuclear envelope.[100] Many substrates are cleaved by combinations of caspases, such as the nuclear mitotic apparatus protein NuMA and the focal adhesion kinase, which are cleaved both by caspase-3 and by caspase-7.[84,101] In addition, there are proteins such as fodrin, the cytoskeletal protein found in plasma membranes, that are cleaved by multiple caspases as well as other proteases such as calpain that are activated during apoptosis.[102,103] Although most cleavages occur by the downstream effector caspases, less frequent are cleavages of substrates by activator caspases, such as the activation of the proapoptotic protein BID by caspase-8 itself (see below).[104,105]

INHIBITORS OF CASPASES

Following the original observations for the recognition of substrates YVAD for caspase-1[10] and DEVD for caspase-3,[94] the corresponding aldehydes were utilized as potent, reversible caspase inhibitors (see refs. 106 and 107). The peptide aldehydes, synthesized with P$_4$ residues specific for their various caspase subclasses, show nanomolar potency against the activated form of the enzyme.[108,109] These inhibitors are much less effective in cells, reflecting their respective difficulties in cell permeability, but this has been overcome by the use of the cell-permeable inhibitor benzyloxycarbonyl-V-A-D(OMe)-fluoromethylketone (zVAD-fmk).[95,110] Because zVAD-fmk is a pancaspase inhibitor and is readily penetrant into cells,[108] inhibition of apoptosis was more extensive than with DEVD or YVAD inhibitors.[111–113] Use of zVAD-fmk has prevented cell death associated with ischemic/reperfusion injury in brain and in the heart[114-118] and to protect against hepatic toxicity.[119] Mitochondrially damaged cells can recover if proteases are inhibited even though cytochrome c has been released. On a cellular level, growth factor-deprived neurons could restore their mitochondrial cytochrome c and functioning if incubated with an Asp-specific irreversible inhibitor.[120] The specificity of these agents extends beyond that of caspases, however, and they can inhibit cellular cathepsins as well.[121] Inhibition of caspase activity by these agents, however, does not totally ensure cell survival; in many cases in which apoptosis is stimulated, cell death can still occur by apoptosis or necrosis even though caspase activity is inhibited.[91,122–124] Cell death probably ensues because of caspase-independent mitochondrial damage.[125]

CASPASE KNOCKOUTS

The importance of caspases and their relative pathways of activation of apoptosis is demonstrated by the phenotypes of the knockouts that have been developed.

Caspase-3 knockouts indicated embryonic and neonatal death had occurred with neurologic abnormalities producing ectopic masses of supernumerary neuronal and glial cells.[126] Whereas there was embryonic stem cell resistance to UV irradiation, there was normal but reduced thymocyte apoptosis by Fas, γ-irradiation, staurosporine, and normal activation of other caspases.[127] While cleavage of PARP occurred normally, indicating the redundancy of active caspases, there was incomplete chromatin condensation and DNA degradation. This was reflective of the necessity for caspase-3–dependent cleavage of the DFF45 DNAse inhibitor; without that cleavage, there was no activation of the apoptotic nuclease (see ref. 96).[127] Furthermore, membrane blebbing was absent in apoptotic hepatocytes of caspase-3–deficient mice because of an inability to cleave the cytoskeletal protein fodrin.[128] Likewise in MCF-7 cells that are normally caspase-3 deficient, apoptosis proceeded without DNA fragmentation and surface blebbing.[129] A separate knockout of the DFF45 protein itself removed the apoptotic nuclease DFF40/CAD from cells and prevented the DNA fragmentation and chromatin condensation associated with apoptotic stimuli, but this had no effect on the activation of caspase-3 or on the resultant apoptotic cell death.[130]

Caspase-9 knockouts are also associated with embryonic lethality and defective brain development with structural perturbations in the cortex and forebrain. Apoptosis in thymocytes stimulated by irradiation and chemotherapeutic drugs was reduced despite a normal release of cytochrome c from the mitochondria. In these caspase-9–deficient cells there was a blockade of caspase-3 activity, and PARP cleavage and DNA fragmentation were inhibited, indicating that caspase-9 was necessary to activate effector caspase activity following these stimuli. By contrast, Fas- and TNFR1-induced activation of caspase-8 and subsequent apoptosis proceeded normally.[34,131] Similar results were found with knockouts of the Apaf-1 protein that activates caspase-9. The mice suffered from embryonical lethality and were found with craniofacial defects and severe hyperproliferation of neural cells as well as retention of interdigital webs. Although cytochrome c release from mitochondria was unaffected in cells from these knockout mice, caspase-3 activation stimulated by a variety of drugs and radiation was inhibited, whereas Fas-induced apoptosis was relatively unaffected.[132,133] In this same pathway, deletion of the mitochondrial protective protein Bcl-X was embryonically lethal and led to extensive cell death of neurons and hematopoietic cells.[134] Similarly, knockouts of the Bcl-2 protein showed early death and renal and melanocyte apoptosis and later lymphocyte death.[135]

Fibroblasts from mice in which caspase-8 was knocked out showed the reciprocal pattern; apoptosis induced by Fas, TNFR1, and death receptor 3 (DR3), but not DR4, was prevented, whereas apoptosis induced by irradiation and drug-induced apoptosis proceeded normally. In these cells there was normal Fas stimulation of JNK (activated by a separate adaptor protein termed Daxx[136]) and normal TNFR1 stimulation of IκBα phosphorylation. Because caspase-8 deletion was embryonically lethal, however, producing impaired heart muscle development and abdominal erythrocyte accumulation (unlike Fas or TNFR1 knockouts), caspase-8 was probably necessary for signaling of a separate unidentified receptor.[137] This latter belief is supported by the observation that knockouts of FADD, the caspase-8 activator within this pathway, showed the same embryonic lethality of cardiac failure and abdominal hemorrhage and the same deficiency in Fas, TNFR1, and DR3, but not DR4 signaling.[138,139]

Study of a FADD-dominant negative transgenic similarly showed the inhibition of Fas-induced apoptosis, but not apoptosis by agents affecting mitochondrial potential. FADD was also shown to be involved in a separate pathway involved in T-cell activation, a pathway not inhibited by CrmA.[140]

A caspase-2 knockout was not embryonically lethal and showed a less dramatic antiapoptotic phenotype, but it did show an excess of germ cells and a reduced apoptosis of oocytes exposed to drugs.[141] Caspase-1 and caspase-11 knockouts, however, showed reductions in interleukin (IL)-1β and IL-18 but only marginal effects on Fas-induced apoptosis and none on other stimulators of apoptosis.[17,18,20,128] These results are consistent with an apoptotic role of only those caspases in the Ced-3 subfamily (FIG. 2), whereas members of the caspase-1 subfamily are probably involved largely in activation of cytoplasmic proteins.

VIRAL AND MAMMALIAN ANTIAPOPTOTIC PROTEINS

One way of determining what proteins or processes are really important in the apoptotic cascade is to look at those steps targeted for inhibition by tumorigenic DNA viruses. Whereas stimulation of cellular DNA replication by the viruses aids viral replication, it also induces activation of tumor suppressor protein p53 which induces apoptosis probably through mitochondrial influences and the activation of caspase-9.[142] Viral antiapoptotic targets range throughout the signaling pathway depicted in FIG. 1 (reviewed in refs. 143 and 144). TNF receptor activation is targeted by poxviruses by production of their soluble TNF Type II receptors (cell response modifier B, CrmB[145]) or by production of a different soluble TNF family member CrmC,[146] both of which act to reduce the ligand inducing apoptosis. An alternative approach is taken by adenoviruses in which expression of the E3/10.4K-14.5K viral proteins induces the proapoptotic receptor Fas to be internalized and degraded.[147–149] In herpesviruses the latent membrane protein 1 (LMP1) or herpesvirus entry mediator HVEM functions like a TNF receptor that activates NF–κB and in so doing upregulates cellular antiapoptotic proteins such as Bcl-2 and the aPS (see below).[150–154] Because of its importance, cellular protein p53 is targeted directly by viruses in various ways. Adenoviruses produce the protein E4orf6 which blocks p53 accumulation and the E1B 55K protein which directly binds to p53 and inactivates it,[155,156] whereas papillomavirus E6 targets p53 for ubiquitination and proteosomal degradation.[157]

Activation of caspases is targeted by a variety of viral proteins. Both herpesviruses and pox viruses encode proteins containing DED protein domains that prevent the binding of caspase-8 to the TNFR1, and the related TNF family death receptors DR3 and DR4.[158,159] These viral proteins and their mammalian counterparts, termed FLIPs (Flice [caspase-8] inhibitor proteins), prevent apoptosis induced only by death receptors and not by alternatively activated mechanisms such as those induced by granzyme B or by chemotherapeutic drugs and irradiation, which are both activated by a caspase-9–dependent mechanism.[160,161] Cell FLIPs discovered in a number of laboratories resemble viral proteins in that they are homologs of caspase-8 that contain DEDs and an inactive caspase domain.[162] A different class of death receptor interacting protein is provided by the adenoviral E3-10.4K/14.5K proteins which interact   both   with   the   Fas   receptor   causing   its   internalization   and downmodulation[149] and with the TNFR1 inhibiting its signal transduction.[163] A separate adenoviral apoptosis inhibitor is the E3-14.7K protein which interacts with cellular proteins associated with Fas and TNFR1 signaling and caspase activation. These proteins include a GTP-binding protein[164,165] as well as two leucine zipper proteins (FIP2 and FIP3) that interact with each other and with the TNF receptor-induced signaling pathway.[166,167] The latter protein is identical with NEMO, the NF–κB essential modulator, a protein necessary for assembly of an activated signalsome kinase complex.[168] The E3-14.7K protein likely is partly antiapoptotic because it indirectly stimulates NF–κB activation and the resultant production of antiapoptotic proteins.

A different class of viral proteins inhibiting caspase activation are the inhibitors of apoptosis proteins (IAPs) originally identified in baculovirus where they prevented insect cell death (see refs. 169 and 170 for a review). Distinguished by having a series of 70 amino acid repeating regions, the baculoviral IAP repeats (BIR), the viral IAP proteins have been found to prevent activation of caspases in their native insect cell hosts.[171] Similar proteins have also been found to be produced endogenously in host cells. The role of native insect cellular IAPs appears also to be directed to the inhibition of activation of caspases.[172,173] Likewise, in mammalian cells, the endogenous IAPs have been found to be associated with the activated TNF receptors[174] where they block the activation of caspase-8, an association and activity that is upregulated by NF–κB activation.[175,176] They also act downstream of mitochondrial release of cytochrome to prevent activation of caspase-9.[177,178] Although the IAP proteins generally have less ability to block apoptosis by preactivated caspases, one member, XIAP, has been shown to block caspase-3 and caspase-7 activity directly via binding to one of its BIR regions.[179,180] The genetic inactivation of a neurally associated IAP member NIAP has been associated with increased spontaneous neural degeneration.[181] A novel IAP-containing protein termed survivin has been identified as prominently expressed in the cytoplasm of a variety of tumor and embryonic cells but not in normal terminally differentiated cells.[182] Survivin is expressed in the G2/M phase of the cell cycle where it binds to microtubules in the mitotic spindle and somehow inhibits the activation of caspase-3 and resultant apoptosis[183] Like other IAPs, survivin has been shown to directly inhibit caspase-3 and caspase-7.[184]

A third class of viral antiapoptotic proteins acting downstream from the IAPs are those proteins that are direct inhibitors of caspase activity. These include the baculoviral inhibitor p35, a potent inhibitor of activated caspases that acts as a pseudosubstrate for caspase activity.[185–188] p35 is a cytosolic, slow-binding, nanomolar inhibitor of a wide range of caspases including -1, -3, -6, -7, -8, and -10, but has little activity on a diverse selection of noncaspase proteases.[189] Because of its generality in caspase inhibition, prevention of apoptosis induced by p35 expression is used to denote causation by activated caspases in the cells. Transgenic mice expressing the p35 protein show an increased resistance to thymocyte apoptosis induced by a variety of stimuli, and this correlated with caspase inhibition in the cells.[190]

Structurally different from p35 but functionally similar are a number of viral inhibitors of caspases that are members of the serpin class of protease inhibitors (see ref. 191 for review). The pox virus early gene product CrmA (cytokine response modifier) was originally identified as a potent inhibitor of IL-1β production by its inhibition of caspase-1.[192] Like p35 CrmA also serves as a caspase-1 pseudosubstrate.[193] The CrmA-related viral proteins SPI-2 and Serp2 were observed to reduce the apoptosis observed in virally infected cells,[194–196] indicating that during viral infection they normally inhibit a variety of caspases associated with apoptosis in addition to caspase-1. Careful analysis of the caspase inhibition by CrmA indicated that in addition to the caspase-1 subfamily, a number of the apoptotic activating caspases (-8, -9, and -10) were potently inhibited.[108] Inhibition at this level would hence prevent initiation of the apoptotic cascade. Unlike p35, however, CrmA is more restrictive in its caspase inhibition; for example, caspase-3, caspase-6, and caspase-7 are much more weakly inhibited by CrmA.[94,108,197] While granzyme B is also inhibited by CrmA,[198] a separate caspase-insensitive serpin proteinase inhibitor, PI-9, is found in cytotoxic lymphocytes and protects them against apoptosis induced by their own granzyme B.[199] A new antiapoptotic protein hepatitis B virus HBx protein has also been shown to potently inhibit caspase-3 activity in an unknown indirect fashion.[200]

MITOCHONDRIA AND APOPTOSIS CONTROL

As has been extensively reviewed,[45,201,202] Bcl-2 and its homologs such as Bcl-x are localized to the outer mitochondrial membrane. They share an overall structural similarity to the DD, DED, and CARD domains with their six-helix bundle conformations. Within the Bcl-2/x structure there is a membrane-spanning region as well as four homologous regions, three of which (Bcl-2 homology region 1, BH2, and BH3) form a large amphipathic groove on the protein surface.[203] In the mitochondrial membrane they function as dimers structurally homologous to ion channel regulators such as diptheria toxin.[204–206] Their major role is to prevent mitochondrial dysfunction by (1) stimulation of ADP/ATP exchange, (2) stabilization of the mitochondrial inner transmembrane potential, preventing mitochondrial hyperpolarization and the resultant reactive oxygen formation, and (3) prevention of the opening of a permeability transition pore (megachannel). The increased mitochondrial permeability ultimately leads to the loss of cytochrome c and a mitochondrial flavoprotein AIF, the release of which subsequently activates Apaf-1 and caspase-9.[207–213] The largest family of viral inhibitors of apoptosis mimics the crucial role played by Bcl-2 family members. These viral inhibitors share homologous regions found in the structure of Bcl-2 and include such proteins as herpesvirus proteins BHRF1[214,215] and HVS,[216] LMW5,[217] and the more distantly related adenoviral E1B-19K protein.[218,219]

A separate proapoptotic cytoplasmic Bcl-2 subfamily includes such members as Bax[220] and Bak.[221,222] These have similar overall structure and translocate to the mitochondria after activation where they form their own homodimers and directly bind to and disrupt the permeability transition pore complex.[223–226] Alternatively, they can form heterodimers with antiapoptotic Bcl-2/x,[227] thus increasing mitochondrial permeability by blocking the antiapoptotic effect of Bcl-2/x. A separate diverse third Bcl-2 subfamily consists of cytoplasmic proteins such as Bik[228,229] or Bad[230,231] that contain only a BH3 region that is homologous in sequence.[45] Members of this group have been found to exert their proapoptotic effects by insertion of their BH3 domain into the corresponding amphipathic groove of the Bcl-2/x, thus inactivating the latter proteins.[232–234] E1B-19K interacts with and blocks apoptosis induced by both the BH1-3–containing Bax and Bak proteins as well as the BH3-containing Bik.[235]

The activity of these proapoptotic Bcl-2 family members is exemplified by the BH3-containing protein BID which was recently characterized in detail.[104,105,236–240] Following stimulation by the TNFR1 death receptor, activated caspase-8 cleaves off the N-terminus of the BID precursor, which has been maintained as inactive and cytoplasmic because its N-terminal domain normally binds into the Bcl-2–like core of the remainder of the protein and masks its potential activity.[241,242] Following its cleavage, BID can insert into mitochondria and induce channel formation directly by homodimerization or indirectly by heterodimerization via binding of its BH3 domain to Bcl-2/x. Thus, despite the lack of overall sequence homology to Bcl-2/x and Bak, members of this third Bcl-x family share the same overall structure and ability to directly form ion channels in the target mitochondria, inducing mitochondrial permeability. The damaged mitochondria release cytochrome c, AIF, caspase-2, and caspase-9[212] (and perhaps caspase-3[243]), which then are activated by Apaf-1. Bcl-2/x may also separately control Apaf-1 activation independently of their mitochondrial effects, because they can bind directly to Apaf-1 via their BH4 regions and control caspase-9 activation.[40,44]

Thus, the activation of effector caspases and the resultant apoptosis are amplified by stimulation of two caspase-activating pathways working together, one of which is Bcl-2/x dependent (caspase-9 and caspase-2) and one that can operate independently of Bcl-2 (caspase-8; see also refs. 82 and 244–246). The relative importance of each of these pathways to apoptosis varies within cells; for example, two related cell types have been identified in which Fas-induced apoptosis works either through caspase-8 activating caspase-3 directly in one cell type or only indirectly by its effects on mitochondria and activation via caspase-9 in the other cell type.[247] This caspase-induced self-amplifying feedback loop leading to apoptosis is also enhanced by direct caspase conversion of antiapoptotic Bcl-2 to a proapoptotic form[248] as well as disruptive effects on mitochondrial permeability.[249]

SUMMARY

It has become apparent over the last several years that the control of apoptosis is mediated by a series of large multiprotein complexes that are activated within the cell. These range from the DISC found at the cell surface where proapoptotic death receptors and adaptor proteins activate caspase-8 and caspase-10 to the apoptosome where Apaf-1, cytochrome c, and perhaps various Bcl-2 family members directly control the activation of caspase-9. The key control point that influences both caspase activation pathways is the mitochondrion, where a variety of pro- and antiapoptotic Bcl-2 family members fine-tune the integrity of the mitochondrial transmembrane potential and permeability barrier. These proteins themselves are regulated in part by influences subsequent to yet another cytoplasmic multiprotein complex, the signalsome, which contains a complex of kinases, adaptor proteins, and ubiquitin-activation components in addition to the NF–κB transcription factor and its inhibitory protein IκBα. The production of Bcl-2, IAPs, antioxidant proteins, and other largely unknown antiapoptotic proteins influences the efficiency of the mitochondrion and modulates the activation of the DISC and apoptosome. The details of that signaling interchange will provide increasing insight into that activation and will provide multiple targets for manipulation by pharmaceuticals.

REFERENCES

1. KERR, J.F.R., A.H. WYLLIE & A.R. CURRIE. 1972. Br. J. Cancer **26:** 239-257.
2. WYLLIE, A.H. 1997. Br. Med. Bull. **53:** 451–465.
3. SAVILL, J. 1997. Br. Med. Bull. **53:** 491–508.
4. FADOK, V.A., D.L. BRATTON, S.C. FRASCH, M.L. WARNER & P.M. HENSON. 1998. Cell Death Differ. **5:** 551–562.
5. STROH, C. & K. SCHULZE-OSTHOFF. 1998. Cell Death Differ. **5:** 997–1000.
6. ENARI, M., H. SAKAHIRA, H. YOKOYAMA, K. OKAWA, A. IWAMATSU & S. NAGATA. 1998. Nature **391:** 43–50.
7. ALNEMRI, E.S., D.J. LIVINGSTON, D.W. NICHOLSON, G. SALVESEN, N.A. THORNBERRY, W.W. WONG & J. YUAN. 1996. Cell **87:** 171.
8. YUAN, J. & H.R. HORVITZ. 1990. Dev. Biol. **138:** 33–41.
9. YUAN, J., S. SHAHAM, S. LEDOUX, H.M. ELLIS & H.R. HORVITZ. 1993. CELL **75:** 641–652.
10. THORNBERRY, N.A., H.G. BULL, J.R. CALAYCAY, K.T. CHAPMAN, A.D. HOWARD, M.J. KOSTURA, D.K. MILLER, S.M. MOLINEAUX, J.R. WEIDNER, J. AUNINS, K.O. ELLISTON, J.A. AYALA, R.J. CASANO, J. CHIN, G.J.-F. DING, L.A. EGGER, E.P. GAFFNEY, G. LIM-JUCO, O.C. PALYHA, S.M. RAJU, A.M. ROLANDO, J.P. SALLEY, T.T. YAMIN, T.D. LEE, J.E. SHIVELY, M. MACCOSS, R.A. MUMFORD, J.A. SCHMIDT & M.J. TOCCI. 1992. Nature **356:** 768–774.
11. CERRETTI, D.P., C.J. KOZLOSKY, B. MOSLEY, N. NELSON, K. VAN NESS, T.A. GREEN-STREET, C.J. MARCH, S.R. KRONHEIM, T. DRUCK, L.A. CANNIZZARO, K. HUEBNER & R.A. BLACK. 1992. Science **256:** 97–100.
12. WILSON, K.P., J.F. BLACK, J.A. THOMSON, E.E. KIM, J.P. GRIFFITH, M.A. NAVIA, M.A. MURCKO, S.P. CHAMBERS, R.A. ALDAPE, S.A. RAYBUCK & D.J. LIVINGSTON. 1994. Nature **370:** 270–275.
13. WALKER, N.P.C., R.V. TALANIAN, K.D. BRADY, L.C. DANG, N.J. BUMP, C.R. FERENZ, S. FRANKLIN, T. GHAYUR, M.C. HACKETT, L.D. HAMMILL, L. HERZOG, M. HUGUNIN, W. HOUY, J.A. MANKOVICH, L. MCGUINESS, E. ORLEWICA, M. PASKIND, C.A. PRATT, P. REIS, A. SUMMANI, M. TERRANOVA, J.P. WELCH, L. XIONG, A. MOLLER, D.E. TRACEY, R. KAMEN & W.W. WONG. 1994. Cell **78:** 343–352.
14. MILLER, D.K., J. MYERSON & J.W. BECKER. 1997. J. Cell Biochem. **64:** 2–10.
15. THORNBERRY, N.A., T.A. RANO, E.P. PETERSON, D.M. RASPER, T. TIMKEY, M. GARCIA-CALVO, V. M. HOUTZAGER, P. A. NORDSTROM, S. ROY, J. P. VAILLANCOURT, K.T. CHAPMAN & D. . NICHOLSON. 1997. J. Biol. Chem. **272:** 17907–17911.
16. ROTONDA, J., D.W. NICHOLSON, K.M. FAZIL, M. GALLANT, Y. GAREAU, M. LABELLE, E.P. PETERSON, D.M. RASPER, R. RUEL, J.P. VAILLANCOURT, N.A. THORNBERRY & J.W. BECKER. 1996. Nature Struct. Biol. **3:** 619–625.
17. KUIDA, K., J.A. LIPPKE, G. KU, M.W. HARDING, D.J. LIVINGSTON, M.S.-S. SU & R.A. FLAVELL. 1995. Science **267:** 2000–2003.
18. LI, P., H. ALLEN, S. BANERJEE, S. FRANKLIN, L. HERZOG, C. JOHNSTON, J. MCDOWELL, M. PASKIND, L. RODMAN, J. SALFELD, E. TOWNE, D. TRACEY, S. WARDWELL, F.-Y. WEI, W. WONG, R. KAMEN & T. SESHADRI. 1995. Cell **80:** 401–411.
19. GHAYUR, T., S. BANERJEE, M. HUGUNIN, D. BUTLER, L. HERZOG, A. CARTER, L. QUIN-TAL, L. SEKUT, R. TALANIAN, M. PASKIND, W. WONG, R. KAMEN, D. TRACEY & H. ALLEN. 1997. Nature **386:** 619–623.

20. WANG, S., M. MIURA, Y.K. JUNG, H. ZHU, E. LI & J. YUAN. 1998. Cell **92:** 501–509.
21. MILLER, D.K. 1997. Semin. Immunol. **9:** 35–49.
22. COHEN, G.M. 1997. Biochem. J. **326:** 1–16.
23. THORNBERRY, N.A. & Y. LAZEBNIK. 1998. Science **281:** 1312–1316.
24. HUMKE, E.W., J. NI & V.M. DIXIT. 1998. J. Biol. Chem. **273:** 15702–15707.
25. HU, S., S.J. SNIPAS, C. VINCENZ, G. SALVESEN & V.M. DIXIT. 1998. J. Biol. Chem. **273:** 29648–29653.
26. AHMAD, M., S.M. SRINIVASULA, R. HEGDE, R. MUKATTASH, T. FERNANDES-ALNEMRI & E.S. ALNEMRI. 1998. Cancer Res. **58:** 5201–5205.
27. ELLIS, R.E., J. YUAN & H.R. HORVITZ. 1991. Annu. Rev. Cell Biol. **7:** 663–698.
28. YANG, X., H.Y. CHANG & D. BALTIMORE. 1998. Science **281:** 1355–1357.
29. HENGARTNER, M.O., R.E. ELLIS & H.R. HORVITZ. 1992. Nature **356:** 494–499.
30. SESHAGIRI, S., W.T. CHANG & L.K. MILLER. 1998. FEBS Lett. **428:** 714.
31. CONRADT, B. & H.R. HORVITZ. 1998. Cell **93:** 519–529.
32. DEL PESO, L., V.M. GONZALEZ & G. NUNEZ. 1998. J. Biol. Chem. **273:** 33495–33500.
33. REED, J.C. 1997. Cell **91:** 559–562.
34. KUIDA, K., T.F. HAYDAR, C.Y. KUAN, Y. GU, C. TAYA, H. KARASUYAMA, M.S. SU, P. RAKIC & R.A. FLAVELL. 1998. Cell **94:** 325–337.
35. ZOU, H., W.J. HENZEL, X. LIU, A. LUTSCHG & X. WANG. 1997. Cell **90:** 405–413.
36. LI, P., D. NIJHAWAN, I. BUDIHARDJO, S.M. SRINIVASULA, M. AHMAD, E.S. ALNEMRI & X. WANG. 1997. Cell **91:** 479.
37. LIU, X., C.N. KIM, J. YANG, R. JEMMERSON & X. WANG. 1996. Cell **86:** 147–57.
38. HOFMANN, K., P. BUCHER & J. TSCHOPP. 1997. Trends Biochem. Sci. **22:** 155–156.
39. HU, Y., L. DING, D.M. SPENCER & G. NUNEZ. 1998. J. Biol. Chem. **273:** 33489–33494.
40. PAN, G., K. O'ROURKE & V.M. DIXIT. 1998. J. Biol. Chem. **273:** 5841–5945.
41. GREEN, D. & G. KROEMER. 1998. Trends Cell Biol. **8:** 267–271.
42. YANG, J., X. LIU, K. BHALLA, C.N. KIM, A.M. IBRADO, J. CAI, T.I. PENG, D.P. JONES & X. WANG. 1997. Science **275:** 1129–1132.
43. KLUCK, R.M., E. BOSSY-WETZEL, D.R. GREEN & D.D. NEWMEYER. 1997. Science **275:** 1132–1136.
44. HU, Y., M.A. BENEDICT, D. WU, N. INOHARA & G. NUNEZ. 1998. Proc. Natl. Acad. Sci. USA **95:** 4386–4391.
45. ADAMS, J.M. & S. CORY. 1998. Science **281:** 1322–1326.
46. ASHKENAZI, A. & V.M. DIXIT. 1998. Science **281:** 1305–1308.
47. TARTAGLIA, L.A., T.M. AYRES, G.H.W. WONG & D.V. GOEDDEL. 1993. Cell **74:** 845–853.
48. HUANG, B., M. EBERSTADT, E.T. OLEJNICZAK, R.P. MEADOWS & S.W. FESIK. 1996. Nature **384:** 638–641.
49. CHINNAIYAN, A.M., K. O'ROURKE, M. TEWARI & V.M. DIXIT. 1995. Cell **81:** 505–512.
50. EBERSTADT, M., B. HUANG, Z. CHEN, R.P. MEADOWS, S.-C. NG, L. ZHENG, M.J. LENARDO & S.W. FESIK. 1998. Nature **392:** 941–945.
51. MUZIO, M.C., A.M., F.C. KISCHKEL, K. O'ROURKE, A. SHEVCHENKO, J. NI, C. SCAFFIDI, J.D. BRETZ, M. ZHANG, R. GENTZ, M. MANN, P.H. KRAMMER, M.E. PETER & V.M. DIXIT. 1996. Cell **85:** 817–827.
52. DUAN, H. & V.M. DIXIT. 1997. Nature **385:** 86–89.
53. AHMAD, M., S.M. SRINIVASULA, L. WANG, R.V. TALANIAN, G. LITWACK, T. FERNANDES-ALNEMRI & E. S. ALNEMRI. 1997. Cancer Res. **57:** 615–619.
54. HARVEY, N.L., A.J. BUTT & S. KUMAR. 1997. J. Biol. Chem. **272:** 13134–13139.
55. GREENBERG, A.H. 1996. Adv. Exp. Med. Biol. **406:** 219–228.
56. YANG, X., H.R. STENNICKE, B. WANG, D.R. GREEN, R.U. JANICKE, A. SRINIVASAN, P. SETH, G.S. SALVESEN & C.J. FROELICH. 1998. J. Biol. Chem. **273:** 34278–34283.
57. ARCH, R. H., R.W. GEDRICH & C.B. THOMPSON. 1998. GENES & DEV. **12:** 2821–2830.

58. MERCURIO, F., H. ZHU, B.W. MURRAY, A. SHEVCHENKO, B.L. BENNETT, J. LI, D.B. YOUNG, M. BARBOSA, M. MANN, A. MANNING & A. RAO. 1997. Science **278:** 860–866.

59. BAEUERLE, P.A. 1998. Current Biol. **8:** R19–22.

60. STANCOVSKI, I. & D. BALTIMORE. 1997. Cell **91:** 299–302.

61. VAN ANTWERP, D.J., S.J. MARTIN, I.M. VERMA & D.R. GREEN. 1998. Trends Cell Biol. **8:** 107–111.

62. BEG, A.A. & D. BALTIMORE. 1996. Science **274:** 782–784.

63. MIAGKOV, A.V., D.V. KOVALENKO, C.E. BROWN, J.R. DIDSBURY, J.P. COGSWELL, S.A. STIMPSON, A.S. BALDWIN & S.S. MAKAROV. 1998. Proc. Natl. Acad. Sci. USA **95:** 13859–13864.

64. WANG, C.Y., M.W. MAYO & A.S. BALDWIN, JR. 1996. Science **274:** 784–787.

65. YAMIN, T.-T., J.M. AYALA & D.K. MILLER. 1996. J. Biol. Chem. **271:** 13273–13282.

66. MUZIO, M., B.R. STOCKWELL, H.R. STENNICKE, G.S. SALVESEN & V.M. DIXIT. 1998. J. Biol. Chem. **273:** 2926–2930.

67. SRINIVASULA, S.M., M. AHMAD, T. FERNANDES-ALNEMRI & E.S. ALNEMRI. 1998. Mol. Cell **1:** 949–57.

68. YANG, X., H.Y. CHANG, & D. BALTIMORE. 1998. Mol. Cell **1:** 319–325.

69. MARTIN, D.A., R.M. SIEGEL, L. ZHENG & M.J. LENARDO. 1998. J. Biol. Chem. **273:** 4345–4349.

70. ROLANDO, A.M., O.C. PALYHA, G.J.-F. DING, A.D. HOWARD & S.M. MOLINEAUX. 1994. J. Cell. Biochem. **18D:** 147.

71. SRINIVASULA, S.M., M. AHMAD, M. MACFARLANE, Z. LUO, Z. HUANG, T. FERNANDES–ALNEMRI & E.S. ALNEMRI. 1998. J. Biol. Chem. **273:** 10107–10111.

72. LIANG, H. & S.W. FESIK. 1997. J. Mol. Biol. **274:** 291–302.

73. CHOU, J.J., H. MATSUO, H. DUAN & G. WAGNER. 1998. CELL **94:** 171–180.

74. HOWARD, A.D., G.J.-F. DING, A.M. ROLANDO, O.C. PALYHA, E.P. PETERSON, F.J. CASANO, E.K. BAYNE, S. DONATELLI, J.M. AYALA, L.A. EGGER, D.K. MILLER, S.M. RAJU, T.T. YAMIN, J. JACKSON, K.T. CHAPMAN, N.A. THORNBERRY, J.A. SCHMIDT, M.J. TOCCI & S.M. MOLINEAUX. 1993. J. Cell. Biochem. **17B:** 113.

75. MACCORKLE, R.A., K.W. FREEMAN & D.M. SPENCER. 1998. Proc. Natl. Acad. Sci. USA **95:** 3655–3660.

76. GU, Y., J. WU, C. FAUCHEU, J.-L. LALANNE, A. DIU, D.J. LIVINGSTON & S.-S. SU. 1995. EMBO J. **14:** 1923–1931.

77. BUTT, A.J., N.L. HARVEY, G. PARASIVAM & S. KUMAR. 1998. J. Biol. Chem. **273:** 6763–6768.

78. COLUSSI, P.A., N.L. HARVEY, L.M. SHEARWIN-WHYATT & S. KUMAR. 1998. J. Biol. Chem. **273:** 26566–26570.

79. CHINNAIYAN, A.M., K. ORTH, K. O'ROURKE, H. DUAN, G.G. POIRIER & V.M. DIXIT. 1996. J. Biol. Chem. **271:** 4573–4576.

80. SRINIVASULA, S.M., M. AHMAD, T. FERNANDES-ALNEMRI, G. LITWACK & E.S. ALNEMRI. 1996. Proc. Natl. Acad. Sci. USA **93:** 14486–14491.

81. TAKAHASHI, A., H. HIRATA, S. YONEHARA, Y. IMAI, K.K. LEE, R.W. MOYER, P.C. TURNER, P.W. MESNER, T. OKAZAKI, H. SAWAI, S. KISHI, K. YAMAMOTO, M. OKUMA & M. SASADA. 1997. Oncogene **14:** 2741–2752.

82. FERRARI, D., A. STEPCZYNSKA, M. LOS, S. WESSELBORG & K. SCHULZE-OSTHOFF. 1998. J. Exp. Med. **188:** 979–984.

83. STENNICKE, H.R., J.M. JURGENSMEIER, H. SHIN, Q. DEVERAUX, B.B. WOLF, X. YANG, Q. ZHOU, H.M. ELLERBY, L.M. ELLERBY, D. BREDESEN, D.R. GREEN, J.C. REED, C.J. FROELICH & G.S. SALVESEN. 1998. J. Biol. Chem. **273:** 27084–27090.

84. HIRATA, H., A. TAKAHASHI, S. KOBAYASHI, S. YONEHARA, H. SAWAI, T. OKAZAKI, K. YAMAMOTO & M. SASADA. 1998. J. Exp. Med. **187:** 587–600.

85. HAN, Z., E.A. HENDRICKSON, T. A. BREMNER & J.H. WYCHE. 1997. J. Biol. Chem. **272:** 13432–13436.
86. HARRIS, J.L., E.P. PETERSON, D. HUDIG, N.A. THORNBERRY & C.S. CRAIK. 1998. J. Biol. Chem. **273:** 27364–27373.
87. FERNANDES-ALNEMRI, T., R.C. ARMSTRONG, J. KREBS, S.M. SRINIVASULA, L. WANG, F. BULLRICH, L.C. FRITZ, J.A. TRAPANI, K.J. TOMASELLI, G. LITWACK & E.S. ALNEMRI. 1996. Proc. Natl. Acad. Sci. USA **93:** 7464–7469.
88. VAN DE CRAEN, M., I. VAN DEN BRANDE, W. DECLERCQ, M. IRMLER, R. BEYAERT, J. TSCHOPP, W. FIERS & P. VANDENABEELE. 1997. Eur. J. Immunol. **27:** 1296–1299.
89. TALANIAN, R.V., X. YANG, J. TURBOV, P. SETH, T. GHAYUR, C.A. CASIANO, K. ORTH & C.J. FROELICH. 1997. J. Exp. Med. **186:** 1323–1331.
90. ANDRADE, F., S. ROY, D. NICHOLSON, N. THORNBERRY, A. ROSEN & L. CASCIOLA-ROSEN. 1998. Immunity **8:** 451–460.
91. TRAPANI, J.A., D.A. JANS, P.J. JANS, M.J. SMYTH, K.A. BROWNE & V.R. SUTTON. 1998. J. Biol. Chem. **273:** 27934–27938.
92. THORNBERRY, N.A. 1998. Curr. Biol. **5:** R97–R103.
93. LAZEBNIK, Y.A., S.H. KAUFMANN, S. DESNOYERS, G.G. POIRIER & W.C. EARNSHAW. 1994. Nature **371:** 346–347.
94. NICHOLSON, D.W., A. ALI, N.A. THORNBERRY, J.P. VAILLANCOURT, C.K. DING, M. GALLANT, Y. GAREAU, P.R. GRIFFIN, M. LABELLE, Y.A. LAZEBNIK, N.A. MUNDAY, S.M. RAJU, M.E. SMULSON, T.–T. YAMIN, V.L. YU & D.K. MILLER. 1995. Nature **376:** 37–43.
95. GREIDINGER, E.L., D.K. MILLER, T.-T. YAMIN, L. CASCIOLA-ROSEN & A. ROSEN. 1996. FEBS Lett. **390:** 299–303.
96. LIU, X., H. ZOU, C. SLAUGHTER & X. WANG. 1997. Cell **89:** 175–184.
97. LIU, X., P. LI, P. WIDLAK, H. ZOU, X. LUO, W.T. GARRARD & X. WANG. 1998. Proc. Natl. Acad. Sci. USA **95:** 8461–8466.
98. SAKAHIRA, H., M. ENARI & S. NAGATA. 1998. Nature **391:** 96–99.
99. JANICKE, R.U., P. NG, M.L. SPRENGART & A.G. PORTER. 1998. J. Biol. Chem. **273:** 15540–15545.
100. LAZEBNIK, Y.A., A. TAKAHASHI, R.D. MOIR, R.D. GOLMAN, G.G. POIRIER, S.H. KAUFMANN & W.C. EARNSHAW. 1995. Proc. Natl. Acad. Sci. USA **92:** 9042–9046.
101. GERVAIS, F.G., N.A. THORNBERRY, S.C. RUFFOLO, D.W. NICHOLSON & S. ROY. 1998. J. Biol. Chem. **273:** 17102–17108.
102. VANAGS, D.M., M.I. PORN-ARES, S. COPPOLA, D.H. BURGESS & S. ORRENIUS. 1996. J. Biol. Chem. **271:** 31075–31085.
103. CRYNS, V.L., L. BERGERON, H. ZHU, H. LI & J. YUAN. 1996. J. Biol. Chem. **271:** 31277–31282.
104. LUO, X., I. BUDIHARDJO, H. ZOU, C. SLAUGHTER & X. WANG. 1998. Cell **94:** 481–490.
105. LI, H., H. ZHU, C.J. XU & J. YUAN. 1998. Cell **94:** 491–501.
106. MILLER, D.K. 1996. *In* Ann. Rep. Med. Chem. Vol. **31:** 249–268. J. A. Bristol, Ed. Academic Press. San Diego, CA.
107. NICHOLSON, D.W. & N.A. THORNBERRY. 1997. Trends Biol. Sci. **22:** 299–306.
108. GARCIA-CALVO, M., E.P. PETERSON, B. LEITING, R. RUEL, D.W. NICHOLSON & N.A. THORNBERRY. 1998. J. Biol. Chem. **273:** 32608–32613.
109. MARGOLIN, N., S.A. RAYBUCK, K.P. WILSON, W. CHEN, T. FOX, Y. GU & D.J. LIVINGSTON. 1997. J. Biol. Chem. **272:** 7223–7228.
110. SLEE, E.A., H. ZHU, S.C. CHOW, M. MACFARLANE, D.W. NICHOLSON & G.M. COHEN. 1996. Biochem. J. **315:** 21–24.
111. Barge, R.M., R. Willemze, P. Vandenabeele, W. Fiers & R. Beyaert. 1997. FEBS Lett. **409:** 207–210.
112. LYNCH, T., J.P. VASILAKOS, K. RASER, K.M. KEANE & B.D. SHIVERS. 1997. Mol. Psychiatry **2:** 227–238.
113. MCCARTHY, J.J., L.L. RUBIN & K.L. PHILPOTT. 1997. J. Cell Sci. **110:** 2165–2173.
114. LODDICK, S.A., A. MACKENZIE & N.J. ROTHWELL. 1996. Neuroreport **7:** 1465–1468.

115. Hara, H., R.M. Friedlander, V. Gagliardini, C. Ayata, K. Fink, Z. Huang, Y. Shimizu-Sasamata & M.A. Moskowitz. 1997. Proc. Natl. Acad. Sci. USA **94:** 2007–2012.
116. Gottron, F.J., H. S. Ying & D.W. Choi. 1997. Mol. Cell Neurosci. **1997:** 159–169.
117. Cheng, Y., M. Deshmukh, A. D'Costa, J.A. Demaro, J.M. Gidday, A. Shah, Y. Sun, M.F. Jacquin, E.M. Johnson & D.M. Holtzman. 1998. J. Clin. Invest. **101:** 1992–1999.
118. Yaoita, H., K. Ogawa, K. Maehara & Y. Maruyama. 1998. Circulation **97:** 276–281.
119. Rodriguez, I., K. Matsuura, C. Ody, S. Nagata & P. Vassalli. 1996. J. Exp. Med. **184:** 2067–2072.
120. Martinou, I., S. Desagher, R. Eskes, B. Antonsson, E. Andre, S. Fakan & J.-C. Martinou. 1999. J. Cell Biol. **144:** 883–889.
121. Schotte, P., W. Declercq, S. Van Huffel, P. Vandenabeele & R. Beyaert. 1999. FEBS Lett. **442:** 117–121.
122. McCarthy, N.J., M.K. Whyte, C.S. Gilbert & G.I. Evan. 1997. J. Cell Biol. **136:** 215–227.
123. Polverino, A.J. & S.D. Patterson. 1997. J. Biol. Chem. **272:** 7013–7021.
124. Lemaire, C., K. Andreau, V. Souvannavong & A. Adam. 1998. FEBS Lett. **425:** 266–270.
125. Finucane, D.M., E. Bossy-Wetzel, N.J. Waterhouse, T.G. Cotter & D.R. Green. 1999. J. Biol. Chem .**274:** 2225–2233.
126. Kuida, K., T.S. Zheng, S. Na, C.-Y. Kuan, D. Yang, H. Karasuyama, P. Rakic & R.A. Flavell. 1996. Nature **384:** 368–384.
127. Woo, M., R. Hakem, M.S. Soengas, G.S. Duncan, A. Shahinian, D. Kagi, A. Hakem, M. McCurrach, W. Khoo, S.A. Kaufman, G. Senaldi, T. Howard, S.W. Lowe & T. . Mak. 1998. Genes Dev. **12:** 806–819.
128. Zheng, T.S., S.F. Schlosser, T. Dao, R. Hingorani, I.N. Crispe, J.L. Boyer & R.A. Flavell. 1998. Proc. Natl. Acad. Sci. USA **95:** 13618–13623.
129. Janicke, R.U., M.L. Sprengart, M.R. Wati & A.G. Porter. 1998. J. Biol. Chem. **273:** 9357–9360.
130. Zhang, J., X. Liu, D.C. Scherer, L. van Kaer, X. Wang & M. Xu. 1998. Proc. Natl. Acad. Sci. USA **95:** 12480–12485.
131. Hakem, R., A. Hakem, G.S. Duncan, J.T. Henderson, M. Woo, M.S. Soengas, A. Elia, J.L. de la Pompa, D. Kagi, W. Khoo, J. Potter, R. Yoshida, S.A. Kaufman, S.W. Lowe, J.M. Penninger & T.W. Mak. 1998. Cell **94:** 339–352.
132. Cecconi, F., G. Alvarez-Bolado, B.I. Meyer, K.A. Roth & P. Gruss. 1998. Cell **94:** 727–737.
133. Yoshida, H., Y.Y. Kong, R. Yoshida, A.J. Elia, A. Hakem, R. Hakem, J. . Penninger & T.W. Mak. 1998. Cell **94:** 739–750.
134. Motoyama, N., F. Wang, K.A. Roth, H. Sawa, K.I. Nakayama, K. Nakayama, I. Negishi, S. Senju, Q. Zhang, S. Fujii & D.Y. Loh. 1995. Science **267:** 1506–1510.
135. Veis, D.J., C.M. Sorenson, S.R. Shutter & S.J. Korsmeyer. 1993. Cell **75:** 229–240.
136. Yang, X., R. Khosravi Far, H.Y. Chang & D. Baltimore. 1997. Cell **89:** 1067–1076.
137. Varfolomeev, E.E., M. Schuchmann, V. Luria, N. Chiannilkulchai, J.S. Beckmann, I.L. Mett, D. Rebrikov, V.M. Brodianski, O.C. Kemper, O. Kollet, T. Lapidot, D. Soffer, T. Sobe, K.B. Avraham, T. Goncharov, H. Holtmann, P. Lonai & D. Wallach. 1998. Immunity **9:** 267–276.
138. Yeh, W.-C., J.L. de la Pompa, M.E. McCurrach, H.-B. Shu, A.J. Elia, A. Shahinian, M. Ng, A. Wakeham, W. Khoo, K. Mitchell, W.S. El-Deiry, W. Lowe, D.V. Goeddel & T.W. Mak. 1998. Science **279:** 1954–1956.

139. ZHANG, J., D. CADO, A. CHEN, N.H. KABRA & A. WINOTO. 1998. Nature **392:** 296–300.
140. WALSH, C.M., B.G. WEN, A.M. CHINNAIYAN, K. O'ROURKE, V.M. DIXIT & S.M. HEDRICK. 1998. Immunity **8:** 439–449.
141. BERGERON, L., G.I. PEREZ, G. MACDONALD, L. SHI, Y. SUN, A. JURISICOVA, S. VARMUZA, K.E. LATHAM, J.A. FLAWS, J.C. SALTER, H. HARA, M.A. MOSKOWITZ, E. LI, A. GREENBERG, J.L. TILLY & J. YUAN. 1998. Genes Dev. **12:** 1304–1314.
142. FEARNHEAD, H.O., J. RODRIGUEZ, E.E. GOVEK, W. GUO, R. KOBAYASHI, G. HANNON & Y.A. LAZEBNIK. 1998. Proc. Natl. Acad. Sci. USA **95:** 13664–13669.
143. O'BRIEN, V. 1998. J. Gen. Virol. **79:** 1833–1845.
144. BARRY, M. & G. MCFADDEN. 1998. Curr. Opin. Immunol. **10:** 422–430.
145. HU, R.-Q., C.A. SMITH & D.J. PICKUP. 1994. Virology **204:** 343–356.
146. SMITH, C.A., F.-Q. HU, T.D. SMITH, C.L. RICHARDS, P. SMOLAK, R.G. GOODWIN & D. J. PICKUP. 1996. Virology **223:** 132–147.
147. SHISLER, J., C. YANG, B. WALTER, C.F. WARE & L.R. GOODING. 1997. J. Virol. **71:** 8299–8306.
148. TOLLEFSON, A.E., T.W. HERMISTON, D.L. LICHTENSTEIN, C.F. COLLE, R.A. TRIP, T. DIMITROV, K. TOTH, C.E. WELLS, P.C. DOHERTY & W.S. WOLD. 1998. Nature **392:** 726–730.
149. ELSING, A. & H. G. BURGER. 1998. Proc. Natl. Acad. Sci. USA **95:** 10072–10077.
150. HENDERSON, S., M. ROWE, C. GREGORY, D. CROOM-CARTER, F. WANG, R. LONG-NECKER, E. KIEFF & A. RICKINSON. 1991. Cell **65:** 1107–1115.
151. LAHERTY, C.D., H.M. HU, A.W. OPIPARI, F. WANG & V.M. DIXIT. 1992. J. Biol. Chem. **267:** 24157–24160.
152. ROWE, M., M. PENG-PILON, D.S. HUEN, R. HARDY, D. CROOM-CARTER & E.R. LUNDGREN. 1994. J. Virol. **68:** 5602–5612.
153. IZUMI, K.M. & E.D. KIEFF. 1997. Proc. Natl. Acad. Sci. USA **94:** 12592–12597.
154. MARSTERS, S.A., T.M. AYRES, M. SKUBATCH, C.L. GRAY, M. ROTHE & A. ASHKENAZI. 1997. J. Biol. Chem. **272:** 14029–14032.
155. QUERIDO, E., R.C. MARCELLUS, A. LAI, R. CHARBONNEAU, J.G. TEOLDORO, G. KETNER & P.E. BRANTON. 1997. J. Virol. **71:** 3788–3798.
156. YEW, P.R., X. LIU & A.J. BERK. 1994. Genes & Dev. **8:** 190–202.
157. SCHEFFNER, M., B.A. WERNESS, J.M. HUIBREGTSE, A.J. LEVINE & P.M. HOWLEY. 1990. Cell **63:** 1129–1136.
158. THOME, M., P. SCHNEIDER, K. HOFMANN, H. FICKENSCHER, E. MEINL, F. NEIPEL, C. MATTMANN, K. BURNS, J.-L. BODMER, M. SCHROTER, C. SCAFFIDI, P.H. KRAMMER, M.E. PETER & J. TSCHOFF. 1997. Nature **386:** 517–521.
159. HU, S., C. VINCENZ, M. BULLER & V.M. DIXIT. 1987. J. Biol. Chem. **272:** 9621–9624.
160. IRMLER, M., M. THOME, M. HAHNE, P. SCHNEIDER, K. HOFMANN, V. STEINER, J.-L. BODMER, M. SCHROTER, K. BURNS, C. MATTMANN, D. RIMOLDI, L.E. FRENCH & J. TSCHOPP. 1997. Nature **388:** 190–195.
161. KATAOKA, T., M. SCHROTER, M. HAHNE, P. SCHNEIDER, M. IRMLER, M. THOME, C.J. FROELICH & J. TSCHOPP. 1998. J. Immunol. **161:** 3936–3942.
162. TSCHOPP, J., M. IRMLER & M. THOME. 1998. Curr. Opin. Immunol. **10:** 552–558.
163. DIMITROV, T., P. KRAJCSI, T.W. HERMISTON, A.E. TOLLEFSON, M. HANNINK & W.S.M. WOLD. 1997. J. Virol. **71:** 2830–2837.
164. LI, Y., J. KANG & M.S. HORWITZ. 1997. J. Virol. **71:** 1576–1582.
165. CHEN, P., J. TIAN, I. KOVESDI & J.T. BRUDER. 1998. J. Biol. Chem. **273:** 5815–5820.
166. LI, Y., J. KANG & M.S. HORWITZ. 1998. Mol. Cell. Biol. **18:** 1601–-1610.
167. LI, Y., J. KANG, J. FRIEDMQAN, L. TARASSISHIN, J. YE, A. KOVALENKO, D. WALLACH & M.S. HORWITZ. 1999. Proc. Natl. Acad. Sci. USA **96:** 1042–1047.
168. YAMAOKA, S., G. COURTOIS, C. BESSIA, S.T. WHITESIDE, R. WEIL, F. AGOU, H.E. KIRK, R.J. KAY & A. ISRAEL. 1998. Cell **93:** 1231–1240.

169. MILLER, L.K. 1997. J. Cell Physiol. **173:** 178–182.
170. DEVERAUX, Q.L. & J.C. REED. 1998. Genes & Dev. **13:** 239–252.
171. SESHAGIRI, S. & L.K. MILLER. 1997. Proc. Natl. Acad. Sci. USA **94:** 13606–13611.
172. KAISER, W.J., D. VUCIC & L.K. MILLER. 1998. FEBS Lett. **440:** 243–248.
173. VUCIC, D., W.J. KAISER & L.K. MILLER. 1998. Mol. Cell. Biol. **18:** 3300–3309.
174. ROTHE, M., M.-G. PAN, W.J. HENZEL, T.M. AYRES & D.V. GOEDDEL. 1995. Cell **83:** 1243–1252.
175. CHU, Z.L., T.A. MCKINSEY, L. LIU, J.J. GENTRY, M.H. MALIM & D.W. BALLARD. 1997. Proc. Natl. Acad. Sci. USA **94:** 10057–10062.
176. WANG, C.Y., M.W. MAYO, R.G. KORNELUK, D.V. GOEDDEL & A.S. BALDWIN, JR. 1998. Science **281:** 1680–1683.
177. DEVERAUX, Q.L., N. ROY, H.R. STENNICKE, T. VAN ARSDALE, Q. ZHOU, S.M. SRINIVASULA, E.S. ALNEMRI, G.S. SALVESEN & J.C. REED. 1998. EMBO J. **17:** 2215–2223.
178. DUCKETT, C.S., F. LI, Y. WANG, K.J. TOMASELLI, C.B. THOMPSON & R.C. ARMSTRONG. 1998. Mol. Cell Biol. **18:** 608–615.
179. ROY, N., Q.L. DEVERAUX, R. TAKAHASHI, G.S. SALVESEN & J.C. REED. 1997. EMBO J. **16:** 6914–6925.
180. DEVERAUX, Q.L., R. TAKAHASHI, G.S. SALVESEN & J.C. REED. 1997. Nature **388:** 300–304.
181. LISTON, P., N. ROY, K. TAMAI, C. LEFEBVRE, S. BAIRD, G. CHERTON-HORVAT, R. FARAHANI, M. MCLEAN, J.-E. IKEDA, A. MACKENZIE & R.G. KORNELUK. 1996. Nature **379:** 349–353.
182. AMBROSINI, G., C. ADIDA & D.C. ALTIERI. 1997. Nat. Med. **3:** 917–921.
183. LI, F., G. AMBROSINI, E.Y. CHU, J. PLESCIA, S. TOGNIN, P.C. MARCHISIO & D.C. ALTIERI. 1998. Nature **396:** 580–584.
184. TAMM, I., Y. WANG, E. SAUSVILLE, D.A. SCUDIERO, N. VIGNA, T. OLTERSDORF & J.C. REED. 1998. Cancer Res. **58:** 5315–5320.
185. BUMP, N.J., K. BRADY, T. GHAYUR, M. HUGUNIN, P. LI, P. LICARI, L.K. MILLER & W.W. WONG. 1995. J. Cell. Biochem. **19B:** 294.
186. XUE, D. & H.R. HORVITZ. 1995. Nature **377:** 248–251.
187. BERTIN, J., S.M. MENDRYSA, D.J. LACOUNT, S. GAUR, J.F. KREBS, R.C. ARMSTRONG, K.J. TOMASELLI & P.D. FRIESEN. 1996. J. Virol. **70:** 6251–6259.
188. MANJI, G.A., R.R. HOZAK, D.J. LACOUNT & P.D. FRIESEN. 1997. J. Virol. **71:** 4509–4516.
189. ZHOU, Q., J.F. KREBS, S.J. SNIPAS, A. PRICE, E.S. ALNEMRI, K.J. TOMASELLI & G.S. SALVESEN. 1998. Biochemistry **37:** 10757–10765.
190. IZQUIERDO, M., A. GRANDIEN, L.M. CRIADO, S. ROBLES, E. LEONARDO, J.P. ALBAR, G.G. DE BUITRAGO & A.C. MARTINEZ. 1999. EMBO J. **18:** 156–166.
191. BIRD, P.I. 1998. Results Probl. Cell Differ. **24:** 63–89.
192. RAY, C.A., R.A. BLACK, S.R. KRONHEIM, T.A. GREENSTREET, P.R. SLEATH, G.S. SALVESEN & D.J. PICKUP. 1992. Cell **69:** 597–604.
193. KOMIYAMA, T. K., C. A. RAY, D. J. PICKUP, A. D. HOWARD, N. A. THORNBERRY, E. P. PETERSON, & G. SALVESEN. 1994. J. Biol. Chem. **269:** 19331-19337.
194. DOBBELSTEIN, M. & T. SHENK. 1996. J. Virol. **70:** 6479-6485.
195. MACEN, J. L., R. S. GARNER, P. Y. MUSY, M. A. BROOKS, P. C. TURNER, R. W. MOYER, F. MCFADDEN, & R. C. BLEACKLEY. 1996. Proc. Natl. Acad. Sci. USA **93:** 9108-9113.
196. MESSUD-PETIT, F., J. GELFI, M. DELVERDIER, M.-F. AMARDEILH, R. PY, G. SUTTER, & S. BERTAGNOLI. 1998. J. Virol. **72:** 7830-7839.
197. ZHOU, Q., S. SNIPAS, K. ORTH, M. MUZIO, V.M. DIXIT & G.S. SALVESEN. 1997. J. Biol. Chem. **272:** 7797–7800.
198. QUAN, L.T., A. CAPUTO, R.C. BLEACKLEY, D.J. PICKUP & G.S. SALVESEN. 1995. J. Biol. Chem. **270:** 10377–10379.

199. BIRD, C.H., V.R. SUTTON, J. SUN, C.E. HIRST, A. NOVAK, S. KUMAR, J.A. TRAPANI & P.I. BIRD. 1998. Mol. Cell Biol. **18:** 6387–6398.
200. GOTTLOB, K., M. FULCO, M. LEVRERO & A. GRAESSMANN. 1998. J. Biol. Chem. **273:** 33347–33353.
201. CHAO, D.T. & S.J. KORSMEYER. 1998. Annu. Rev. Immunol. **16:** 395–419.
202. TSUJIMOTO, Y. 1998. Genes Cells **3:** 697–707.
203. MUCHMORE, S.W., M. SATTLER, H. LIANG, R.P. MEADOWS, J.E. HARLAN, H.S. YOON, D. NETTESHEIM, B.S. CHANG, C.B. THOMPSON, S.-L. WONG, S.-C. NG & S.W. FESIK. 1996. Nature **381:** 335–341.
204. SCHENDEL, S.L., Z. XIE, M.O. MONTAL, S. MATSUYAMA, M. MONTAL & J.C. REED. 1997. Proc. Natl. Acad. Sci. USA **94:** 5113–5118.
205. MINN, A.J., P. VELEZ, S.L. SCHENDEL, H. LIANG, S.W. MUCHMORE, S.W. FESIK, M. FILL & C.B. THOMPSON. 1997. Nature **385:** 353–357.
206. SCHLESINGER, P.H., A. GROSS, X.M. YIN, K. YAMAMOTO, M. SAITO, G. WAKSMAN & S.J. KORSMEYER. 1997. Proc. Natl. Acad. Sci. USA **94:** 11357–11362.
207. GREEN, D.R. & J.C. REED. 1998. Science **281:** 1309–1312.
208. SUSIN, S.A., N. ZAMZAMI & G. KROEMER. 1998. Biochim. Biophys. Acta **1366:** 151–165.
209. CAI, J. & D.P. JONES. 1998. J. Biol. Chem. **273:** 11401–11404.
210. MATSUYAMA, S., Q. XU, J. VELOURS & J.C. REED. 1998. Molec. Cell **1:** 327–336.
211. HAMPTON, M.B., B. FADEEL & S. ORRENIUS. 1998. Ann. N.Y. Acad. Sci. **854:** 328–335.
212. SUSIN, S.A., H.K. LORENZO, N. ZAMZAMI, I. MARZO, B.E. SNOW, G.M. BROTHERS, J. MANGION, E. JACOTOT, P. COSTANTINI, M. LOEFFLER, N. LAROCHETTE, D.R. GOODLETT, R. AEBERSOLD, D.P. SIDEROVSKI, J.M. PENNINGER & G. KROEMER. 1999. Nature **397:** 441–446.
213. VANDER HEIDEN, M.G., N.S. CHANDEL, P.T. SCHUMACKER & C.B. THOMPSON. 1999. Molec. Cell **3:** 159–167.
214. PEARSON, G.R., J. LUKA, L. PETTI, J. SAMPLE, M. BIRKENBACH, D. BRAUN & E. KIEFF. 1987. Virology **160:** 151–161.
215. SUBRAMANIAN, T., B. TARODI & G. CHINNADURAI. 1995. Curr. Topics Microbiol. Immunol. **199:** 153–161.
216. DERFUSS, T., H. FICKENSCHER, M.S. KRAFT, G. HENNING, D. LENGENFELDER, B. FLECKENSTEIN & E. MEINL. 1998. J. Virol. **72:** 5897–5904.
217. NEILAN, J.G., Z. LU, C.L. AFONSO, G.F. KUTISH, M.D. SUSSMAN & D.L. ROCK. 1993. J. Virol. **67:** 4391–4394.
218. CHIOU, S.-K., C.-C. TSENG, L. RAO & E. WHITE. 1994. J. Virol. **68:** 6553–6566.
219. HUANG, D.C., S. CORY & A. STRASSER. 1997. Oncogene **14:** 405–414.
220. OLTVAI, Z.N., C.L. MILLIMAN & S.J. KORSMEYER. 1993. Cell **74:** 609–619.
221. KIEFER, M.C., M.J. BRAUER, V.C. POWERS, J.J. WU, S.R. UMANSKY, L.D. TOMEI & P.J. BARR. 1995. Nature **374:** 736–739.
222. JURGENSMEIER, J.M., S. KRAJEWSKI, R.C. ARMSTRONG, G.M. WILSON, T. OLTERSDORF, L.C. FRITZ, J.C. REED & S. OTTILIE. 1997. Mol. Biol. Cell **8:** 325–339.
223. WOLTER, K.G., Y.T. HSU, C.L. SMITH, A. NECHUSHTAN, X.G. XI & R.J. YOULE. 1997. J. Cell Biol. **139:** 1281–1292.
224. JURGENSMEIER, J.M., Z. XIE, Q. DEVERAUX, L. ELLERBY, D. BREDESEN & J.C. REED. 1998. Proc. Natl. Acad. Sci. USA **95:** 4997–5002.
225. GROSS, A., J. JOCKEL, M.C. WEI & S.J. KORSMEYER. 1998. EMBO J. **17:** 3878–3885.
226. MARZO, I., C. BRENNER, N. ZAMZAMI, J.M. JURGENSMEIER, S.A. SUSIN, H.L.A. VIEIRA, M.-C. PREVOST, K.Z. XIE, S. MATSUYAMA, J.C. REED & G. KROEMER. 1998. Science **281:** 2027–2031.
227. MAHAJAN, N.P., K. LINDER, G. BERRY, G.W. GORDON, R. HEIM & B. HERMAN. 1998. Nat. Biotechnol. **16:** 547–552.

228. AVERY, R. G. EBB, T. SUBRAMANIAN, T. CHITTENDEN, R.J. LUTZ & G. CHINNADURAI. 1995. Oncogene **11:** 1921–1928.

229. ELANGOVAN, B. & G. CHINNADURAI. 1997. J. Biol. Chem. **272:** 24494–24498.

230. YANG, E., J. ZHA, J. JOCKEL, L.H. BOISE, C.B. THOMPSON & S.J. KORSMEYER. 1995. Cell **80:** 285–291.

231. KELEKAR, A., B.S. CHANG, J.E. HARLAN, S.W. FESIK & C.B. THOMPSON. 1997. Mol. Cell Biol. **17:** 7040–7046.

232. COSULICH, S.C., V. WORRALL, P.J. HEDGE, S. GREEN & P.R. CLARKE. 1997. Curr. Biol. **7:** 913–920.

233. SATTLER, M., H. LIANG, D. NETTESHEIM, R.P. MEADOWS, J.E. HARLAN, M. EBERSTADT, H.S. YOON, S.B. SHUKER, B.. CHANG, A.J. MINN, C.B. THOMPSON & S.W. FESIK. 1997. Science **275:** 983–986.

234. NARITA, M., S. SHIMIZU, T. ITO, T. CHITTENDEN, R.J. LUTZ, H. MATSUDA & Y. TSUJIMOTO. 1998. Proc. Natl. Acad. Sci. USA **95:** 14681–14686.

235. WHITE, E. 1996. Genes Dev. **10:** 1–15.

236. GROSS, A., X.M. YIN, K. WANG, M.C. WEI, J. JOCKEL, C. MILLIMAN, H. ERDJUMENT-BROMAGE, P. TEMPST & S.J. KORSMEYER. 1999. J. Biol. Chem. **274:** 1156–1163.

237. HAN, Z., K. BHALLA, P. PANTAZIS, E.A. HENDRICKSON & J.H. WYCHE. 1999. Mol. Cell Biol. **19:** 1381–1389.

238. KUWANA, T., J.J. SMITH, M. MUZIO, V. DIXIT, D.D. NEWMEYER & S. KORNBLUTH. 1998. J. Biol. Chem. **273:** 16589–16594.

239. STEEMANS, M., V. GOOSSENS, M. VAN DE CRAEN, F. VAN HERREWEGHE, K. VANCOMPERNOLLE, K. DE VOS, P. VANDENABEELE & J. GROOTEN. 1998. J. Exp. Med. **188:** 2193–2198.

240. SRINIVASAN, A., F. LI, A. WONG, L. KODANDAPANI, R. SMIDT, JR., J.F. KREBS, L.C. FRITZ, J.C. WU & K.J. TOMASELLI. 1998. J. Biol. Chem. **273:** 4523–4529.

241. CHOU, J.J., H. LI, G.S. SALVESEN, J. YUAN & G. WAGNER. 1999. Cell **96:** 615–624.

242. MCDONNELL, J.M., D. FUSHMAN, C.L. MILLIMAN, S.J. KORSMEYER & D. COWBURN. 1999. Cell **96:** 625–634.

243. MANCINI, M., D.W. NICHOLSON, S. ROY, N.A. THORNBERRY, E.P. PETERSON, L.A. CASCIOLA-ROSEN & A. ROSEN. 1998. J. Cell Biol. **140:** 1485–1495.

244. BRADHAM, C.A., T. QIAN, K. STREETZ, C. TRAUTWEIN, D.A. BRENNER & J.J. LEMASTERS. 1998. Mol. Cell Biol. **18:** 6353–6364.

245. SUSIN, S.A., H.K. LORENZO, N. ZAMZAMI, I. MARZO, C. BRENNER, N. LAROCHETTE, M.C. PREVOST, P.M. ALZARI & G. KROEMER. 1999. J. Exp. Med. **189:** 381–394.

246. EARNSHAW, W.C. 1999. Nature **397:** 387–388.

247. SCAFFIDI, C., S. FULDA, A. SRINIVASAN, C. FRIESEN, F. LI, K.J. TOMASELLI, K.M. DEBATIN, P.H. KRAMMER & M.E. PETER. 1998. EMBO J. **17:** 1675–1687.

248. CHENG, E.H., D.G. KIRSCH, R.J. CLEM, R. RAVI, M.B. KASTAN, A. BEDI, K. UENO & J.M. HARDWICK. 1997. Science **278:** 1966–1968.

249. MARZO, I., S.A. SUSIN, P.X. PETIT, L. RAVAGNAN, C. BRENNER, N. LAROCHETTE, N. ZAMZAMI & G. KROEMER. 1998. FEBS Lett. **427:** 198–202.

250. CASCIOLA-ROSEN, L., D.W. NICHOLSON, T. CHONG, K.R. ROWAN, N.A. THORNBERRY, D.K. MILLER & A. ROSEN. 1996. J. Exp. Med. **183:** 1957–1964.

251. WATERHOUSE, N., S. KUMAR, Q. SONG, P. STRIKE, L. SPARROW, G. DREYFUSS, E.S. ALNEMRI, G. LITWACK, M. LAVIN & D. WATTERS. 1996. J. Biol. Chem. **271:** 29335–39341.

252. RHEAUME, E., L.Y. COHEN, F. UHLMANN, C. LAZURE, A. ALAM, J. HURWITZ, R.-P. SEKALY & F. DENIS. 1997. EMBO J. **16:** 6346–6354.

253. UBEDA, M. & J.F. HABENER. 1997. J. Biol. Chem. **272:** 19562–19568.

254. SAMEJIMA, K., P.A. SVINGEN, G.S. BASI, T. KOTTKE, P.W. MESNER, JR., L. STEWART, F. DURRIEU, G.G. POIRIER, E.S. ALNEMRI, J.J. CHAMPOUX, S.H. KAUFMANN & W.C.

EARNSHAW. 1999. J. Biol. Chem. **274:** 4335–4340.

255. HSU, H.-L. & N.-H. YEH. 1996. J. Cell Sci. **109:** 277–288.

256. WEAVER, V.M., C.E. CARSON, P.R. WALKER, N. CHALY, B. LACH, Y. RAYMOND, D.L. BROWN & M. SIKORSKA. 1996. J. Cell Sci. **109:** 45–56.

257. KOTHAKOTA, S., T. AZUMA, C. REINHARD, A. KLIPPEL, J. TANG, K. CHU, T.J. MCGARRY, M.W. KIRSCHNER, K. KOTHS, D.J. KWIATKOWSKI & L.T. WILLIAMS. 1997. Science **278:** 294–298.

258. MASHIMA, T., M. NAITO, N. FUJITA, K. NOGUCHI & T. TSURUO. 1995. Biochem. Biophys. Res. Commun. **217:** 1185–1192.

259. BRANCOLINI, C., M. BENEDETTI & C. SCHNEIDER. 1995. EMBO J. **14:** 5179–5190.

260. EMOTO, Y., Y. MANOME, G. MEINHARDT, H. KISAKI, S. KHARBANDA, M. ROBERTSON, T. GHAYUR, W.W. WONG, R. KAMEN, R. WEICHSELBAUM & D. KUFE. 1995. EMBO J. **14:** 6148–6156.

261. GHAYUR, T., M. HUGUNIN, R.V. TALANIAN, S. RATNOFSKY, C. QUINLAN, Y. EMOTO, P. PANDEY, R. DATTA, S. KHARBANDA, H. ALLEN, R. KAMEN, W. WONG & D. KUFE. 1996. J. Exp. Med. **184:** 2399–2404.

262. DATTA, R., H. KOJIMA, K. YOSHIDA & D. KUFE. 1997. J. Biol. Chem. **272:** 20317–20320.

263. RUDEL, T. & G.M. BOKOCH. 1997. Science **276:** 1571–1574.

264. CRYNS, V.L., Y. BYUN, A. RANA, H. MELLOR, K.D. LUSTIG, L. GHANEM, P.J. PARKER, M.W. KIRSCHNER & J.Y. YUAN. 1997. J. Biol. Chem. **272:** 29449–29453.

265. DEAK, J.C., J.V. CROSS, M. LEWIS, Y. QIAN, L.A. PARROTT, C.W. DISTELHORST & D.J. TEMPLETON. 1998. Proc. Natl. Acad. Sci. USA **95:** 5595–5600.

266. GRAVES, J.D., Y. GOTOH, K.E. DRAVES, D. AMBROSE, D.K. HAN, M. WRIGHT, J. CHERNOFF, E.A. CLARK & E.G. KREBS. 1998. EMBO J. **17:** 2224–2234.

267. LEE, K.-K., M. MURAKAWA, E. NISHIDA, S. TSUBUKI, S.-I. KAWASHIMA, K. SAKAMAKI & S. YONEHARA. 1998. Oncogene **16:** 3029–3037.

268. LEVKAU, B., H. KOYAMA, E.W. RAINES, B.E. CLURMAN, B. HERREN, K. ORTH, J.M. ROBERTS & R. ROSS. 1998. Mol. Cell **1:** 553–563.

269. GERVAIS, J.L., P. SETH & H. ZHANG. 1998. J. Biol. Chem. **273:** 19207–19212.

270. WIDMANN, C., S. GIBSON & G.L. JOHNSON. 1998. J. Biol. Chem. **273:** 7141–7147.

271. WANG, X., J.-T. PAI, E.A. WIEDENFELD, J.C. MEDINA, C.A. SLAUGHTER, J.L. GOLDSTEIN & M.S. BROWN. 1995. J. Biol. Chem. **270:** 18044–18050.

272. ERHARDT, P., K.J. TOMASELLI & G.M. COOPER. 1997. J. Biol. Chem. **272:** 15049–15052.

273. RAVI, R., A. BEDI, E.J. FUSCHS & A. BEDI. 1998. Cancer Res. **58:** 882–886.

274. JANICKE, R.U., P.A. WALKER, X.Y. LIN & A.G. PORTER. 1996. EMBO J. **15:** 6969–6978.

275. NA, S., T.-H. CHUANG, A. CUNNINGHAM, T.G. TURI, J.H. HANKE, G.M. BOKOCH & D.E. DANLEY. 1996. J. Biol. Chem. **271:** 11209–11213.

276. SANTORO, M.F., R.R. ANNAND, M.M. ROBERTSON, Y.-W. PENG, M.J. BRADY, J.A. MANKOVICH, M.C. HACKETT, T. GHAYUR, G. WALTER, W.W. WONG & D.A. GIEGEL. 1998. J. Biol. Chem. **273:** 13119–13128.

277. 7WISSING, D., H. MOURITZEN, M. EGEBLAD, G.G. POIRIER & M. JAATTELA. 1997. Proc. Natl. Acad. Sci. USA **94:** 5073–5077.

278. HARVEY, K.F., N.L. HARVEY, J.M. MICHAEL, G. PARASIVAM, N. WATERHOUSE, E.S. ALNEMRI, D. WATTERS & S. KUMAR. 1998. J. Biol. Chem. **273:** 13524–13530.

279. WELLINGTON, C.L., L.M. ELLERBY, A.S. HACKAM, R.L. MARGOLIS, M.A. TRIFIRO, R. SINGARAJA, K. MCCUTCHEON, G.S. SALVESEN, S.S. PROPP, M. BROMM, K.J. ROWLAND, T. ZHANG, D. RASPER, S. ROY, N. THORNBERRY, L. PINSKY, A. KAKIZUKA, C.A. ROSS, D.W. NICHOLSON, D.E. BREDESEN & M.R. HAYDEN. 1998. J. Biol. Chem. **273:** 9158–9167.

280. GRUNBERG, J., J. WALTER, H. LOETSCHER, U. DEUSCHLE, H. JACOBSEN & C. HAASS. 1998. Biochemistry **37:** 2263–2270.
281. LEE, N., H. MACDONALD, C. REINHARD, R. HALENBECK, A. ROULSTON, T. SHI & L.T. WILLIAMS. 1997. Proc. Natl. Acad. Sci. USA **94:** 13642–13647.
282. BEYAERT, R., V.J. KIDD, S. CORNELIS, M. VAN DE CRAEN, G. DENECKER, J.M. LAHTI, R. GURURAJAN, P. VANDENABEELE & W. FIERS. 1997. J. Biol. Chem. **272:** 11694–11697.
283. KING, P. & S. GOODBOURN. 1998. J. Biol. Chem. **273:** 8699–8704.
284. THOMPSON, J.D., D.G. HIGGINS & T.J. GIBSON. 1994. Nucleic Acids Res. **22:** 4673–4680.

Strategies to Adapt Adenoviral Vectors for Targeted Delivery

DAVID T. CURIEL[a]

Gene Therapy Center, University of Alabama at Birmingham, Birmingham, Alabama 35294-3300, USA

ABSTRACT: The utility of current generation adenoviral vectors for targeted, cell-specific gene delivery is limited by the promiscuous tropism of the parent virus. To address this issue, we have developed both genetic and immunologic methods to alter viral tropism. Immunologic retargeting has been achieved via conjugates comprised of an antifiber knob Fab and a targeting moiety consisting of a ligand or antireceptor antibody. Gene delivery by this approach has been accomplished via a variety of cellular pathways including receptors for folate, FGF, and EGF. In addition to cell-specific gene delivery, this strategy has allowed enhanced gene delivery to target cells lacking the native adenoviral receptor, CAR. Of note, this specific and extended gene delivery allowed enhanced survival in murine models of human carcinoma via cancer gene therapy. Genetic strategies to alter adenoviral tropism have included both fiber modification and fiber replacement. In the former, we have identified the HI loop of fiber as a propitious locale for introduction of heterologous peptides. Incorporation of an RGDC peptide at this locale allowed gene delivery via cellular integrins with dramatic efficiency augmentations. As a strategy to achieve both new tropism as well as to ablate native tropism, methods have been developed to replace the fiber protein with heterologous motif which preserves the key trimeric quaternary structure of fiber and allows for propagation. Such a fiber-replacement virus has been rescued and has demonstrated capacities consistent with its utility as a novel vector agent. These strategies have allowed the achievement of cell-specific gene delivery via adenoviral vectors and thus have the potential to enhance the utility of this vector agent.

INTRODUCTION

For the effective application of gene therapy strategies to human disease, Anderson[1] suggested certain criteria should be met, namely, that vectors should deliver a therapeutic gene specifically to a target cell, that resultant gene expression should be at an appropriate level and for an appropriate period of time, and that delivery and expression of the therapeutic gene should be achieved within an acceptable safety margin.[1] These criteria remain largely unmet. However, in recent years disappointment in the results of clinical trials has forced a refocus on the basics of vector design, resulting in steady advancements in vector technology, which now show promise for more successful gene therapy.

---

[a]Address for correspondence: David T. Curiel, MD, Director, Gene Therapy Center, University of Alabama at Birmingham, 1824 Sixth Avenue South, Room WTI 620, Birmingham, Alabama 35294-3300 USA. Phone, 205/934-8627; fax, 205-975-7476.
e-mail, david.curiel@ccc.uab.edu

Development of vectors that have *in vivo* efficacy is critical, because many diseases for which gene therapy can rationally be considered require direct *in situ* gene delivery and cannot feasibly be addressed by an *ex vivo* approach. Replication incompetent adenovirus is a potential candidate vector for clinical gene therapy based on several key attributes, including ease of production to high titer, infection of both dividing and nondividing cells, and systemic stability, which has allowed for efficient *in vivo* gene expression.[2] However, the virus has several important limitations including its widespread tropism, stimulation of inflammatory and immune responses, and short-term transgene expression.[3–5] This article focuses chiefly on the issue of targeted gene delivery to address the limitations brought about by native viral tropism. To date, several groups have sought to exploit the fundamental advantages of adenovirus by using it in specific contexts where the recognized limitations were judged to be less important. For example, it was thought that the issue of the widespread tropism of the virus could be circumvented by administering the vector by direct injection, particularly in the context of tumors. However, in phase I human trials, dissemination beyond the injected site was found. Application to "compartmentalized" disease has also met with problems. For example, poor gene transfer efficiency has been noted following administration into the pleural space for therapy of mesothelioma[6] (S.M. Albelda, unpublished data), and in the peritoneum, effective use of antitumor gene therapy has been limited by concurrent gene transfer of the liver with subsequent toxicity.[7] Further limitations have arisen in the application to pulmonary disease. Here, prior clinical experience had indicated that the virus had a natural tropism for the respiratory tract; therefore, direct administration of vector to the airways for cystic fibrosis therapy seemed a rational approach.[8–12] In reality, the achieved levels of gene transfer were lower than expected, because differentiated airway epithelial cells lack sufficient adenoviral receptors and the integrins required for viral internalization.[13–16] Therefore, even in these apparently favorable anatomic locations there is a strong case for developing a vector with cell-specific targeting properties. Despite the limitations of adenovirus, its basic advantages, particularly its *in vivo* efficacy, justify using this virus as a starting point in the development of improved vector systems.

ADENOVIRAL ENTRY PATHWAY

Strategies for retargeting viral vectors were first applied to retroviruses and were based on a sound understanding of viral entry mechanisms.[17] The entry mechanisms of adenovirus, including the recent identification of primary adenoviral receptors, are now well understood and allow for a rational approach to the targeting of adenoviral vectors (FIG. 1).

The adenovirus is an unenveloped icosahedral particle with 12 fibers projecting from the surface.[18] During the assembly phase of viral replication, fiber monomers trimerize in the cytoplasm, then bind to a viral penton base protein that is subsequently incorporated into the viral capsid. At the distal tip of each fiber monomer is a globular region referred to as the knob domain. It is this knob region that binds to cellular adenoviral receptors, initially anchoring the virus to the cells. Two cellular receptors for adenovirus were recently described. The coxsackie/adenoviral receptor

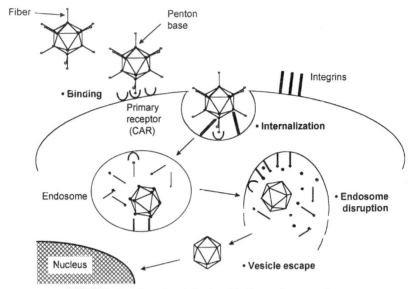

FIGURE 1. Adenovirus infection: binding and entry pathway.

(CAR)[3,19] binds both adenovirus and group B coxsackie viruses. The murine and human receptors are 365 and 352 amino acids, respectively, and 91% identical. The extracellular region appears to contain two immunoglobulin-like domains. In a separate report, viral binding to the $\alpha 2$ domain of major histocompatability complex class 1 was also shown.[20] Following attachment, viral entry requires a second step, which involves the interaction between Arg-Gly-Asp (RGD) motifs in the penton base with cell surface integrins $\alpha v \beta 3$ or $\alpha v \beta 5$, which then leads to receptor-mediated endocytosis of the virion.[21] In the endosome the virus undergoes a stepwise disassembly, and endosomal lysis occurs (a process mediated by the penton base and low endosomal pH), followed by transport of the viral DNA to the cell nucleus. This endosomolysis step is critical for efficient gene delivery, and the ability of the adenovirus to effect endosomal escape is a key factor in its efficiency as a vector. Importantly, viral entry and endosomal escape are functionally uncoupled[22]; thus, entry via a non-native, cell-specific pathway does not appear to compromise downstream delivery of DNA to the nucleus. Based on the foregoing, a logical place to start in the development of a targeted adenoviral vector is manipulation of the knob domain. Several groups are now developing strategies to impart targeting ability to adenoviral vectors. The strategies currently being developed may be categorized as "immunologic" or "genetic."

IMMUNOLOGIC RETARGETING

Immunologic retargeting strategies are based on the use of bispecific conjugates, typically a conjugate between an antibody directed against a component of the virus

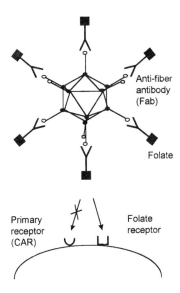

Anti-fiber
antibody
(Fab)

Folate

Primary
receptor
(CAR)

Folate
receptor

FIGURE 2. Schema for altering adenoviral tropism by an immunologic targeting approach. A retargeting moiety formed by conjugating folate to the Fab fragment of an anti-knob antibody is used to direct adenoviral binding to the folate receptor.

and a targeting antibody or ligand. True targeting requires simultaneous abolition of native targeting and introduction of new tropism; therefore, Douglas and colleagues[23] developed a neutralizing monoclonal antibody against the knob region of adenovirus. This was achieved by immunizing mice with adenovirus and recombinant knob protein, then developing hybridomas that produced antibodies capable of neutralizing native adenoviral infection (as determined by a cytopathic effect assay using HeLa cells). The Fab fragment of an antibody generated in this way (1D6.14) was then conjugated to folate to effect targeting to the folate receptor. Folate was chosen because the folate receptor is upregulated on several tumor types and the receptor internalizes after ligand binding.[24] Using this conjugate, adenoviral infection was redirected away from the native receptor to the folate receptor (FIG. 2). The gene transfer efficiency of this approach was approximately 70% of that seen with the native virus, which contrasted to the experience with retroviral retargeting where redirection had generally resulted in a dramatic fall in infectivity.[17] Although binding of the complex to cells was clearly mediated by folate, the mechanism of viral internalization was not established. In this regard, folate is normally internalized by potocytosis and enters the cell via a caveolus.[25] Normally the size of this caveolus would be too small to encompass the folate-virus complex, but whether it could enlarge under these circumstances or whether viral entry was effected by the usual integrin-mediated pathway is unknown. Using a slightly different approach, Wickham and colleagues[26] developed an adenovirus that contained a FLAG domain introduced into the penton base region and then used a bispecific antibody directed against FLAG and αv integrins to direct binding to integrins on endothelial and smooth muscle cells. Because the retargeting bispecific conjugate was larger than the viral fiber, it was hypothesized that the conjugate would be functionally available for binding by extending outward past the knob domain. In this way, by using integrins as the attachment target on these cells that express low levels of CAR, gene delivery was enhanced.

Further development in the immunologic retargeting approach was reported by Watkins and colleagues.[27] This group generated a bacteriophage library displaying single chain antibodies (sFvs) derived from the spleen of a mouse immunized against adenoviral knob. From this library a suitable neutralizing anti-knob sFv was isolated, and a fusion protein between this and epidermal growth factor (EGF) was then produced. This "adenobody" was successfully used to retarget adenoviral gene delivery, resulting in enhanced gene transfer of EGF receptor (EGFR)-expressing cells. Interestingly, this study showed that retargeting in this way appeared to bypass the need for the penton base/cell integrin interaction for internalization of the virus. This was shown by using an excess of an RGD-containing peptide that competes with penton for binding to integrins. This peptide reduced native viral gene transfer, but it had no effect on the gene transfer levels achieved with the retargeted vector complex, thus implying that in the latter case, viral entry was achieved by EGF receptor-mediated internalization. Taking a different approach to EGF receptor targeting, we used a conjugate between 1D6.14 Fab and a monoclonal antibody that binds to EGFR (mAb 425).[28,29] Using this approach, we demonstrated retargeted delivery to two murine fibroblast cell lines, one stably expressing human EGFR, the other expressing a mutant of EGFR that does not internalize (C.R. Miller, unpublished data). Therefore, depending on the target selected, it may be possible to exploit internalization mechanisms of either the targeted receptor itself or, if a noninternalizing target is selected, the native integrin pathway. The potential for overcoming a lack of integrins in some settings or the ability to target to noninternalizing cell surface molecules if integrins are sufficient implies a very broad potential applicability of retargeted vectors.

After the initial demonstration that immunologic retargeting of adenovirus could be achieved, further studies have explored the potential for therapeutic application of this approach. These applications might be considered in the context of several worthwhile goals of targeting with differing levels of stringency, including general nonspecific enhancement of delivery to a broad range of cell types, gene transfer of previously untransducible cells (relevant to both *ex vivo* and *in vivo* applications), targeting to enhance gene delivery and potentially reduce toxicity in a loco-regional or compartmental context, and cell-specific gene delivery following intravenous administration of vector.

At the lowest level of stringency, retargeting approaches to achieve enhanced gene delivery, even in the absence of a clear specificity advantage, are worthwhile in compartmentalized disease contexts. Such approaches at the very least should allow for the use of smaller doses of virus, thus potentially reducing direct viral toxic effects, dissemination from the administration site, and innate immune responses, which are clearly dose dependent. In this regard we used basic fibroblast growth factor (FGF2) as a targeting ligand, based on the knowledge that FGF receptors are upregulated in many tumor types. A conjugate between 1D6.14 Fab and FGF2 was used to retarget adenoviral infection of different tumor lines with varying baseline levels of susceptibility to adenoviral infection. Enhancements in gene transfer from 2- to greater than 10-fold were seen (B.E. Rogers, unpublished data).

With regard to the gene transfer of resistant cells, Kaposi's sarcoma (KS) is an example of a disease in which gene therapy applications have been limited in part because of the poor transducibility of this tumor (J.A. Campain, unpublished data). Goldman and colleagues[30] used the FGF2 retargeting approach to investigate retargeted gene delivery to previously untransfectable KS cell lines. The results demonstrated a dramatic increase in gene transfer. Furthermore, the potential therapeutic utility was shown by transfecting cells with a retargeted adenovirus carrying the gene for herpes simplex thymidine kinase (AdCMVHSV-TK). These cells were then far more susceptible to killing by the subsequent administration of the pro-drug ganciclovir than were cells that had been infected with the untargeted virus. T lymphocyte is another cell type that is resistant to adenoviral infection because of the lack of both CAR and αv integrins. Thus, Wickham and colleagues[31] successfully retargeted adenoviral vectors by using a conjugate between the anti-FLAG antibody and anti-CD3, thereby achieving significantly enhanced gene transfer.[31] Thus, this study indicates that the benefits of targeting can also be exploited in contexts relevant to *ex vivo* therapy.

The ability to increase the number of genetically modified cells without resorting to an increase in viral dose is extremely important in view of the direct cytotoxic effects of adenovirus. For example, in the vasculature, when gene transfer is limited by a relatively low level of CAR expression,[26] gene transfer efficiency increases with escalating viral dose over a fairly narrow range, then it dramatically falls as cytotoxicity supervenes and leads to a loss of infected cells. For example, Schulick and colleagues[32] found maximal gene transfer efficiency in vascular smooth muscle cells of approximately 40% with 5×10^{10} pfu, which decreased to zero at 10^{11} pfu; similar results were found in the endothelium.[33] Using the bispecific anti-FLAG/anti-integrin approach, Wickham[26] achieved seven- to ninefold enhancement of endothelial cell gene transfer. As FGF receptor expression is upregulated in proliferating vasculature and is therefore relevant to several pathologic processes including tumor angiogenesis, we examined the effect of FGF2 targeting of adenoviral gene delivery to proliferating endothelial cells. Here, approximately 30-fold enhancement in luciferase expression was seen. Flow cytometry analysis of cells transfected with a β-galactosidase encoding vector demonstrated that FGF2 retargeting led to both an increase in the number of genetically modified cells and an increase in the amount of gene expression per cell. By contrast, when FGF2 retargeting was used in the infection of quiescent, confluent cells, transgene expression was actually reduced, indicating a degree of cell-specific targeting based on the level of expression of the targeted receptor (P.N. Reynolds, unpublished data).

Toxicity at high viral doses has also been seen in murine carcinoma models, in which escalating the dose of a herpes simplex thymidine kinase encoding virus (HSV-TK) eventually led to death from toxicity before complete tumor eradication could be achieved.[7] Also, in the context of HSV-TK, increasing the amount of transgene expression per cell (rather than the number of genetically modified cells) by manipulation of promoters did not increase the therapeutic effect once a threshold level of expression was achieved.[34] Thus, Rancourt and colleagues investigated the use of FGF2 retargeting of AdCMVHSV-TK in a murine model of ovarian carcinoma (C. Rancourt, unpublished data). First, FGF receptor expression on the ovarian carcinoma line SKOV3.ip1 was confirmed by radiolabeled FGF binding. Then, enhancement of adenovirally mediated gene delivery to these cells using FGF2 retargeting *in vitro* with the luciferase reporter gene was demonstrated. Next, validation of the retargeting approach *in vivo* was obtained. Tumors were established in nude mice by intraperitoneal inoculation with SKOV3.ip1 cells, followed in 5 days by a peritoneal injection of AdCMVLuc either alone or with FGF2 retargeting. Mice were sacrificed, and luciferase expression in the tumors was quantified. Tumors from mice that had received the retargeted vector had a 10-fold greater level of luciferase expression. Thus, these results importantly established that immunologic retargeting was efficacious *in vivo*. Tumors were then established in mice as before, followed by intraperitoneal injection of either placebo, AdCMVHSV-TK alone, or AdCMVHSV-TK with FGF2 retargeting (with viral doses of 10^8 and 10^9 pfu). Mice were then divided into two groups, received either ganciclovir or placebo for 14 days, and were monitored for survival. The mice that did not receive ganciclovir had no survival advantage over the mice that received no gene therapy. When survival curves for mice that received ganciclovir were analyzed, two important results emerged (FIG. 3). First, a statistically significant increase in survival occurred with FGF2 retargeting than with the untargeted vector at each dose of virus. Second, the

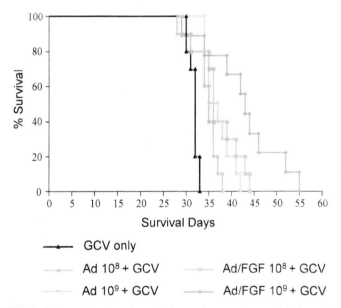

FIGURE 3. Retargeting adenovirus to enhance therapeutic gene delivery enhances survival in a murine model of ovarian carcinoma. Mice with peritoneal ovarian tumors received intraperitoneal injections of placebo or adenovirus carrying the herpes simplex thymidine kinase gene (10^8 or 10^9 pfu), either unmodified virus (Ad) or virus complexed to a retargeting moiety (formed by conjugating FGF2 to anti-knob Fab) (Ad/FGF). Mice were then treated with ganciclovir (GCV) and survival was monitored. Mice treated with retargeted adenovirus had a significant increase in median survival. Ad (10^8 pfu) vs Ad/FGF (10^8 pfu), $p = 0.0025$; Ad (10^9 pfu) vs Ad/FGF (10^9 pfu), $p = 0.007$.

survival curve for mice treated with 10^8 pfu of virus with FGF2 retargeting was the same as that for mice treated with 10^9 pfu of untargeted vector. Thus, FGF2 retargeting effected a 10-fold reduction in viral dose for the same therapeutic outcome. These results thus indicate a potential for increasing the clinical utility and therapeutic index of adenoviral vectors by using a retargeting approach.

Successful targeting following intravenous administration of a targeted adenoviral vector has yet to be reported. In this context, one major hurdle to overcome is hepatic uptake of injected virus, which accounts for greater than 90% of the injected dose. Although initially this problem was considered to be due in part to nonspecific uptake related to entrapment of virus in hepatic sinusoids, recent evidence suggests that this is a receptor-mediated phenomenon and therefore it is potentially addressed by modification of native viral tropism. To this end, Zinn and colleagues[35] investigated the *in vivo* distribution of technetium-labeled adenovirus serotype 5 (Ad5) knob. They found that most of it became localized to the liver 10 minutes after injection. Importantly, this localization could be inhibited by prior injection of an excess of unlabeled Ad5 knob, but not by an excess of serotype 3 (Ad3) knob (which binds to a different receptor), indicating the specificity of hepatic uptake. When labeled Ad5 knob was complexed with 1D6.14 Fab before injection, hepatic uptake was markedly reduced, providing further evidence of the receptor-dependent nature of the uptake and a degree of stability of the Fab to knob bond in the bloodstream.

In summary, developments thus far using immunologic retargeting strategies have established several important principles. Modification of tropism was successfully achieved, indicating that true cell-specific delivery is possible. Evidence to date suggests that limitations in gene transfer due to a deficiency in either CAR, αv integrins, or both may be overcome by retargeting. Not only is efficiency of gene delivery with retargeted complexes comparable to that of wild-type vector, but also in many cases it has resulted in substantial improvement in gene delivery, which is itself a worthwhile goal. Retargeted complexes are efficacious *in vivo*, at least in a compartmental context. The use of a retargeted vector has been shown to enhance a therapeutic endpoint, and finally, the limitations of intravenous application of these vectors, imposed by hepatic uptake of virus, appear to be a receptor-mediated phenomenon and may therefore also be overcome by retargeting. The full potential of immunologic retargeting, however, is yet to be defined, and there are certain practical and theoretic limitations to this approach. Large scale production of bispecific antibody conjugates of consistent configuration is difficult when using the heterobifunctional crosslinkers that have so far been reported. Also, clearance of retargeting complexes and activation of the complement system may limit *in vivo* application. Although further protein engineering refinements, such as the fusion protein "adenobody" approach, may address some of these issues, the stability of the targeting complex-virion bond following systemic delivery remains of concern, especially when attempting intravenous administration. Thus, development of another approach, genetic retargeting, is also being pursued.

GENETIC RETARGETING

In view of the practical and theoretic limitations of the immunologic approach to retargeting just mentioned, development of targeted vectors by genetic manipulation of the virus itself has proceeded alongside the immunologic strategies. In addition, the immunologic targeting approach is not likely to be sufficient for application to the controlled replicating viral vector systems being developed to improve gene delivery to malignant tumors. In these systems, precise targeting of both the initial viral dose and the progeny viruses is particularly important and only achievable by genetic modifications.

Based on the knowledge of native viral binding, a rational place to begin in the development of genetically targeted vectors is with the knob domain, and most strategies have so far focused on this region. The question of whether viral tropism could be modified genetically was initially addressed by Krasnykh and colleagues.[36] A chimeric adenovirus containing the serotype 3 knob on the adenovirus 5 fiber shaft and capsid was produced by homologous recombination in 293 cells, using a modification of the shuttle and rescue plasmid technique developed by Graham.[37] Because Ad5 and Ad3 recognize different receptors, the tropism of the chimeric vector could be assessed by blocking infection of cells with an excess of free Ad5 or Ad3 recombinant knob. This confirmed that an 'Ad5' vector possessing Ad3 tropism had been produced. A similar strategy was reported by Stevenson and colleagues[38] who also demonstrated differences in the gene transfer efficiency of various cell lines depending on whether wild-type or chimeric fiber vectors were used.[38] After the initial proof of principle, incorporation of specific targeting ligands was investigated.

When modifying the knob domain, important structural constraints must be addressed. Because fibers must trimerize to allow attachment to the penton base for subsequent capsid formation, any modification of the fiber must not perturb trimerization.[39] Incorporation of a small ligand (gastrin-releasing peptide) at the carboxy terminal of fiber and subsequent generation of trimers of this chimeric fiber were initially reported by Michael and colleagues.[40] It has since been discovered that there are limits to the size of peptides that can be used in this way. Although the limits probably relate to the actual sequence used rather than its length alone, trimerization is much less likely to occur with ligands longer than 25–30 amino acids. On the other hand, deletion of just 1 amino acid from the carboxy terminal leads to failure of trimerization. Despite these limitations, the addition of small peptide ligands may have utility. For example, we recently added a moiety containing 6 histidine residues (6-His) to the knob carboxy terminal, successfully rescued the virus, and confirmed the binding availability of the 6-His moiety using nickel column chromatography. This virus may be used to address concerns about the stability of the bond between adenoviral vectors and immunologic retargeting complexes. Theoretically, using an immunologic retargeting complex containing an anti-6His antibody, followed by the use of nickel MMPP technology, might allow the formation of a stable covalent bond between the virus and the targeting complex.[41] Wickham[42] recently reported a number of carboxy terminal modifications, including one containing an RGD motif (21 amino acids) to target cell surface integrins and one containing seven lysine residues to target cell surface heparan sulfates. Production of virus with longer carboxy terminal additions was also attempted. A virus containing a 32 amino acid peptide for targeting the laminin receptor was produced, but it failed to bind its target receptor, whereas a virus containing a 27 amino acid E-selectin binding peptide could not be produced. Neither of the successfully produced viruses had any modification to native tropism; therefore, their potential application is in the context of enhancing delivery to otherwise poorly transfectable cells, rather than true cell-specific targeting.

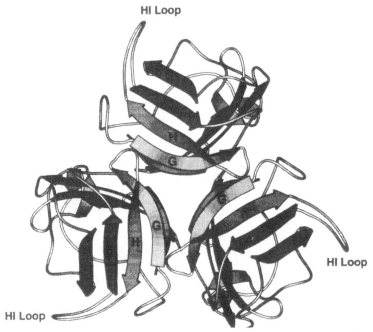

FIGURE 4. The knob trimer showing the position of the HI loop. Reprinted, with permission, from Xia *et al.,*[43] p. 42.

Nevertheless, enhanced vascular delivery using the polylysine virus was demonstrated *in vivo* in a vascular injury model and may have utility in the therapy of angioplasty restenosis. The RGD-containing virus enhanced gene delivery to endothelial and smooth muscle cells *in vitro.*

In view of the limitations involved in attaching ligands to the carboxy terminal, other regions of the knob may ultimately prove to be better sites for ligand incorporation. In this regard, we investigated the HI loop region of the knob. X-ray crystallographic modeling of the three-dimensional structure of trimeric knob indicates that the HI loop is located on the outer aspect in an area potentially available for interaction with receptors (FIG. 4).[43,44] Also, this region does not appear to be directly involved in trimerization, contains mostly hydrophilic amino acids, and is different lengths in different Ad serotypes, suggesting less rigid structural constraints than at the carboxy terminal. As initial proof of concept we successfully incorporated a FLAG epitope into the HI loop[45] using a technique of recombinant virus generation involving homologous recombination in *Escherichia coli.*[46] Affinity binding to an M2 matrix column confirmed that this epitope was available for binding in the context of the intact virion. Other ligands with more relevant targeting potential have now been incorporated, including a cyclic RGD peptide (which has affinity for tumor vasculature)[47] and somatostatin. The size constraints of ligand incorporation at this site are yet to be determined; therefore, incorporation of large ligands such as EGF and sFvs is currently being investigated. However, it is likely that the sheer size of an sFv will require an alternate strategy such as complete replacement of the entire knob domain.

Ultimately, for true targeting to be achieved, modification to ablate native tropism will need to be addressed. It may be that incorporation of large ligands into the HI loop will simultaneously ablate native tropism by steric hindrance; however, if this is not the case, further modifications will be required. In this regard, receptor binding epitopes within the knob that may be suitable for mutagenesis strategies have been identified by Boulanger.[48] Clearly, if complete replacement of the knob with a targeting and trimerization moiety could be achieved, it would simultaneously ablate native tropism. An integral part of any such strategy will be the use of permissive cell lines possessing the relevant target receptor to allow rescue and propagation of the virus.

Genetic modification strategies are not limited to the fiber. Wickham[49] introduced modifications into the penton base for targeting to cell-specific integrins. Hexon capsid proteins might also be exploited for targeting. An attractive aspect of this approach is the number of hexon proteins, 720, compared to the 36 knob regions; therefore, hexon modification might have the potential for higher affinity binding. Such a strategy, however, will still have to take into account the need to ablate native knob-dependent binding and to address the stoichiometric issues relating to the fiber projecting out from the capsid, to ensure physical accessibility of the ligands introduced into the hexon.

As progress is being made in the development of retargeted vectors, the importance of identifying truly cell-specific ligands has been highlighted. Although there are many established ligands and antibodies that may be candidates in certain settings, in many cases, such as mature airway epithelium, truly specific targets have yet to be discovered; therefore, further target definition is required. This is especially relevant in the context of those genetic retargeting strategies that attempt to target with small peptide ligands. In this regard, the use of bacteriophage panning techniques have shown potential utility in target definition.[47,50,51] Bacteriophage can be engineered to express peptide sequences of various lengths and configurations (e.g., linear or cyclic) on their surface. Libraries of phage can be generated that express all possible sequences of peptide of a defined length or configuration. Using this library we can pan against target proteins, cells, or even organs and tissues *in vivo*. By isolating from the library the phage that has affinity for the target of interest, serial rounds of panning can ultimately identify peptide sequences that show particular affinity for the target. For example, using this approach *in vivo*, Pasqualini and colleagues[52] identified a double cyclic RGD-containing peptide with particular affinity for tumor vasculature. Similar strategies are also being used to define sFvs with targeting potential.

In summary, it has clearly been shown that viral tropism can be modified by genetic strategies. Concurrent ablation of native tropism has not yet been achieved however. The targeting ligands that have been successfully introduced at this stage are limited to short peptides, and incorporation of larger ligands may require new approaches. Nevertheless, progress in this area has been rapid, and the results to date, coupled with the immunologic retargeting results, indicate that development of a systemically stable, cell-specific vector is a very realistic aim.

ACKNOWLEDGMENTS

We appreciate the secretarial support of Connie H. Weldon. The work cited in this manuscript was conducted at the Gene Therapy Center, University of Alabama at Birmingham and was supported by the following grants: National Institutes of Health grants RO1CA74242 (DTC), RO1CA68245 (DTC), and HL50255 (DTC); American Heart Association grant 965075-1W (DTC); a grant from the US Department of Defense (DTC); and a grant from the American Lung Association (DTC).

REFERENCES

1. ANDERSON W.F. & J.C. FLETCHER. 1980. Sounding boards. Gene therapy in human beings: When is it ethical to begin? N. Engl. J. Med. **303:** 1293–1297.
2. BRODY S.L. & R.G. CRYSTAL. 1994. Adenovirus-mediated in vivo gene transfer. Ann. N.Y. Acad. Sci. **716:** 90–101.
3. TOMKO R.P., R. XU & L. PHILIPSON. 1997. HCAR and MCAR: The human and mouse cellular receptors for subgroup C adenoviruses and group B coxsackieviruses. Proc. Natl. Acad. Sci. **94:** 3352–3356.
4. YANG, Y., K.U. JOOSS, Q. SU et al. 1996. Immune responses to viral antigens versus transgene product in the elimination of recombinant adenovirus-infected hepatocytes in vivo. Gene Ther. **3:** 137–144.
5. YANG, Y., Q. LI, H.C. ERTL et al. 1995. Cellular and humoral immune responses to viral antigens create barriers to lung-directed gene therapy with recombinant adenoviruses. J. Virol. **69:** 2004–2015.
6. ESANDI, M.C., G.D. VAN SOMEREN, A.J. VINCENT et al. 1997. Gene therapy of experimental malignant mesothelioma using adenovirus vectors encoding the HSVtk gene. Gene Ther. **4:** 280–287.
7. YEE, D., S.E. MCGUIRE, N. BRUNNER et al. 1996. Adenovirus-mediated gene transfer of herpes simplex virus thymidine kinase in an ascites model of human breast cancer. Hum. Gene Ther. **7:** 1251–1257.
8. BELLON, G., L. MICHEL-CALEMARD et al. 1997. Aerosol administration of a recombinant adenovirus expressing CFTR to cystic fibrosis patients: A phase I clinical trial. Hum. Gene Ther. **8:** 15–25.
9. CRYSTAL, R.G., N.G. MCELVANEY, M.A. ROSENFELD et al. 1994. Administration of an adenovirus containing the human CFTR cDNA to the respiratory tract of individuals with cystic fibrosis. Nat. Genet. **8:** 42–51.
10. KNOWLES, M.R., K.W. HOHNEKER, Z. ZHOU et al. 1995. A controlled study of adenoviral-vector-mediated gene transfer in the nasal epithelium of patients with cystic fibrosis [see comments]. N. Engl. J. Med. **333:** 823–831.
11. ZABNER, J., L.A. COUTURE, R.J. GREGORY et al. 1993. Adenovirus-mediated gene transfer transiently corrects the chloride transport defect in nasal epithelia of patients with cystic fibrosis. Cell **75:** 207–216.
12. ZABNER, J., B.W. RAMSEY, D.P. MEEKER et al. 1996. Repeat administration of an adenovirus vector encoding cystic fibrosis transmembrane conductance regulator to the nasal epithelium of patients with cystic fibrosis. J. Clin. Invest. **97:** 1504–1511.
13. GOLDMAN, M., Q. SU & J.M. WILSON. 1996. Gradient of RGD-dependent entry of adenoviral vector in nasal and intrapulmonary epithelia: Implications for gene therapy of cystic fibrosis. Gene Ther. **3:** 811–818.
14. GOLDMAN, M.J. & J.M. WILSON. 1995. Expression of alpha v beta 5 integrin is necessary for efficient adenovirus-mediated gene transfer in the human airway. J. Virol. **69:** 5951–5958.
15. GRUBB, B.R., R.J. PICKLES, H. YE et al. 1994. Inefficient gene transfer by adenovirus vector to cystic fibrosis airway epithelia of mice and humans. Nature **371:** 802–806.

16. ZABNER, J., P. FREIMUTH, A. PUGA *et al.* 1997. Lack of high affinity fiber receptor activity explains the resistance of ciliated airway epithelia to adenovirus infection. J. Clin. Invest. **100:** 1144–1149.
17. COSSET, F.L. & S.J. RUSSELL. 1996. Targeting retrovirus entry. Gene Ther. **3:** 946–956.
18. SHENK, T. 1996. Adenoviridae: The viruses and their replication. *In* Fields Virology B.N. Fields, D.M. Knipe & P.M. Howley, Eds. 3rd Ed. :2111–2148. Lippincott-Raven. Philadelphia.
19. BERGELSON, J.M., J.A.CUNNINGHAM, G. DROGUETT *et al.* 1997. Isolation of a common receptor for Coxsackie B viruses and adenoviruses 2 and 5. Science **275:** 1320–1333.
20. HONG, S.S., L. KARAYAN, J. TOURNIER *et al.* 1997. Adenovirus type 5 fiber knob binds to MHC Class I alpha-2 domain at the surface of human epithelial and B lymphoblastoid cells. EMBO J. **16:** 2294–2306.
21. WICKHAM, T.J., P. MATHIAS, D.A. CHEREH *et al.* 1993. Integrins alpha v beta 3 and alpha v beta 5 promote adenovirus internalization but not virus attachment. Cell **73:** 309–319.
22. MICHAEL, S.I., C.H. HUANG, M.U. ROMER *et al.* 1993. Binding-incompetent adenovirus facilitates molecular conjugate-mediated gene transfer by the receptor-mediated endocytosis pathway. J. Biol. Chem. **268:** 6866–6869.
23. DOUGLAS, J.T., B.E. ROGERS, M.E. ROSENFELD *et al.* 1996. Targeted gene delivery by tropism-modified adenoviral vectors. Nat. Biotech. **14:** 1574–1578.
24. WEITMAN, S.D., R.H. LARK, L.R. CONEY *et al.* 1992. Distribution of the folate receptor GP38 in normal and malignant cell lines and tissues. Cancer Res. **52:** 3396–3401.
25. ANDERSON, R.G., B.A. KAMEN, K.G. ROTHBERG *et al.* 1992. Potocytosis: Sequestration and transport of small molecules by caveolae. Science **255:** 410–411.
26. WICKHAM, T.J., D.M. SEGAL, P.W. ROELVINK *et al.* 1996. Targeted adenovirus gene transfer to endothelial and smooth muscle cells by using bispecific antibodies. J. Virol. **70:** 6831–6838.
27. WATKINS, S.J., V.V. MESYANZHINOV, L.P. KUROCHKINA *et al.* 1997. The adenobody approach to viral targeting: Specific and enhanced adenoviral gene delivery. Gene Ther. **4:** 1004–1012.
28. MURTHY, U., A. BASU, U. *et al.* 1987. Binding of an antagonistic monoclonal antibody to an intact and fragmented EGF-receptor polypeptide. Arch. Biochem. Biophys. **252:** 549–560.
29. WERSALL, P., I. OHLSSON, P. BIBERFELD *et al.* 1997. Intratumoral infusion of the monoclonal antibody, mAb 425, against the epidermal-growth-factor receptor in patients with advanced malignant glioma. Cancer Immunol. Immunother. **44:** 157–64.
30. GOLDMAN, C.K., B.E. ROGERS, J.T. DOUGLAS *et al.* 1997. Targeted gene delivery to Kaposi's sarcoma cells via the fibroblast growth factor receptor. Cancer Res. **57:** 1447–1451.
31. WICKHAM, T.J., G.M. LEE, J.A. TITUS *et al.* 1997. Targeted adenovirus-mediated gene delivery to T cells via CD3. J. Virol. **71:** 7663–7669.
32. SCHULICK, A.H., K.D. NEWMAN, R. VIRMANI *et al.* 1995. In vivo gene transfer into injured carotid arteries. Optimization and evaluation of acute toxicity. Circulation **91:** 2407–2414.
33. SCHULICK, A.H., G. DONG, K.D. NEWMAN *et al.* 1995. Endothelium-specific in vivo gene transfer. Circ. Res. **77:** 475–485.
34. ELSHAMI, A.A., J.W. COOK, K.M. AMIN *et al.* 1997. The effect of promoter strength in adenoviral vectors containing herpes simplex virus thymidine kinase on cancer gene therapy in vitro and in vivo. Cancer Gene Ther. **4:** 213–221.

35. ZINN, K.R., C. SMYTH, H.-G. LIU et al. 1998. Imaging and tissue biodistribution of 99-m-Tc-labeled adenovirus knob (serotype 5). Gene Ther. **5.** In press.

36. KRASNYKH, V.N., G.V. MIKHEEVA, J.T. DOUGLAS et al. 1996. Generation of recombinant adenovirus vectors with modified fibers for altering viral tropism. J. Virol. **70:** 6839–6846.

37. GRAHAM, F. & L. PREVEC. 1991. Manipulation of adenovirus vectors. In Methods in Molecular Biology. E.J. Murray & J.M. Walker, Eds. Vol. 7. Gene Transfer and Expression Techniques. :109–129. Humana Press. Clifton, NJ.

38. STEVENSON, S.C., M. ROLLENCE, J. MARSHALLNEFF et. al. 1997. Selective targeting of human cells by a chimeric adenovirus vector containing a modified fiber protein. J. Virol. **71:** 4782–4790.

39. NOVELLI, A. & P.A. BOULANGER. 1991. Deletion analysis of functional domains in baculovirus-expressed adenovirus type 2 fiber. Virology **185:** 365–376.

40. MICHAEL, S.I., J.S. HONG, D.T. CURIEL et al. 1995. Addition of a short peptide ligand to the adenovirus fiber protein. Gene Ther. **2:** 660–668.

41. FANCY, D.A., K. MELCHER, S.A. JOHNSTON et al. 1996. New chemistry for the study of multiprotein complexes: the six-histidine tag as a receptor for a protein crosslinking reagent. Chem. Biol. **3:** 551–559.

42. WICKHAM, T.J., E. TZENG, L.L. SHEARS et al. 1997. Increased in vitro and in vivo gene transfer by adenovirus vectors containing chimeric fiber proteins. J. Virol. **71:** 8221–8229.

43. XIA, D., L. HENRY, R.D. GERARD et al. 1995. Structure of the receptor binding domain of adenovirus type 5 fiber protein. In The Molecular Repertoire of Adenoviruses 1. W. Doerfler & P. Bohm, Eds. : 39–46. Springer-Verlag. Berlin.

44. XIA, D., L.J. HENRY, R.D. GERARD et al. 1994. Crystal structure of the receptor-binding domain of adenovirus type 5 fiber protein at 1.7 A resolution. Structure **2:** 1259–1270.

45. KRASNYKH, V., I. DMITRIEV, G. MIKHEEVA et al. 1998. Characterization of an adenovirus vector containing a heterologous peptide epitope in the HI loop of the fiber knob. J. Virol. In press.

46. CHARTIER, C., E. DEGRYSE, M. GANTZIER et al. 1996. Efficient generation of recombinant adenovirus vectors by homologous recombination in Escherichia coli. J. Virol. **70:** 4805–4810.

47. PASQUALINI, R., E. KOIVUNEN, E. RUOSLAHTI et al. 1997. Alpha v integrins as receptors for tumor targeting by circulating ligands. Nat. Biotech. **15:** 542–546.

48. HONG, S.S. & P. BOULANGER. 1995. Protein ligands of the human adenovirus type 2 outer capsid identified by biopanning of a phage-displayed peptide library on separate domains of wild-type and mutant penton capsomers. EMBO J. **14:** 4714–4727.

49. WICKHAM, T.J., M.E. CARRION & I. KOVESDI. 1995. Targeting of adenovirus penton base to new receptors through replacement of its RGD motif with other receptor-specific peptide motifs. Gene Ther. **2:** 750–756.

50. BARRY, M.A., W.J. DOWER & S.A. JOHNSTON. 1996. Toward cell-targeting gene therapy vectors: selection of cell-binding peptides from random peptide-presenting phage libraries. Nat. Med. **2:** 299–305.

51. PASQUALINI, R. & E. RUOSLAHTI. 1996. Organ targeting in vivo using phage display peptide libraries. Nature **380:** 364–366.

52. NERI, D., B. CARNEMOLLA, A. NISSIM et al. 1997. Targeting by affinity-matured recombinant antibody fragments of an angiogenesis associated fibronectin isoform. Nat. Biotech. **15:** 1271–1275.

Homeodomain-Derived Peptides

In and Out of the Cells

ALAIN PROCHIANTZ[a]

Ecole Normale Supérieure, CNRS UMR 8542, 46, rue d'Ulm,
75230 Paris Cedex 05, France

ABSTRACT: The internalization of homeodomains and of homeopeptides derived from the third helix of the homeodomain of Antennapedia, a *Drosophila* transcription factor, is used by some investigators to target exogenous hydrophilic compounds into live cells. In addition to this very practical aspect of drug delivery, translocation across biologic membranes of peptides subsequently addressed to the cell cytoplasm and nucleus raises several questions. A first series of questions pertains to the mechanism of translocation. Thanks to the synthesis of several peptides derived from the third helix of the Antennapedia homeodomain, we began to investigate the mechanism of translocation and we have shown that it is not dependent upon the presence of a chiral receptor and probably involves the formation of inverted micelles. A second series of questions is related to the physiologic significance of the phenomenon. In a first approach, we demonstrated that some full-length homeoproteins are internalized and secreted *in vitro*. The mechanism of internalization is probably similar to that of the homeodomain or of its third helix, but secretion involves a different mechanism which requires an association with specialized intracellular membranous structures. The existence of specific mechanisms for homeoprotein internalization and secretion suggests that this class of transcription factors may have important signaling properties.

INTRODUCTION

Homeoproteins define a class of transcription factors involved in multiple biologic processes, primarily but not only during development,[1] and characterized by their DNA-binding domain, the homeodomain. The homeodomain is highly conserved across homeoproteins and across species (reviewed in ref. 2). Its long sequence of 60 amino acids is composed of three α-helices. Homeoproteins are expressed in all tissues, including the central nervous system, where they are responsible for the early differentiation of large morphologic domains. For example, the genetic deletion of *Engrailed-1*, a homeogene expressed in the midbrain/hindbrain, leads to nearly total disappearance of this territory in the mouse (reviewed in refs. 3 and 4). In addition to their early patterning function, homeogenes have a role late in development. Indeed, mutations in homeogenes can modify the specificity of axonal pathways[5–7] and synapse formation.[8–10] Accordingly, they are expressed throughout development and, in fact, in adulthood, suggesting a possible role in the morphologic plasticity that characterizes the developing and adult vertebrate nervous system.

[a]Phone, 0033 (0)1 44 32 39 26; fax, 0033 (0)1 44 32 39 88.
e-mail, prochian@wotan.ens.fr

TRANSLOCATING HOMEODOMAINS

To investigate the function of homeoproteins in neurite outgrowth, we adapted a protocol aimed at antagonizing the activity of endogenous homeoproteins through the mechanical internalization of homeodomains into postmitotic neurons.[11–13] During the latter experiments we accidently discovered that the homeodomain of Antennapedia, a *Drosophila* transcription factor, is internalized by cells in culture. [13–16]

This capture takes place at 4° and 37°C, it does not depend on classical endocytosis, and the homeodomain is directly addressed to the cytoplasm and eventually to the nucleus of the cells. We then generated several point mutations in the homeodomain[16,17] and described modifications leading to different properties. Some mutants, still internalized but deprived of their specific DNA-binding properties, were instrumental in showing that the stimulatory effect of the Antennapedia homeodomain on neurite elongation takes place at the transcriptional level.[14,16,17] However, in the context of this conference, the most interesting modification is the removal of two aminoacids, a tryptophan and a phenylalanine, present in positions 48 and 49 of the homeodomain, thus within the third helix.[16] Indeed, that this mutated homeodomain was incapable of translocating across biologic membranes suggested that the third helix might be responsible in part for the unexpected translocating properties of the entire homeodomain.

PENETRATINS

We thus chemically synthesized the third helix and followed its internalization by live cells in culture thanks to an added biotine residue. This peptide of 16 residues which corresponds almost exactly to the third helix of the homeodomain (amino acids 43 to 58 of the homeodomain), was internalized with an efficiency comparable to that of the entire homeodomain.[18] Because shorter peptides (15 amino acids long) failed to translocate across the membrane, it was proposed that the 16 amino-acid long polypeptide is necessary and sufficient for the internalization of the entire Antennapedia homeodomain. It was therefore termed Penetratin-1 and used as a matrix for the synthesis of several other peptides. FIGURE 1 presents a few examples of the peptides that have been produced and tested for translocation.

With the exception of Phe48,56 in which the two tryptophan residues have been replaced by two phenylalanins, all peptides in FIGURE 1 are internalized at 4°C and 37°C,[19] thus defining the penetratin family (also called Trojan peptides[20]). All of them are addressed directly to the cytoplasm of cells from which they can be retrieved without apparent degradation. Contrary to Penetratin-1, some variants, in particular those with one or three prolines, do not travel from the cytoplasm to the nucleus and may therefore be used for more specific cytoplasmic targeting. Translocation across the plasma membrane is not concentration dependent (at least between 10 pM and 100 μM), and toxicity is rare below 10 μM.

To investigate the presence of a chiral receptor, we synthesized two peptides, a peptide in which the order of amino acids is reversed (58–43 instead of 43–58) and a peptide entirely composed of D-enantiomers. The two peptides are internalized, thus almost certainly precluding the presence of a chiral receptor. This is an impor-

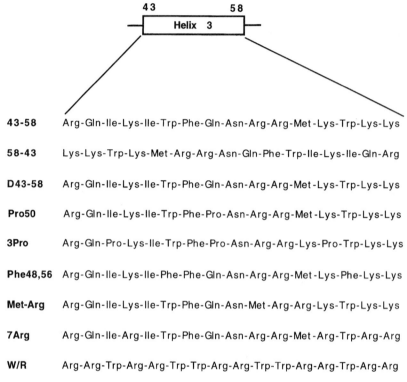

FIGURE 1. Amino acid sequences of the Antennapedia third helix (43–58) and of its derived peptides. All peptides presented in this table except Phe48,56 retain the ability to cross the cytoplasmic membrane.

tant property as it might explain why penetratins translocate across the plasma membrane of all cell types tested to this day, even though translocation can be modulated by the presence of highly charged macromolecules, such as polysialic acid.[15]

Penetratin-1 is poorly structured in water but adopts a helical structure in a hydrophobic environment.[18] We therefore wanted to know if a helical conformation, adopted in the hydrophobic environment of the membrane, was necessary. To this end, helicity was broken by introducing one or three proline residues within the sequence (FIG. 1). Because these two peptides are internalized, we concluded that translocation across the plasma membrane does not require a helical conformation.[19]

INVERTED MICELLES?

Interestingly, a peptide in which the two tryptophan residues (positions 43 and 58) have been replaced by two phenylalanins is not internalized[18] (FIG. 1). This peptide was used to compare its interactions with brain phospholipids with those of Penetratin-1. It was observed, by ^{31}P-NMR, that Penetratin-1 but not the non-

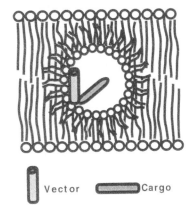

FIGURE 2. A model for Antennapedia third helix and cargo internalization. The peptides interact with charged phospholipids on the outer side of the membrane. Destabilization of the bilayer results in the formation of inverted micelles that travel across the membrane and eventually open on its cytoplasmic side. Note that in this model the peptides never leave an aqueous environment and can thus accommodate a cargo.

internalized variant provokes the formation of inverted micelles (ref. 21 and unpublished observations). In support of the inverted micelle hypothesis, fluorescence and ^{1}H-NMR spectroscopies demonstrated that the conformational flexibility of the peptide backbones is compatible with their adaptation to the concave surface of SDS micelles and to the convex surface of a reverse micelle.[21]

We are therefore encouraged to propose a model of internalization in which (FIG. 2) the peptides, localized in the reverse micelle, travel across the plasma membrane within a hydrophilic pocket. The direct association of the peptides with the membrane probably involves electrostatic interactions which, in SDS micelles, can be due to SDS itself[21] and, in natural membranes, may require the presence of charged phospholipids, gangliosides, glycosaminoglycans, or polysialic acid. It is noteworthy in this context that polysialic acid increases the rate of internalization of the Antennapedia homeodomain by a factor of four.[15] A similar model based on inverted micelle formation has been proposed for the translocation of apocytochrome c into mitochondria.[22]

USE OF PENETRATINS TO INTERNALIZE HYDROPHILIC CARGOES INTO LIVE CELLS

In the inverted micelle model, the peptides remain inside a hydrophilic environment. As schematized in FIGURE 2, it was therefore plausible that hydrophilic molecules linked to penetratins can be internalized by live cells. This was proven to be the case, and several applications of this finding have been developed and recently reviewed.[20,23] Many oligonucleotides, peptides, and phosphopeptides have been internalized *in vitro* (reviewed in ref. 20). For example, specific phosphopeptides interacting with the SH2 domains of Grb2 or PLCγ were developed to block the signaling pathways of FGF or EGF receptors in a highly specific manner.[24,25] Another interesting application is the *in vitro* blockage of the interaction between p16 and cyclin-dependent kinases.[26]

It is worth mentioning that Penetratins have also been used *in vivo*. The first *in vivo* application was the induction of the T-cell response by specific antigenic peptides linked to the homeodomain of Antennapedia and internalized by antigen-presenting cells.[27] The principle of the experiment was to address the epitope into the cell cytoplasm to allow its presentation in the MHC-I context. In the latter study, in contrast with *in vitro* priming, *in vivo* immunization was possible only when the peptide was associated with negative charges under the form of SDS or polysialic acid. We speculate that the role of negative charges is to protect the peptides from degradation and to allow their diffusion within the organism.

The second *in vivo* application was with peptide nucleic acids (PNAs). PNAs are oligonucleotides in which the sugar-phosphate backbone has been replaced with a neutral peptide backbone. This modification confers to the molecules the specificity of antisense oligonucleotides and the resistance of peptides. Unfortunately, PNAs are only poorly internalized by live cells, and this has limited, until now, their use *in vitro* and *in vivo*. Recently, it was shown the PNAs directed against type-1 galanin receptor (Gal-R1) and linked to Penetratin-1 are internalized *in vivo*. Following internalization, they specifically downregulate the synthesis of Gal-R1 and the physiologic activity of galanin.[28]

THE PARACRINE HYPOTHESIS

The third helix is a highly conserved structure among homeodomains,[2] suggesting that translocation might represent an intrinsic property of many homeodomains and homeoproteins. This was verified for the homeodomains of Fushi tarazu, Engrailed, Hoxa-5-, Hoxc-8, and for full-length homeoproteins (Engrailed, Hoxa-5, and Hoxc-8) (refs. 29–31 and unpublished experiments). It was shown in particular that Hoxa-5 is internalized by neurons in culture and targeted to their nuclei.[29] Internalization occurs at very low concentrations (in the pM range), is not inhibited at 4°C, and requires the presence of the homeodomain. It is therefore likely that the mechanisms responsible for Hoxa-5 internalization are similar to those described for homeodomains and penetratins. On this basis, we proposed that homeoproteins may have unsuspected paracrine activity.[32]

To test this hypothesis we expressed the Engrailed homeoprotein in COS-7 cells cocultured with rat neurons. The Engrailed homeoprotein is secreted by expressing cells, captured by the neurons, and addressed to neuronal nuclei.[31] Engrailed homeoprotein was retrieved intact from the neurons, demonstrating that the full-length transcription factor can transfer from producing to receiving cells. We then mutated the protein and identified a sequence of 11 amino acids overlapping the second and third helices of the homeodomain and necessary for Engrailed secretion.

USE OF PENETRATINS TO IDENTIFY GENETIC PATHWAYS

To identify target genes in the genetic pathway of Engrailed homeoprotein, we have developed an approach that combines induction gene trap in embryonic stem (ES) cells[33,34] with the ability of extracellularly applied homeodomains to gain direct access to the cytoplasm and nucleus of cells in culture. Once in the nucleus, translocated homeodomains interfere with the transcriptional activity of endogenous homeoproteins. Because Engrailed homeoprotein is expressed in undifferentiated ES cells,[35] this technology was applied to screen ES cells for genes active in the *Engrailed* genetic pathway, allowing us to identify several genes, in particular *BPAG1*, as candidate targets of Engrailed proteins.[36]

It is noteworthy that this technology is not limited to homeoprotein and that through the internalization of a polypeptide capable of interacting with intracellular effectors expressed in ES cells, one could, in principle, identify genes up- or down-regulated in response to the intracellular interaction between the bait and its target, be it protein or nucleic acid.

CONCLUSIONS

The internalization of proteins or peptides across biologic membranes is not limited to homeoproteins or homeoprotein-derived peptides. In addition to toxins, which have been the focus of several studies,[37] other proteins share similar properties, including TAT transcription factor, lactoferrin, Herpes VP22 protein, and FGF-2.[32,38-40] It is also noteworthy that if one adds to all known homeodomain third helices and their variants (as in FIG. 1) their reverse helices, the list of sequences possibly internalized by live cells might rapidly become long enough to allow the identification of conserved structural traits. The obvious hope is that the availability of a large series of peptides with translocating properties will lead to the synthesis of peptidomimetic molecules which, needless to say, will be of invaluable pharmaceutical interest.

ACKNOWLEDGMENTS

The help of EC through grants Biomed 950524 and Biotech 960146 is acknowledged.

REFERENCES

1. KRUMLAUF, R. 1994. Hox genes in vertebrate development. Cell **78:** 191–201.
2. GEHRING, W.J., Y.Q. QIAN, M. BILLETER, K. FURUKUBO-TOKUNAGA, A.F. SCHIER, D. RESENDEZ-PEREZ, M. AFFOLTER, G. OTTING & K. WÜTHRICH. 1994. Homeodomain-DNA recognition. Cell **78:** 211–223.
3. JOYNER, A.L. 1996. *Engrailed, Wnt* and *Pax* genes regulate midbrain-hindbrain development. Trends Genet. **12:** 15–20.
4. JOYNER, A.L. & M. HANKS. 1991. The engrailed genes: Evolution of function. Semin. Dev. Biol. **2:** 435–445.
5. DOE, C.Q. & M.P. SCOTT. 1988. Segmentation and homeotic gene function in the developing nervous system of Drosophila. Trends Neurosci. **11:** 101–107.
6. DOE, C.Q., S. SMOUSE & C.S. GOODMAN. 1988. Control of neuronal fate by the *Drosophila* segmentation gene even-skipped. Nature **333:** 376–378.
7. LE MOUELLIC, H., Y. LALLEMAND & P. BRULET. 1992. Homeosis in the mouse induced by a null mutation in the *Hox-3.1* gene. Cell **69:** 251-264.
8. MILLER, D.M., M.M. SHEN, C.E. SHAMU, T.R. BURGLIN, G. RUVKIN, M.L. DUBOIS, M. GHEE & L. WILSON. 1992. C. elegans *unc-4* genes encode a homeoprotein that determines the pattern of synaptic input to specific motor neurons. Nature **355:** 841-845.
9. TIRET, L., H. LE MOUELLIC, M. MAURY & P. BRÛLET. 1998. Increased apoptosis of motoneurons and altered somatotopic maps in the brachial spinal cord of Hoxc-8-deficient mice. Development **125:** 279–291.

10. WHITE, J.G., E. SOUTHGATE & J.N. THOMSON. 1992. Mutations in *Caenorhabditis elegans unc-4* gene alter the synaptic input to ventral cord motor neurons. Nature **355:** 838–841.32.

11. AYALA, J., N. TOUCHOT, A. ZAHRAOUI, A. TAVITIAN & A. PROCHIANTZ. 1990. The product of *rab2*, a small GTP binding protein, increases neuronal adhesion and neurite growth *in vitro*. Neuron **4:** 797–805.

12. BORASIO, G.D., J. JOHN, A. WITTINGHOFER, Y.-A. BARDE, M. SENDTNER & R. HEUGMAN. 1989. Ras p21 protein promotes survival and fiber outgrowth of cultured embryonics neurons. Neuron **2:** 1087-1096.

13. JOLIOT, A., C. PERNELLE, H. DEAGOSTINI-BAZIN & A. PROCHIANTZ. 1991. Antennapedia homeobox peptide regulates neural morphogenesis. Proc. Natl. Acad. Sci. USA **88:** 1864-1868.

14. BLOCH-GALLEGO, E., I. LE ROUX, A.H. JOLIOT, M. VOLOVITCH, C.E. HENDERSON & A. PROCHIANTZ. 1993. Antennapedia homeobox peptide enhances growth and branching of embryonic chicken motoneurons in vitro. J. Cell Biol. **120:** 485-492.

15. JOLIOT, A. H., A. TRILLER, M. VOLOVITCH, C. PERNELLE & A. PROCHIANTZ. 1991. α-2,8-Polysialic acid is the neuronal surface receptor of Antennapedia homeobox peptide. New Biol. **3:** 1121-1134.

16. LE ROUX, I., A.H. JOLIOT, E. BLOCH-GALLEGO, A. PROCHIANTZ & M. VOLOVITCH. 1993. Neurotrophic activity of the Antennapedia homeodomain depends on its specific DNA-binding properties. Proc. Natl. Acad. Sci. USA **90:** 9120–9124.

17. LE ROUX, I., S. DUHARCOURT, M. VOLOVOTCH, A. PROCHIANTZ & E. RONCHI. 1995. Promoter-specific regulation of genes expression by an exogenously added homeodomain that promotes neurite growth. FEBS Lett. **368:** 311–314.

18. DEROSSI, D., A.H. JOLIOT, G. CHASSAING & A. PROCHIANTZ. 1994. The third helix of Antennapedia homeodomain translocates through biological membranes. J. Biol. Chem. **269:** 10444–10450.

19. DEROSSI, D., S. CALVET, A. TREMBLEAU, A. BRUNISSEN, G. CHASSAING & A. PROCHIANTZ. 1996. Cell internalization of the third helix of the Antennapedia homeodomain is receptor-independent. J. Biol. Chem. **271:** 18188–18193.

20. DEROSSI, D., G. CHASSAING & A. PROCHIANTZ. 1998. Trojan peptides: The penetratin system for intracellular delivery. Trends Cell Biol. **8:** 84–87.

21. BERLOSE, J.P., O. CONVERT, D. DEROSSI, A. BRUNISSEN & G. CHASSAING. 1996. Conformational and associative behaviours of the third helix of Antennapedia homeodomain in membrane-mimetic environments. Eur. J. Biochem. **242:** 372–386.

22. DEKRUIJFF, B., P.R. CULLIS, A.J. VERKLEIJ, M.J. HOPE, C.J.A. VANECHTELD, T.F. TARASCHI, P. VANHOOGEVEST, J.A. KILLIAN, A. RIETVEL & A.T.M. VANDERSTEEN. 1985. Modulation of lipid polymorphism by lipid-protein interactions. *In* Progress in Protein-Lipid Interactions: 89–142. Elsevier Science Publishers B.V. Netherlands.

23. PROCHIANTZ, A. 1996. Getting hydrophilic compounds into cells: Lessons from homeopeptides. Curr. Opin. Neurobiol. **6:** 629–634.

24. Hall, H., E.J. Williams, S.E. Moore, F.S. Walsh, A. Prochiantz & P. Doherty. 1996. Inhibition of FGF-stimulated phosphatidylinositol hydrolysis and neurite outgrowth by a cell-membrane permeable phosphopeptide. Curr. Biol. **6:** 580–587.

25. WILLIAMS, E.J., D.J. DUNICAN, P.J. GREEN, F.V. HOWELL, D. DEROSSI, F.S. WALSH & P. DOHERTY. 1997. Selective inhibition of growth factor-stimulated mitogenesis by a cell-permeable Grb2-binding peptide. J. Biol. Chem. **272:** 22349–22354.

26. FAHRAEUS, R., J.M. PARAMIO, K.L. BALL, S. LAIN & D.P. LANE. 1996. Inhibition of pRb phopshorylation and cell-cycle progresion by a 20-residue peptide derived from p16 CDKN2/INK4A. Curr. Biol. **6:** 84–91.

27. SCHUTZE-REDELMEIER, M.P., H. GOURMIER, F. GARCIA-PONS, M. MOUSSA, A.H. JOLIOT, M. VOLOVITCH, A. PROCHIANTZ & F. LEMONNIER. 1996. Introduction of

exogenous antigen into the MHC Class I processing and presentation pathway by *Drosophila* Antennapedia homeodomain primes cytotoxic T cells *in vivo*. J. Immunol. **157:** 650–655.

28. POOGA, M., U. SOOMETS, M. HÄLLBRINK, A. VALKNA, K. SAAR, K. REZAEI, U. KAHL, J.-X. HAO, X.-J. XU, Z. WIESENFELD-HALLIN, T. HÖKFELD, T. BARTFAI & Ü. LANGEL. 1998. Cell penetrating PNA constructs down regulate galanin receptor expression and modify pain transmission *in vivo*. Nature Biotech. **16:** 857–861.

29. CHATELIN, L., M. VOLOVITCH, A.H. JOLIOT, F. PEREZ & A. PROCHIANTZ. 1996. Transcription factor Hoxa-5 is taken up by cells in culture and conveyed to their nuclei. Mech. Dev. **55:** 111–117.

30. JOLIOT, A., A. TREMBLEAU, G. RAPOSO, S. CALVET, M. VOLOVITCH & A. PROCHIANTZ. 1997. Association of engrailed homeoproteins with vesicles presenting caveolae-like properties. Development **124:** 1865–1875.

31. JOLIOT, A., A. MAIZEL, D. ROSENBERG, A. TREMBLEAU, S. DUPAS, M. VOLOVITCH & A. PROCHIANTZ. 1998. Identification of a signal sequence necessary for the unconventional secretion of Engrailed homeoprotein. Curr. Biol. **8:** 856–863.

32. PROCHIANTZ, A. & L. THEODORE. 1995. Nuclear/growth factors. BioEssays **17:** 39–45.

33. FORRESTER, L.M., A. NAGY, M. SAM, A. WATT, L. STEVENSON, A. BERNSTEIN, A.L. JOYNER & W. WURST. 1996. An induction gene trap screen in embryonic stem cells: Identification of genes that respond to retinoic acid in vitro. Proc. Natl. Acad. Sci. USA **93:** 1677–1682.

34. HILL, D.P. & W. WURST. 1993. Screening for novel pattern formation genes using trap approaches. Methods Enzymol. **225:** 664–681.

35. DAVIS, C.A., D.P. HOLMYARD, K.J. MILLEN & A.J. JOYNER. 1991. Examining pattern formation in mouse, chicken and frog embryos with an En-specific antiserum. Development **111:** 287–298.

36. MAINGUY, G., H. ERNØ, M.L. MONTESINOS, B. LESAFFRE, W. WURST, M. VOLOVITCH & A. PROCHIANTZ. 1999. Regulation of epidermal pemphigoid antigen 1 (BRAG1e) synthesis by homeoprotein transcription factors. J. Invest. Dermatol. **113:** 643–650.

37. AULLO, P., M. GIRY, S. OLSNES, M.R. POPOFF, C. KOCKS & P. BOQUET. 1993. A chimeric toxin to study the role of 21 kDa GTP binding protein Rho in the control of actin microfilament assembly. EMBO J. **12:** 921–931.

38. ELLIOTT, G. & P. O'HARE. 1997. Intercellular trafficking and protein delivery by a herpesvirus structural protein. Cell **88:** 223–233.

39. HE, J. & P. FURMANSKI. 1995. Sequence specificity and transcriptional activation in the binding of lactoferrin to DNA. Nature **373:** 721–724.

40. VIVES, E., P. BRODIN & B. LEBLEU. 1997. A truncated HIV-1 Tat protein basic domain translocates through the plasma membrane and accumulates in the cell nucleus. J. Biol. Chem. **272:** 16010–16017.

In Vitro Evaluation of a Novel 2,6,9-Trisubstituted Purine Acting As a Cyclin-Dependent Kinase Inhibitor

NICOLE GIOCANTI,[a] RAMIN SADRI,[a] MICHEL LEGRAVEREND,[b] ODILE LUDWIG,[b] EMILE BISAGNI,[b] SOPHIE LECLERC,[c] LAURENT MEIJER,[c] AND VINCENT FAVAUDON[a,d]

[a]*U 350 INSERM and* [b]*UMR 176 CNRS, Institut Curie, Centre Universitaire, 91405 Orsay, France*

[c]*UPR 9042 CNRS, Station Biologique, 29682 Roscoff, France*

The frequent deregulation of cell cycle progression in cancer[1] has prompted an active search for kinase inhibitors with high affinity and specificity for cyclin-dependent kinases (Cdks). Three major classes of Cdk-targeting drugs have been identified to date, including butyrolactone I,[2] polyhydroxylated flavones such as flavopiridol,[3] and substituted purines.[4] The first substituted purine derivative acting as a selective Cdk inhibitor, olomoucine, has been identified from screening against Cdk1/cyclin B complex.[5] Olomoucine competitively inhibits Cdk1, Cdk2, Cdk5, and, to a lesser extent, Erk1.[5]

Recent results have pointed to unexpected pharmacologic properties of 2,6,9-trisubstituted purines derived from the olomoucine lead structure.[6,7] To investigate the question in more detail, we developed a program for synthesis and evaluation of new compounds in this series. Twenty-seven derivatives were synthesized and assayed for specific inhibition of Cdk1/cyclin B from starfish oocytes and human recombinant Cdk5/p35 complex. In agreement with earlier results,[5] data showed that a strong correlation exists between inhibitory efficiencies against Cdk1 and Cdk5. In contrast, all compounds were only marginally active against Erk1 and Erk2 kinases. One compound in the series, ML-1437, proved much more active than olomoucine against purified Cdk1/cyclin B, Cdk5/p35, and Cdk2/cyclin E. It also showed pronounced cytotoxicity against human cervix carcinoma HeLa cells *in vitro,* even on short exposure. Growing IMR-90 (human normal fibroblasts), LoVo (human colon adenocarcinoma), and SQ-20B (human head and neck squamous carcinoma) cells gave similar results, but drug resistance increased rapidly as cells (SQ-20B and IMR-90) reached confluence. These results suggest that the affinity for Cdks and the cytotoxic potential of the drugs are interrelated (FIG. 1, TABLE 1).

With the exception of pronounced lengthening of S phase transit during early-S in synchronized HeLa cells, ML-1437 at subtoxic concentration proved unable to produce reversible arrest of the cell cycle progression. When observed, arrest in the G1 and G2 phases of the cell cycle correlated with induced cell death, and chronic exposure to lethal doses of the drug resulted in massive micronucleation in relation to mitotic cell death, with no evidence of endoreduplication (polyploidization) or ap-

[d]Corresponding author: Vincent Favaudon, Institut Curie-Recherche, Labs. 110-112, Centre Universitaire, 91405 Orsay Cedex, France. Phone, 33 1 69 86 31 88; fax, 33 1 69 86 31 87.
e-mail, Vincent.Favaudon@curie.u-psud.fr

TABLE 1. Kinase inhibition in enzyme assays and *in vitro* cytotoxicity of olomoucine and ML-1437

	IC_{50} (μM) for Kinase Inhibition				IC_{50} (μM) for HeLa Cell Survival	
	Cdk1	Cdk2	Cdk5	Erk1	24-H Contact	2-H Contact
Olomoucine	3.0	7.0	3.0	≈20	43	>400
ML-1437	0.16	0.65	0.16	≈20	6.7	25.3

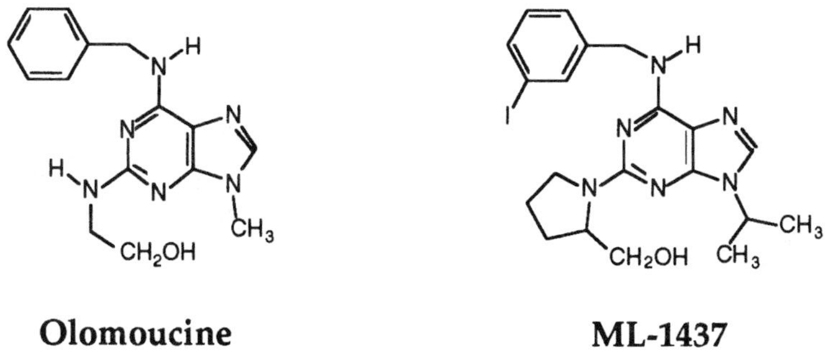

Olomoucine   **ML-1437**

FIGURE 1. Chemical structure of ML-1437 and of the parent compound, olomoucine.

optosis. Lovastatin-synchronized SQ-20B cells demonstrated increased cytotoxic response to ML-1437 in early-G1, but no straightforward cell cycle phase specificity of the cytotoxic response to the drug was observed in thymidine-synchronized HeLa cells. On the other hand, short exposure to olomoucine or ML-1437 concomitantly with radiation resulted in marked protection against radiation-induced cell kill selectively at low radiation doses.

Together, our data suggest that the Cdk2/cyclinE and/or Cdk2/cyclin A complexes are major, but not lethal targets of trisubstituted purines in living cells. Moreover, in agreement with Buquet-Fagot *et al.*,[8] we found that olomoucine and ML-1437 inhibit nucleoside import in the course of an equilibrium reaction, with K_d values in the same range as those for Cdks in acellular extracts. This notwithstanding, the large increase in the cytotoxic potential for ML-1437 relative to olomoucine is very encouraging for finding new antitumor agents, especially as the cytotoxicity of this drug was specific for the growing cell fraction and proved effective from the time of early contact with the drug in all cell lines. Conversely, olomoucine derivatives were recently shown to protect central and peripheral neurons from apoptotic cell death,[7] presumably through Cdk5 inhibition.[9,10]

REFERENCES

1. BARTKOVA, J., J. LUKAS & J. BARTEK. 1997. Aberrations of the G1- and G1/S-regulating genes in human cancer. *In* Progress in Cell Cycle Research, Vol. 3. L. Meijer, S. Guidet, & E.M. Philippe, Eds.: 211–220. Plenum Press. New York.

2. KITAGAWA, M., T. OKABE, H. OGINO *et al.* 1993. Butyrolactone I, a selective inhibitor of cdk2 and cdc2 kinase. Oncogene **8:** 2425–2432.
3. CARLSON, B.A., M.M. DUBAY, E.A. SAUSVILLE, L. BRIZUELA & P.J. WORLAND. 1996. Flavopiridol induces G(1) arrest with inhibition of cyclin-dependent kinase (CDK) 2 and CDK4 in human breast carcinoma cells. Cancer Res. **56:** 2973-2978.
4. MEIJER, L. & S.-H. KIM. 1997. Chemical inhibitors of cyclin-dependent kinases. Methods Enzymol. **283:** 113–128.
5. VESELY, J., L. HAVLICEK, M. STRNAD *et al.* 1994. Inhibition of cyclin-dependent kinases by purine analogues. Eur. J. Biochem. **224:** 771–786.
6. WALKER, D.H., P.A. PARKER & R.M. LAETHEM. 1998. Cell cycle arrest induced by the CDK inhibitor olomoucine protects normal, but not tumor cells, from killing by cytotoxic anticancer drugs. Proc. Am. Assoc. Cancer Res. **39:** 1678.
7. MAAS, J.W., S. HORSTMANN, G.D. BORASIO, J.M.H. ANNESER, E.M. SHOOTER & P.J. KAHLE. 1998. Apoptosis of central and peripheral neurons can be prevented with cyclin-dependent kinase/mitogen-activated protein kinase inhibitors. J. Neurochem. **70:** 1401–1410.
8. BUQUET-FAGOT, C., F. LALLEMAND, M.-N. MONTAGNE & J. MESTER. 1997. Effects of olomoucine, a selective inhibitor of cyclin-dependent kinases, on cell cycle progression in human cancer cell lines. Anti-Cancer Drugs **8:** 623–631.
9. HENCHCLIFFE, C. & R.E. BURKE. 1997. Increased expression of cyclin-dependent kinase 5 in induced apoptotic neuron death in rat substantia nigra. Neurosci. Lett. **230:** 41–44.
10. ZHANG, Q., H.S. AHUJA, Z.F. ZAKERI & D.J. WOLGEMUTH. 1997. Cyclin-dependent kinase 5 is associated with apoptotic cell death during development and tissue remodeling. Dev. Biol. **183:** 222–233.

Homologous Recombination between Heterologs during Repair of a Double-Strand Break

Suppression of Translocations in Normal Cells

CHRISTINE RICHARDSON, MARY ELLEN MOYNAHAN, AND MARIA JASIN

Cell Biology and Genetics Program, Memorial Sloan-Kettering Cancer Center and Cornell University Graduate School of Medical Sciences, 1275 York Avenue, New York, New York 10021, USA

The faithful repair of DNA damage such as chromosomal double-strand breaks (DSBs) is necessary for the maintenance of genomic integrity. Aberrantly repaired DSBs are expected to result in chromosomal rearrangements, including translocations, which promote mutagenesis, transformation, or even cell lethality. Specific DNA sequences including repetitive elements observed near breakpoints of recurring translocations have been implicated in the aberrant repair of DSBs, possibly by promoting homologous recombination between two otherwise heterologous chromosomes.[1,2] In addition, exposure to DNA damaging agents, including chemotherapeutic agents such as topoisomerase II inhibitors, has been implicated in creating or stabilizing the initial break that leads to chromosomal instability[3] possibly by inhibition of normal repair and thus enhancement of inappropriate recombination with new chromosome partners.[4] Therefore, it seems that human cells with a large fraction of repetitive DNA should be at high risk for genome rearrangements especially following exposure to DNA-damaging agents. We are investigating the mechanisms used by the cell during repair of DSBs, especially those that may result in aberrant repair and the recurring chromosomal rearrangements identified in many solid tumors and lymphoid malignancies.

Because chromosome breaks are the most potent inducers of recombination known in mammalian cells,[5–8] we directly determined the potential of homologous DSB repair to lead to chromosomal translocations using mouse ES cells. To do this, we developed a system to analyze recombination between neomycin gene (*neo*) repeat substrates on two heterologous chromosomes. Specifically, chromosomes 14 and 17 were each marked with a defective *neo* gene with a total length of homology approximately 1.1 kb (FIG. 1). The *neo* repeat on chromosome 17 contains a cleavage site for a rare-cutting endonuclease, I-*Sce* I.[9] Homologous recombination between the two chromosomes at the *neo* loci may restore a functional *neo* gene. A simple gene conversion without crossing-over will maintain the parental configuration of alleles, but gene conversion with crossing-over will result in a chromosomal translocation event.

Although spontaneous recombination events were undetectable (frequency < 1×10^{-9}), recombination was induced >1,000-fold when a single DSB was intro-

184   ANNALS NEW YORK ACADEMY OF SCIENCES

TABLE 1. Summary of DSB-induced interchromosomal recombination products[a]

	Number of Clones
Short tract gene conversion	170
Long tract gene conversion	4
Reciprocal or nonreciprocal translocation	0

[a]The major interchromosomal recombination product was a short tract gene conversion (STGC) product, observed in 98% of the clones. In the remaining clones, long tract gene conversion (LTGC) events were seen in which at least a few kb downstream of the break site on chromosome 17 was converted to sequences from chromosone 14. There was no evidence for translocations in any of the clones.

duced in the *neo* gene on chromosome 17. An I-*Sce* I expression vector, pCBASce, was electroporated into several independently derived parental cell lines containing the *neo* gene elements, and *neo*[+] colonies were selected in G418. Following induction of a DSB, G418[R] colonies were readily obtained from all cell lines with an average frequency of recombination of 3.5×10^{-6}. These data demonstrate that a single DSB can stimulate recombination between loci on nonhomologous chromosomes at least three orders of magnitude, from less than 1×10^{-9} to more than 1×10^{-6}. Ninety-eight per cent of the G418[R] clones had undergone short tract gene conversion (STGC) events using the small region of homology from the donor *neo* allele on chromosome 14 to repair the broken *neo* allele on chromosome 17 (TABLE 1) with no other alterations to either chromosomal locus. A small portion of clones (4 of 174) were consistent with conversion extending beyond the 3' end of the donor *neo* gene on chromosome 14 into a region of heterology (TABLE 1). To distinguish between LTGCs and translocations, we used FISH of metaphase chromosome spreads and observed two intact chromosome 14s and two intact chromosome 17s in each of

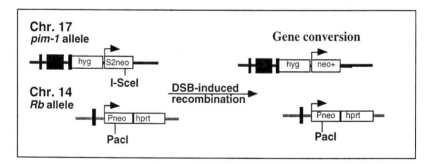

FIGURE 1. Substrates for DSB-induced interchromosomal recombination. Two defective neo genes were targeted to mouse chromosomes 14 and 17. On chromosome 17, neo was linked to a selectable hygro gene within a pim-1 locus targeting construct. The I-Sce I DSB recognition site is located within this neo gene. On chromosome 14, neo was linked to a selectable hprt gene within an Rb locus targeting construct. This neo donor allele contains an upstream Pac I mutation to render it also nonfunctional. Following induction of a DSB, a simple gene conversion without crossing-over will maintain the parental configuration of alleles, as shown, but gene conversion with crossing-over will result in a chromosomal translocation event.

the clones with no evidence of reciprocal or nonreciprocal translocations (TABLE 1). Additionally, we did not detect a patch of chromosome 14 within one of the repaired chromosome 17s that would be expected for extensive conversion tracts.

Thus, although the cell is capable of using homologous sequences on a heterologous chromosome for repair of a single DSB, crossover events that would result in genome rearrangements are suppressed in normal cells. These data suggest that the use of homologous sequences from a new chromosome partner is not a sufficient initiating event to result in chromosomal translocations. The lack of crossover events supports a model coupling recombination to replication of the correcting sequences on chromosome 14 and then reannealing to homologous sequences on chromosome 17 or, in the rare LTGC event, to downstream nonhomologous sequences. This model suggests that crossovers, leading to chromosomal translocations, may be part of an alternate or aberrant repair pathway. In support of this, studies with global DNA damaging agents have demonstrated that genome rearrangements are induced by mechanisms other than conservative homologous recombination.[10–12] The lack of observed translocations underscores the fact that the cell makes every effort to maintain genomic integrity while repairing a DSB. Many recently identified homologs of known yeast proteins involved in homologous recombination and repair are yet to be examined for their role in human and mouse DSB-induced recombination. In addition, genes involved in sensing DNA damage or directing signals for its repair in normal cells may be responsible for suppression of aberrant events.[13] With the defined genetic system presented here, it should now be possible to determine the components involved in interchromosomal recombination in mammalian cells and also to unravel the safeguards that prevent the occurrence of translocation events.

REFERENCES

1. JEFFS, A.R. *et al.* 1998. The BCR gene recombines preferentially with Alu elements in complex BCR-ABL translocations of chronic myeloid leukemia. Hum. Mol. Gen. **7:** 767–776.
2. MORRIS, C. *et al.* 1996. BCR gene recombines with genomically distinct sites on band 11q13 in complex BCR-ABL translocations of chronic myeloid leukemia. Oncogene **12:** 677–685.
3. ROSS, W. *et al.* 1984. Role of topoisomerase II in mediating epipodophyllotoxin-induced DNA cleavage. Cancer Res. **44:** 5857–5860.
4. IKEDA, H. 1995. DNA topoisomerase-mediated illegitimate recombination. Adv. Pharmacol. **29:** 147–150.
5. CHOULIKA, A. *et al.* 1995. Induction of homologous recombination in mammalian chromosomes by using the I-SceI system of *Saccharomyces cerevisiae*. Mol. Cell. Biol. **15:**1963–1973.
6. LIANG, F. *et al.* 1998. Homology-directed repair is a major double-strand break repair pathway in mammalian cells. Proc. Natl. Acad. Sci. **95:** 5172–5177.
7. ROUET, P. *et al.* 1994. Introduction of double-strand breaks into the genome of mouse cells by expression of a rare-cutting endonuclease. Mol. Cell. Biol. **14:** 8096–8106.
8. SARGENT, R.G. *et al.* 1997. Repair of site-specific double-strand breaks in a mammalian chromosome by homologous and illegitimate recombination. Mol. Cell. Biol. **17:** 267–277.
9. COLLEAUX, L. *et al.* 1998. Recognition and cleavage site of the intron-encoded omega transposase. Proc. Natl. Acad. Sci. **85:** 6022–6026.
10. PHILLIPS, J.W. *et al.* 1994. Illegitimate recombination induced by DNA double-strand breaks in a mammalian chromosome. Mol. Cell. Biol. **14:** 5794–5803.

11. CHEN, C. *et al.* 1998. Chromosomal rearrangements occur in *S. cerevisiae* rfa1 mutator mutants due to mutagenic lesions processed by double-strand-break repair. Mol. Cell **2:** 9–22.

12. HABER, J.E. *et al.* 1996. Lack of chromosome territoriality in yeast: Promiscuous rejoining of broken chromosome ends. Proc. Natl. Acad. Sci. USA **93:** 13949–13954.

13. LEVINE A.J. 1997. p53, the cellular gatekeeper for growth and division. Cell **88:** 323–331.

Selection of Genetic Suppressor Elements Conferring Resistance to DNA Topoisomerase II Inhibitors

C. DELAPORTE, L. GROS, S. FREY, D. COCCARD, L. CAVAREC,[a] A. DUBAR,[b] A. GUDKOV,[c] AND A. JACQUEMIN-SABLON

CNRS UMR 1772, Unité de Biochimie-Enzymologie, Institut Gustave Roussy, 39 rue Camille Desmoulins, 94805 Villejuif, France

[a] CNRS UMR 1569

[b] INSERM U362

[c] University of Illinois

Type II DNA topoisomerases are dimeric enzymes that have been implicated in a variety of cellular functions and are essential for the survival of eukaryotic cells. In addition to their physiologic function, topoisomerases II are the target of some of the most frequently used antitumor agents in human cancer chemotherapy. Despite their structural diversity, these agents all have in common their capacity to increase the number of cleavable complexes present on the cell genome at a given time. The cleavable complex is a covalent enzyme-DNA complex formed as an intermediate during the catalytic cycle of topoisomerase II. In this complex, both strands of the DNA molecule are interrupted, and each enzyme subunit is attached to newly formed 5' termini by a phosphotyrosyl bond. In normal conditions, these complexes are present in low steady-state concentrations. However, if their number increases significantly, they behave as DNA lesions, which may provoke various deleterious effects. Antitumor topoisomerase II inhibitors can increase the number of cleavable complexes either by inhibiting the religation of cleaved DNA or by enhancing the rate of DNA cleavage.[1]

Although the drug-target interaction is an essential step in the mechanism of action of cytotoxic agents, it is now widely admitted that the cellular response to these agents depends on a variety of genetically controlled mechanisms that can be divided into two groups: (1) genes acting upstream of the drug-target interaction to control the cellular accumulation and intracellular metabolism of the drug; (2) genes acting downstream of the drug-target interaction to control the transmission, through a complex pathway, of a signal that will finally determine the cell response, that is, apoptosis, cell cycle arrest, or resistance. Alterations of several genes involved in these different pathways may then result in a drug resistance phenotype.

Our experimental model is a Chinese hamster cell line (DC-3F), from which a variant was selected for a high level of resistance to 9-OH-ellipticine (9-OH-E). Previous studies showed that during a very long selection process, these cells (DC-3F/ 9-OH-E) accumulated genetic alterations that may contribute to their resistance phenotype.[2] The goal of this work is to identify and characterize the genes that are involved in the resistance to topoisomerase II inhibitors by selecting genetic suppressor elements that confer resistance to 9-OH-E in the DC-3F cells.

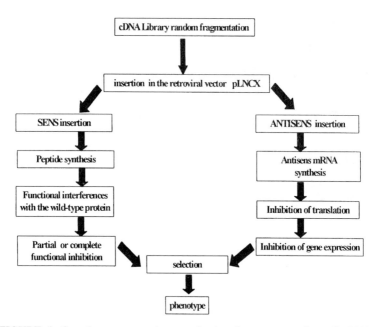

FIGURE 1. Genetic suppressor element selection, from a mammalian cell cDNA population, makes it possible to identify the genes that are involved in selectable cellular phenotypes. Three types of genes can be identified: genes already known to be involved in drug resistance; genes already known, but not as drug resistance genes; and new genes.

Gene identification by selection of genetic suppressor elements (GSE) was first described by Roninson et al.[3] Fragments of cDNA (300–500 bp) are inserted in a retroviral vector. These vectors are then used to infect drug-sensitive cells, in this case DC-3F cells, and then drug-resistant clones are selected. There are two possibilities (FIG.1): If the fragment is in the sens orientation, it will be translated in the cell to produce a peptide corresponding to a functional region of a protein and eventually to inhibit the function of this protein; alternatively, the fragment may be in the antisens orientation and, in that case, an antisens RNA will be produced, which eventually will inhibit the expression of the homologous gene. If either one of these effects confers resistance to the drug, the cells containing the corresponding fragment will then be selected. From the selected cells, the GSEs can be isolated by PCR and sequenced. It is then possible to identify the genes to which they are homologous. At least in principle, this technique allows us to identify any gene the inactivation of which leads to the selected phenotype. It may be a gene known to be involved in the resistance process, a gene that was known but not as possibly involved in the resistance process, or a completely new gene.

A Chinese hamster GSE library, representing 2.5×10^7 genetic events, was prepared as described by Gudkov et al.[4] Fragments inserted in the vector pLNCX were transfected in the packaging cells, BOSC 23. The virus present in the medium supernatant was used to infect the DC-3F cells, followed by 9-OH-E selection. Inserts

TABLE 1. Sequence homologies

insert	Best homology found	score	E value	Database
1-9	Mouse brain cDNA	194	5.10^{-48}	gb/R75025
1-10	No homology found	/	/	/
1-16/2	snRNP Core Sm protein homologue Sm-X5	52	3.10^{-5}	gb/AF050157
1-29/1	Soares testis Homo Sapiens cDNA clone	129	10^{-28}	gb/AA432211
1-41*	/	/	/	/
1-46/2*	/	/	/	/
1-59/3	Soares mouse mammary gland cDNA clone	163	9.10^{-39}	gb/AA759607
1-106/3	No homology found	/	/	/
1-122/2	No homology found	/	/	/
2-6	No homology found	/	/	/

*1-41 and 1-46/2 are concatenated forms of 1-9

The *Advanced Blast* algorithm was used for homology search in the different sequence databases (NR : Genebank, EMBL, DDBJ or dbEST)

from surviving cells were religated in pLNCX and submitted to a second round of selection. At that step, a major increase in the number of survivors relative to control was observed, indicating enrichment in active GSEs.

Polymerase chain reaction (PCR) analysis of the integrated proviral inserts from 166 surviving clones allowed us to identify 10 nonidentical GSE sequences. Four of them were recloned in pLNCX in the same position and orientation as in the original plasmid, and they were tested for the ability to confer resistance to 9-OH-E. Three were found to induce the resistance, indicating that they are active GSEs.

Sequences of the 10 cloned GSEs were analyzed for homology to known nucleic acids and proteins (TABLE 1). No significant homologies were found for five of them, whereas three others presented a strong homology with sequences previously identified in mouse or human organs.

Clone 1-9, the most frequently detected, was further analyzed. By probing the DC-3F cDNA library with this GSE, three cDNA were cloned. Their amino acid sequences showed strong homology with protein arginine *N*-methyltransferases.

ACKNOWLEDGMENT

This work was supported in part by the Ligue Nationale Française contre le Cancer and the Association pour la Recherche contre le Cancer.

REFERENCES

1. FROELICH-AMMON, S.J. & N. OSHEROFF. 1995. Topoisomerase poisons: Harnessing the dark side of enzyme mechanism. J. Biol. Chem. **270:** 21429–21432.

2. LARSEN, A.K. & A. JACQUEMIN-SABLON. 1989. Multiple resistance mechanisms in Chinese hamster cells resistant to 9-Hydroxyellipticine. Cancer Res. **49:** 7115–7119.
3. RONINSON, I.B. *et al.* 1995. Genetic suppressor elements: New tools for molecular biology. Cancer Res. **55:** 4023–4028.
4. Gudkov, A.V. *et al.* 1994. Cloning mammalian genes by expression selection of genetic suppressor elements: Association of kinesin with drug resistance and cell immortalization. Proc Natl. Acad. Sci. USA **91:** 3744–3748.

BAP1, a Candidate Tumor Suppressor Protein That Interacts with BRCA1

DAVID E. JENSEN AND FRANK J. RAUSCHER, III[a]

The Wistar Institute, 3601 Spruce St., Philadelphia, Pennsylvania 19104, USA

BAP1 (BRCA1-ASSOCIATED PROTEIN-1)

Attempts to identify a biochemical function of the Breast/Ovarian Cancer Susceptibility Gene, BRCA1, have focused on identifying its protein partners. Recent studies have yielded a novel RING finger/BRCT-domain–containing protein, BARD1, of unknown function,[1] the hRAD51 protein, which is involved in DNA recombination/repair,[2] DNA Polymerase II,[3] and the second Breast Cancer Susceptibility Gene, BRCA2.[4] We have identified a novel protein, BAP1, that binds to the wild-type BRCA1 RING finger domain but not to mutated RING fingers (i.e., those found in breast tumors from women with heritable breast cancer) or other closely related RING fingers.[5] BAP1 is a novel, nuclear-localized enzyme that displays the signature motifs and has the activity of a ubiquitin carboxy-terminal hydrolase. BAP1 is a 90-kD protein (729 a.a.) that binds to BRCA1 *in vitro* and *in vivo*, cleaves ubiquitin from a model substrate (similar to other members of this family), and enhances the growth-suppressive properties of BRCA1.[5] Our data suggest that the BAP1 carboxy-terminus is tethered to the BRCA1 RING finger domain, leaving the UCH catalytic domain free to interact with ubiquitinated (or ubiquitin-like) substrates. The human BAP1 locus was mapped to chromosome 3p21.3, a region of the genome that is routinely deleted or rearranged in many cancers. Indeed, we have found rearrangements, deletions, and missense mutations of BAP1 in small cell and non-small cell lung cancer cell lines and, more recently, in breast cancer tumor samples, suggesting that BAP1 may be a tumor suppressor gene.

THE UBIQUITIN SYSTEM

The identification of BAP1 as a ubiquitin hydrolase implicates the ubiquitin-proteasome pathway as a potential direct effector and/or regulator of BRCA1 function(s). Regulated ubiquitination of proteins and subsequent proteasome-dependent proteolysis plays a role in almost every cellular growth, differentiation, and homeostatic process.[6] The pathway is regulated both at the level of substrate specificity and at the level of proteolytic deubiquitination and ubiquitin hydrolysis. The latter enzymes are ubiquitin-specific, thiol proteases that have been broadly classified into two families, the ubiquitin-specific proteases (UBPs) and the ubiquitin carboxy-terminal hydrolases (UCHs).

[a]Phone, 215/898-0995; fax, 215/898-3929.
e-mail, rauscher@wistar.upenn.edu

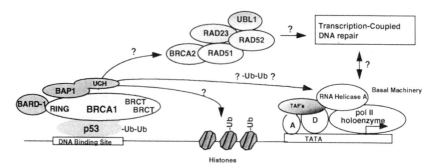

FIGURE 1. BAP1 may affect several biochemical pathways. The enzymatic activity of BAP1 could be involved in any of several processes including, but certainly not limited to, (1) the deubiquitination of histones leading to chromatin rearrangement; (2) the deubiquitination of various transcription factors (e.g., p53) or proteins of the basal machinery (assuming the ubiquitination of some of these elements); and/or (3) the hydrolysis of ubiquitin-like proteins from any of the aforementioned factors/proteins as well as the BRCA2-hRAD51 complex which probably contains proteins from this pathway.

The UBP family members are 50–300 kD, cytoplasmic, or nuclear-localized proteins that generally cleave ubiquitin or ubiquitin-conjugates from large substrates and whose enzymatic activity can be found directly associated with the 26S proteasome. The UCH family has traditionally been characterized as a set of small (25–30 kD) cytoplasmic proteins that prefer to cleave ubiquitin from ubiquitin-conjugated small substrates and may also be involved in the cotranslational processing of pro-ubiquitin. UCH family members are strongly and differentially expressed in neuronal, hematopoietic, and germ cells in many species, and like the UBPs, UCHs show considerable tissue specificity and developmentally timed regulation.[7]

BAP1 AND CELL FUNCTION

BAP1, the newest member of the UCH family, considerably expands the potential roles of this family of proteases, because it is the first large, nuclear-localized UCH to be identified. BAP1's association with BRCA1 could suggest that BRCA1 is regulated like other tumor suppressor proteins that are known to be ubiquitinated (leading to their degradation). This scenario suggests that BAP1 would stabilize the BRCA1 protein and protect it from proteasome-mediated degradation. However, we have found no evidence that BRCA1 is ubiquitinated, suggesting that proteasome-mediated degradation of BRCA1 is probably not part of its regulation (D. Jensen and F.J. Rauscher, unpublished results). Alternatively, BRCA1 could modulate BAP1's activity on other proteins, including other tumor suppressor proteins. In this scenario, BRCA1 could function as an assembly or scaffold molecule for regulated assembly of multiprotein complexes. For example, BRCA1 and p53 have been shown to associate,[8] and it is known that p53 protein levels are regulated through the ubiquitin/proteasome pathway.[9] Therefore, it is possible that BRCA1, BAP1, and p53 may exist (albeit transiently) within the same complex and may crucially determine control of the cells' response to DNA damage (FIG. 1).

This concept, which broadly implicates BRCA1 pathways in DNA repair processes, is further supported by the association of BRCA1[2] (and BRCA2[10]) with the RAD51 protein and by the recent finding that BRCA1 null cells are deficient in transcription-coupled repair.[11] The RAD51/52-dependent DNA repair pathway is highly regulated and includes many proteins, some of which may be potential substrates for BAP1-mediated ubiquitin hydrolysis. RAD23, which associates with the RAD51/52 complex, contains an aminoterminal ubiquitin-like domain, which is required for RAD23 function and double-strand break repair.[12] Recently, the RAD51/52 complex was shown to contain both a ubiquitin-like protein, UBL-1,[13] and a ubiquitin-like conjugating enzyme, hUBC9/UBE2I.[14] Therefore, it now appears that the BRCA1/BRCA2-RAD51 DNA repair complex contains the elements necessary to conjugate a ubiquitin-like molecule to proteins of the complex. Furthermore, because BAP1 associates with BRCA1, it is exciting to speculate that BAP1 might be a new member of this ubiquitin-like pathway.

These models for the potential actions of BAP1 provide a multitude of directions for the search for its biochemical function(s). Given that BAP1 is an enzyme and that it is associated with the BRCA1 complex of proteins, its loss or inactivation could affect a variety of signaling pathways in the cell and, furthermore, this loss/mutation may account for some familial breast cancers or other cancers that are not accounted for by mutation of the BRCA1 gene.

REFERENCES

1. WU, L.C., Z.W. WANG, *et al.* 1996. Identification of a RING protein that can interact in vivo with the BRCA1 gene product. Nature Genet. **14:** 430–440.
2. SCULLY, R., J. CHEN *et al.* 1997. Association of BRCA1 with Rad51 in mitotic and meiotic cells. Cell **88:** 265–275.
3. SCULLY, R., S.F. ANDERSON *et al.* 1997. BRCA1 is a component of the RNA polymerase II holoenzyme. Proc. Natl. Acad. Sci. USA **94:** 5605–5610.
4. CHEN, J., D.P. SILVER *et al.* 1998. Stable interaction between the products of the BRCA1 and BRCA2 tumor suppressor genes in mitotic and meiotic cells. Mol. Cell **2:** 317–328.
5. JENSEN, D.E., M. PROCTOR *et al.* 1998. BAP1: A novel ubiquitin hydrolase which binds to the BRCA1 RING finger and enhances BRCA1-mediated cell growth suppression. Oncogene **16:** 1097–1112.
6. HOCHSTRASSER, M. 1996. Ubiquitin-dependent protein degradation. Ann.. Rev. Genet. **30:** 405–439.
7. WILKINSON, K.D., S. DESHPANDE & C.N. LARSEN. 1992. Comparisons of neuronal (PGP 9.5) and non-neuronal ubiquitin C-terminal hydrolases. Biochem. Soc. Trans. **20:** 631–637.
8. ZHANG, H., K. SOMASUNDARAM *et al.* 1998. BRCA1 physically associates with p53 and stimulates its transcriptional activity. Oncogene **16:** 1713–1721.
9. SCHEFFNER, M., J.M. HUIBREGTSE, R.D. VIERSTRA & P.M. HOWLEY. 1993. The HPV-16 E6 and E6-AP complex functions as a ubiquitin-protein ligase in the ubiquitination of p53. Cell **75:** 495–505.
10. WONG, A.K.C., R. PERO *et al.* 1997. RAD51 interacts with the evolutionarily conserved BRC motifs in the human breast cancer susceptibility gene brca2. J. Biol. Chem. **272:** 31941–31944.
11. GOWEN, L.C., A.V. AVRUTSKAYA *et al.* 1998. BRCA1 required for transcription-coupled repair of oxidative DNA damage. Science **281:** 1009–1012.

12. WATKINS, J.F., P. SUNG, L. PRAKASH & S. PRAKASH. 1993. The *Saccharomyces cerevisiae* DNA repair gene RAD23 encodes a nuclear protein containing a ubiquitin-like domain required for biological function. Mol. Cell. Biol. **13:** 7757–7765.
13. SHEN, Z., P.E. PARDINGTON-PURTYMUN *et al.* 1996. UBL1, a human ubiquitin-like protein associating with human RAD51/RAD52 proteins. Genomics **36:** 271–279.
14. JOHNSON, E.S. & G. BLOBEL. 1997. Ubc9p is the conjugating enzyme for the ubiquitin-like protein Smt3p. J. Biol. Chem. **272:** 26799–267802.

Histone Deacetylase Inhibitor Activates the p21/WAF1/Cip1 Gene Promoter through the Sp1 Sites

Y. SOWA,[a,c] T. ORITA,[c] S. HIRANABE-MINAMIKAWA,[c] K. NAKANO, [a,b]
T. MIZUNO,[c] H. NOMURA,[c] AND T. SAKAI[a,d]

[a]Department of Preventive Medicine and [b]Second Department of Surgery, Kyoto Prefectural University of Medicine, Kamigyo-ku, Kyoto 602-8566, Japan
[c]Chugai Research Institute for Molecular Medicine, Inc., 153-2, Nagai, Niihari, Ibaraki 300-4101, Japan

p21/WAF1/Cip1 protein potently inhibits various cyclin-dependent kinases[1–3] that regulate the cell cycle, thereby supposedly inducing cell cycle arrest.[1,4] The p21/WAF1/Cip1 gene was first identified as a p53-inducible gene,[5] but more recently its induction was shown to occur via p53-independent mechanisms in various cell lines stimulated for differentiation and growth arrest. We previously showed that the pleiotropic agent sodium butyrate inhibited proliferation and induced p21/WAF1/Cip1 expressions in the p53-negative human cell lines WiDr and MG63, derived from colon cancer and osteosarcoma, respectively.[6] Although butyrate is known to be pleiotropic, it has been suggested that it is a rather unspecific inhibitor of histone deacetylase, also affecting some other enzymes.[7] In comparison, trichostatin A (TSA), which differs in chemical structure, is antimycotic, and induces differentiation in Friend leukemia cells, was recently shown to be a specific inhibitor of histone deacetylase at much lower concentrations *in vivo* and *in vitro*.[8] To elucidate the role

[d]Author for correspondence. Phone, +81-75-251-5339; fax, +81-75-241-0792.
e-mail, tsakai@basic.kpu-m.ac.jp

FIGURE 1. (**A**) Effect of TSA on the growth of MG63 cells. One day after inoculation, TSA was added at 10 (○), 50 (△), 100 (□), 500 (◇) or 1,000 (▽) ng/ml, and cell growth was compared with that in control culture (●). (**B**) Effects of TSA on distribution of cellular DNA content in MG63 cells. After incubation with or without 500 ng/ml TSA for 24 hours, cells were collected and their isolated nuclei were analyzed by flow cytometry. (**C**) Dose response of TSA on the p21/WAF1/Cip1 protein. Cells were exposed to either medium alone (0) or medium containing 10, 50, 100, 500, and 1,000 ng/ml TSA for 24 hours, and then expression of p21/WAF1/Cip1 protein was examined. (**D**) Time course effects of TSA on p21/WAF1/Cip1 protein. Cells were exposed to medium containing 500 ng/ml TSA and harvested at 2, 4, 6, 8, 10, 12, and 24 hours after the start of TSA treatment, and then expression of p21/WAF1/Cip1 protein was examined. (**E**) Time course effects of TSA on p21/WAF1/Cip1 mRNA. Cells were cultured with either medium alone (-) or medium containing 500 ng/ml TSA (+) and collected at the indicated time points (0, 1, 3, 6, 12, and 24 hours) after stimulation for total RNA isolation, and then expression of p21/WAF1/Cip1 mRNA was examined.

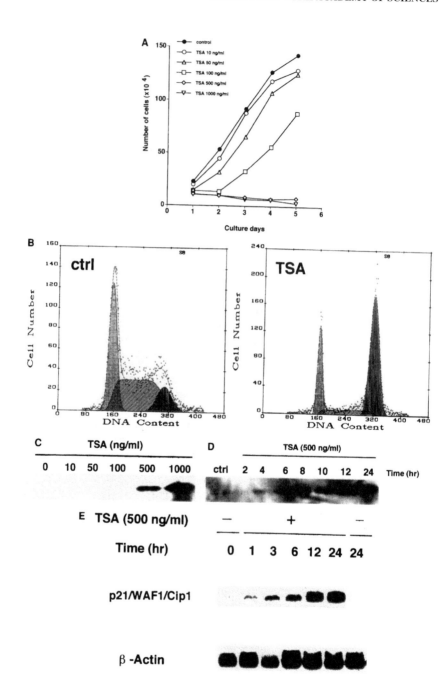

FIGURE 1. *See legend on preceding page.*

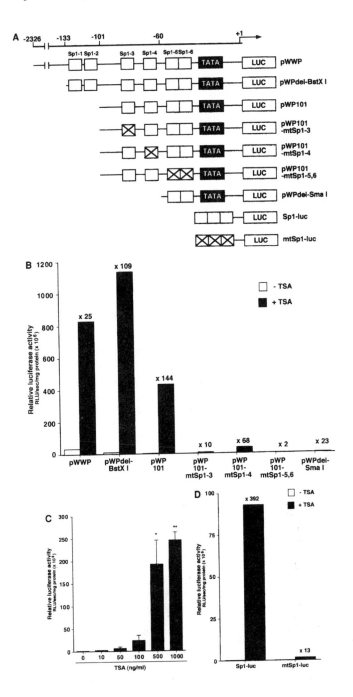

FIGURE 2. *See legend on following page.*

of histone hyperacetylation in the regulation of p21/WAF1/Cip1 gene expression, we examined the effects of TSA on the expression of p21/WAF1/Cip1 in MG63 cells; the status of the p53 gene is negative.

Our results demonstrate that hyperacetylated histone H4 and expressions of p21/WAF1/Cip1 are induced on TSA treatment in MG63 cells. When using a series of mutant p21/WAF1/Cip1 promoter constructs, we found that two Sp1 sites at −82 and −69 relative to the transcription start site are involved in activation of the p21/WAF1/Cip1 promoter by TSA. Also, the Sp1-luc plasmid containing SV40 promoter-derived three consensus Sp1 binding sites was markedly activated by TSA compared to the mutant Sp1-luc plasmid, indicating that a consensus Sp1 site is essential for activation by TSA. These results indicate that TSA activates the p21/WAF1/Cip1 promoter through Sp1 sites in a p53-independent manner.

Electrophoretic mobility shift assay (EMSA) using MG63 cells revealed that Sp1 and Sp3 can specifically interact with this main TSA-responsive element at the p21/WAF1/Cip1 promoter. However, the intensity and mobility pattern of the retarded bands were not changed by TSA, which means that TSA activation of the p21/WAF1/Cip1 promoter does not appear to be due to increasing the binding of Sp1 or Sp3 itself.

SUMMARY

Trichostatin A (TSA), a specific histone deacetylase inhibitor, induces histone hyperacetylation and modulates the expression of some genes. We examined the effects of TSA on MG63 cells. TSA induced growth arrest and expression of the p21/WAF1/Cip1 protein. A close correlation between the level of histone acetylation and induction of the p21/WAF1/Cip1 protein was detected. Using several mutant p21/WAF1/Cip1 promoter fragments, mutation of either of two Sp1 sites at −82 or −69 of the p21/WAF1/Cip1 promoter reduced the responsiveness to TSA. This finding indicates that TSA activates the p21/WAF1/Cip1 promoter through the Sp1 sites in a p53-independent manner.

FIGURE 2. (A) Schematic representation of full size, deleted, and mutated p21/WAF1/Cip1 promoter-luciferase plasmids and three tandem repeats of consensus Sp1 sites and mutant Sp1 sites driving luciferase plasmids used in transfection assays. *Open boxes* show locations of the Sp1 elements of the promoter. **(B)** Deletion and mutation analysis of activation of the p21/WAF1/Cip1 promoter by TSA in MG63 cells. Constructed plasmids were transiently transfected into MG63 cells, and luciferase activities were measured after 24 hours of treatment with (*closed bar*) or without (*open bar*) 500 ng/ml TSA. Fold induction by TSA is calculated to compare with the activities of the control (without TSA treatment). **(C)** Dose response of TSA on p21/WAF1/Cip1 promoter activity. Cells were transiently transfected with the pWPdel-BstX I reporter plasmid, and luciferase activity was measured after treatment with either medium alone or various concentrations of TSA for 24 hours. **(D)** Activation of promoter activity of Sp1-luc in MG63 cells. Cells were transiently transfected with either the Sp1-luc reporter plasmid or mtSp1-luc, and luciferase activities were measured after 24 hours of treatment with (*closed bar*) or without (*open bar*) 500 ng/ml TSA for 24 hours. Fold induction by TSA is calculated to compare with the activities of the control (without TSA treatment).

REFERENCES

1. HARPER, J.W. *et al.* 1993. The p21 Cdk-interacting protein Cip1 is a potent inhibitor of G1 cyclin-dependent kinases. Cell **75:** 805–816.
2. XIONG, Y. *et al.* 1993. p21 is a universal inhibitor of cyclin kinases. Nature (Lond.) **366:** 701–704.
3. GU, Y. *et al.* 1993. Inhibition of CDK2 activity in vivo by an associated 20K regulatory subunit. Nature (Lond.) **366:** 707–710.
4. DULIC, V. *et al.* 1994. P53-dependent inhibition of cyclin-dependent kinase activities in human fibroblasts during radiation-induced G1 arrest. Cell **76:** 1013–1023.
5. EL-DEIRY, W.S. *et al.* 1993. WAF1, a potential mediator of p53 tumor suppression. Cell **75:** 817–825.
6. NAKANO, K. *et al.* 1997. Butyrate activates the WAF1/Cip1 gene promoter through Sp1 sites in a p53-negative human colon cancer cell line. J. Biol. Chem. **272:** 22199–22206.
7. KRUH, J. 1982. Effects of sodium butyrate, a new pharmacological agent, on cells in culture. Mol. Cell. Biochem. **42:** 65–82.
8. YOSHIDA, M. *et al.* 1990. Potent and specific inhibition of mammalian histone deacetylase both in vivo and in vitro by trichostatin A. J. Biol. Chem. **265:** 17174–17179.

Selective Induction of Cyclin-Dependent Kinase Inhibitors and Their Roles in Cell Cycle Arrest Caused by Trichostatin A, an Inhibitor of Histone Deacetylase

YOUNG BAE KIM,[a] MINORU YOSHIDA, AND SUEHARU HORINOUCHI

Department of Biotechnology, Graduate School of Agriculture and Life Sciences, The University of Tokyo, Bunkyo-ku, Tokyo 113-8657, Japan

Trichostatin A (TSA) is a microbial metabolite that specifically inhibits mammalian histone deacetylase and causes accumulation of highly acetylated histone molecules at nanomolar concentrations.[1] Inhibition of histone deacetylase (HDAC) by TSA causes several effects such as the induction of differentiation and apoptosis, or alteration of transcription.[1] One of those prominent effects of TSA is its long-term growth inhibiton and arrest of the cell cycle at the G1 phase in mammalian cells.[1] Recently, several potent antitumor agents such as FR901228[2] and oxamflatin[3] were shown to be novel HDAC inhibitors. However, the molecular mechanism by which HDAC inhibitor induced cell cycle arrest and antitumor activity remains to be elucidated. To understand this mechanism, we screened for cell cycle regulators whose expression is affected by TSA treatment using reverse transcriptase–polymerase chain reaction (RT-PCR) and Western blot analysis. During these series of experiments, we found marked changes in expression of several cell cycle regulating factors and inactivation of cdk2 activity, resulting in hypophosphorylation of pRB.[4]

TSA INDUCES EXPRESSION OF CDK INHIBITORS (CKIS)

The effects of TSA on gene expression of various cell cycle regulators were examined by comparing untreated and treated cells using semiquantitative RT-PCR. We found that expression of p21[WAF1] in various cell lines was greatly upregulated in response to TSA in a dose-dependent manner, whereas that of p27[Kip1] was unaffected. An increase in the amount of p21[WAF1] was also shown by Western blotting even in cells lacking functional p53, such as T24, HL60, and SV40-transformed WI38. Another CKI, p16[INK4A], was also upregulated by TSA at higher concentrations than those for p21[WAF1]. By contrast, Cdks and cyclins were not dramatically increased by TSA. These results suggest that histone hyperacetylation induces specific activation

[a]Address for correspondence: Young Bae Kim, Department of Biotechnology, Graduate School of Agriculture and Life Sciences, the University of Tokyo, Yayoi 1-1-1, Bunkyo-ku, Tokyo 113-8657, Japan. Phone, +81-3-3812-2111 ext. 5124; fax, +81-3-3812-0544.
e-mail, aa67122@hongo.ecc.u-tokyo.ac.jp

of p21^{WAF1} transcription independent of p53. In all cell lines, induction of p21^{WAF1} started 6 hours after TSA treatment at 200 ng/ml. These increases in protein and mRNA levels of p21^{WAF1} correlated well with the decrease in proliferating cells incorporating BrdU following accumulation of hyperacetylated histones. Removal of TSA caused a decrease in the p21^{WAF1} protein level following a rapid decrease in the histone acetylation level, which allowed cells to resume the cell cycle. These results suggest that histone acetylation/deacetylation plays an important role in transcriptional regulation of p21^{WAF1} and that its overexpression is responsible for the specific cell cycle arrest induced by the histone hyperacetylating agents. It is still possible that the increase in p16^{INK4A} plays some role in cell cycle arrest by TSA.

CHANGES IN EXPRESSION OF CYCLINS AND OTHER GENES

In contrast to the induction of CKIs, expression of cyclin A was downregulated, whereas the amounts of CDKs were almost unchanged on TSA treatment. This downregulation of cyclin A showed the perfect reverse pattern to the induction of p21^{WAF1}. Because expression of cyclin A is thought to be necessary to enter S phase,[4] it seems likely that the decrease in cyclin A is also involved in TSA-induced cell cycle arrest. However, it is also possible that this downregulation is secondary,because Cdk activity in G1 phase is required for cyclin A expression.[5] As a result of the inactivation of Cdk2 by overproduction of p21^{WAF1}, cyclin A expression may be downregulated. Expression of D-type cyclins also decreased but not significantly. On the other hand, cyclin E was induced on TSA treatment. This derepression of cyclin E may come from alleviation of transcriptional repression by E2F, a transcriptional factor recruiting HDAC through binding with pRB.[6]

Treatment with TSA also affected the expression of several other genes that are involved in cell migration, cell adhesion, and/or cytoskeletal reconstitution. It caused upregulation of gelsolin, a putative tumor suppressor gene,[7] and fibronectin, an extracellular matrix protein.[8] The induction of these genes might explain the morphologic changes and stress fiber formation of tumor cells cause by TSA.[1,9]

CONCLUDING REMARKS

Changes in gene expression in HeLa cells by TSA are summarized in TABLE 1. Other HDAC inhibitors such as trapoxin, oxamflain,[3] and FR901228 (Y.B. Kim, unpublished data) caused essentially the same pattern of expression. Among CKIs induced by TSA, the increase in the amount of p21^{WAF1} correlated best with the onset of cell cycle arrest and the reduction of Cdk2 activity, resulting in hypophosphorylation of pRB.[10] These results suggest that overproduction of p21^{WAF1} on TSA treatment is responsible, at least in part, for the induced cell cycle arrest. Because MTS family members involving p16^{INK4A} are frequently lost or mutated in human tumor cells,[11] chemical induction of CKIs by HDAC inhibitors may compensate for the functional loss of the tumor suppressors. In addition to these results, overexpression of gelsolin and fibronectin would also contribute to the antitumor activity of HDAC inhibitors synergistically with the changes in expression of the cell cycle regulators.

TABLE 1. Changes in gene expression by TSA[a]

Group	Gene	Change caused by TSA treatment
CKI	p21^{WAF1}	++++[b]
	p27^{Kip1}	±[c]
	p16^{INK4A}	+++
	p15^{INK4B}	ND
	p57^{Kip2}	ND
Cyclins	Cyclin A	___[d]
	Cyclin B	±
	Cyclin C	−
	Cyclin D	± (−)
	Cyclin E	+++
Cdks	cdc2	±
	cdk2	±
	cdk4	±
	cdk6	±
Others	Gelsolin	++
	Fibronectin	+
	p53	± (−)
	pRB	± (+)

[a]Detected by RT-PCR and/or Western blot. [b]Upregulated. [c]Not significantly changed. [d]Down-regulated. ND, not detected.

REFERENCES

1. YOSHIDA, M., S. HORINOUCHI & T. BEPPU. 1995. Trichostatin A and trapoxin: Novel chemical probes for the role of histone acetylation in chromatin structure and function. Bioessays **17:** 423–430.
2. NAKAJIMA, H., Y.B. KIM, H. TERANO et al. 1998. FR901228, a potent antitumor antibiotic, is a novel histone deacetylase inhibitor. Exp. Cell Res. **241:** 126–133.
3. KIM, Y.B., K.-H. LEE, K. SUGITA et al. 1998. Oxamflatin is a novel antitumor compound that inhibits mammalian histone deacetylase. Oncogene **18:** 2461–2470.
4. KING, R.W., P.K. JACKSON & M.W. KIRSCHNER. 1994. Mitosis in transition. Cell **79:** 563–571.
5. ZERFASS-THOME, K., A. SCHULZE, W. ZWERSCHKE et al. 1997. p27KIP1 blocks cyclin E-dependent transactivation of cyclin A gene expression. Mol. Cell. Biol. **17:** 407–415.
6. MAGNAGHI, J.L., R. GROISMAN, I. NAGUIBNEVA et al. 1998. Retinoblastoma protein represses transcription by recruiting a histone deacetylase. Nature **391:** 601–605.
7. FUJITA, H., L.E. LAHAM, P.A. JANMEY et al. 1995. Functions of [His321]gelsolin isolated from a flat revertant of ras- transformed cells. Eur. J. Biochem. **2295:** 615–620.
8. AKIYAMA, S.K. & K.M. YAMADA. 1987. Fibronectin. Adv. Enzymol. Relat. Areas Mol. Biol. **59:** 1–57.
9. SONODA, H., K. NISHIDA, T. YOSHIOKA et al. 1996. Oxamflatin: A novel compound which reverses malignant phenotype to normal one via induction of JunD. Oncogene **13:** 143–149.

10. LEPLEY, D.M. & J.C. PELLING. 1997. Induction of p21/WAF1 and G1 cell-cycle arrest by the chemopreventive agent apigenin. Mol Carcinog **19:** 74–82.
11. CALDAS, C., S.A. HAHN, C.L. DA *et al.* 1994. Frequent somatic mutations and homozygous deletions of the p16(MTS1) gene in pancreatic adenocarcinoma. Nat. Genet. **8:** 27–32.

Identification of a Novel Nuclear Export Signal Sensitive to Oxidative Stress in Yeast AP-1–Like Transcription Factor

NOBUAKI KUDO,[a] HIROSHI TAOKA, MINORU YOSHIDA, AND SUEHARU HORINOUCHI

Department of Biotechnology, Graduate School of Agriculture and Life Sciences, The University of Tokyo, Bunkyo-ku, Tokyo 113, Japan

Leptomycin B (LMB) is an antitumor antibiotic that causes arrest of the cell cycle.[1,2] Recently, it was found to inhibit nuclear export of proteins bearing nuclear export signal (NES) such as human immunodeficiency virus type I (HIV-1).[3] The target molecule of LMB in fission yeast has genetically been suggested to be CRM1, a protein structurally conserved in eukaryotes.[4] CRM1 was shown to be a receptor for the leucine-rich NESs of proteins and was renamed exportin 1.[5–8] We showed that LMB directly binds CRM1 and inhibits the association of CRM1 with NES-bearing proteins, resulting in the nuclear accumulation of NES-bearing proteins that should be exported to the cytoplasm.[9] Therefore, LMB is a useful probe for determining the presence or absence of an NES in a protein of interest.

IDENTIFICATION OF A NOVEL NES SENSITIVE TO OXIDATIVE STRESS IN PAP1

Pap1, a fission yeast homolog of AP-1, is a transcription factor that directs expression of stress-activated genes.[10] Because genetic analysis suggested that Pap1 was negatively regulated by CRM1,[11] we hypothesized that Pap1 contains a functional NES by which Pap1 is excluded from the nucleus. To analyze the subcellular localization of Pap1, we expressed GFP-fused Pap1 and its mutants in fission yeast (FIG. 1A). Pap1 was localized normally in the cytoplasm but translocated into the nucleus when CRM1 was inactivated by LMB or a temperature-sensitive mutation. Deletion of the C-terminal cysteine-rich domain (CRD) consisting of 57-amino acids resulted in nuclear accumulation of Pap1, whereas a GST-GFP-fused CRD alone was localized exclusively in the cytoplasm in a CRM1-dependent manner. The CRD also was exported by the CRM1/exportin 1–mediated system in mammalian cells in an LMB-sensitive way, as a purified GST-CRD-GFP fusion protein was rapidly translocated to the cytoplasm when it was microinjected into the nucleus. We found that

[a]Address for correspondence: Nobuaki Kudo, Department of Biotechnology, Graduate School of Agriculture and Life Sciences, The University of Tokyo, Yayoi 1-1-1, Bunkyo-ku, Tokyo 113, Japan. Phone, +81-3-5841-5124; fax, +81-3-5841-5337.
e-mail, kudo@bio.m.u-tokyo.ac.jp

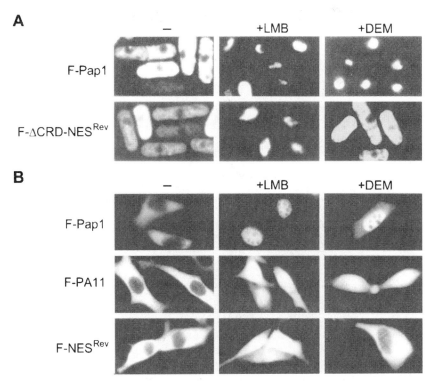

FIGURE 1. CRM1/exportin 1-dependent nuclear export of Pap1 and its inhibition by oxidative stress. (**A**) Subcellular localization of GFP-fused Pap1 (F-Pap1) and Pap1 containing Rev NES instead of CRD (F-ΔCRD-NES^{Rev}) in fission yeast. Changes in the localization of the fusion proteins were observed after treating with 50 ng/ml LMB for 0.5 hour or 2 mM DEM for 1 hour. (**B**) Nuclear export and DEM response of F-Pap1, GFP-PA11 (F-PA11) and GFP-Rev NES (F-NES^{Rev}) in NIH3T3 cells. Changes in the subcellular localization were observed after treating with 5 ng/ml LMB for 1 hour or 0.8 mM DEM for 2 hours.

Pap1-mediated transcriptional activation was induced depending on the nuclear accumulation of Pap1, indicating that Pap1 function is controlled by its subcellular localization. Deletion and mutational analyses identified several important amino acids in a 19-amino acid region (named PA11, residues 515-533 in the CRD), which serves as an NES (FIG. 2). We identified cysteine residues as important residues for the NES activity, in addition to hydrophobic amino acids, typical of the classical leucine-rich NES. The presence of at least one of the two cysteine residues (Cys-523 and Cys-532) was essential for the nuclear export. We next analyzed the mechanism by which Pap1 is activated in response to oxidative stress. Pap1 relocalized to the nucleus upon diethyl maleate (DEM) treatment (FIG. 1A). The nuclear export of Pap1 was inhibited by DEM. Pap1 containing Rev NES instead of CRD failed to response to DEM, suggesting that the Pap1 NES is unique in that it is sensitive to oxidative stress.

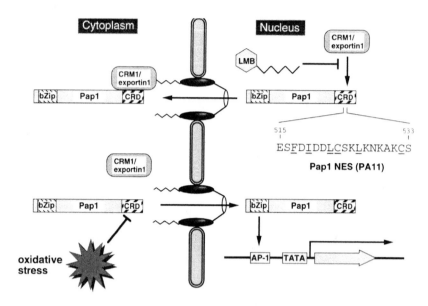

FIGURE 2. Schematic diagram for nuclear export and oxidative stress response of Pap1. The important residues for Pap1 NES (PA11) are underlined.

OXIDATIVE STRESS RESPONSE OF PAP1 IS CONSERVED IN MAMMALIAN CELLS

To test whether the nuclear export of the Pap1 NES is also sensitive to DEM in animal cells, we expressed GFP-Pap1 and GFP-PA11 in mammalian cells. As shown in FIGURE 1B, DEM treatment induced rapid nuclear translocation of Pap1 and PA11, as did LMB. However, GFP-fused Rev NES was insensitive to DEM. These results indicate that Pap1 NES can fully respond to oxidative stress not only in yeast but also in mammalian cells.

CONCLUSION

We show that Pap1 contains a novel NES sensitive to oxidative stress. The NES was an atypical leucine-rich sequence with important cysteine residues and was sufficient for the response to oxidative stress. We could not separate the DEM response from NES function by site-directed mutagenesis, indicating that the amino acid residue(s) that is responsible for the response is present in the NES sequence. We demonstrated that the Pap1 NES was fully functional in mammalian cells. Thus, the Pap1 NES is the first example containing important cysteine residues, the function of which is inhibited by oxidative stress through an evolutionalrily conserved mechanism.

REFERENCES

1. KOMIYAMA, K. *et al.* 1985. Antitumor activity of leptomycin B. J. Antibiot. **38:** 427–429.
2. YOSHIDA, M. *et al.* 1990. Effects of leptomycin B on the cell cycle of fibroblasts and fission yeast cells. Exp. Cell Res. **187:** 150–156.
3. WOLFF, B. *et al.* 1997. Leptomycin B is an inhibitor of nuclear export: inhibition of nucleo-cytoplasmic translocation of the human immunodeficiency virus type 1 (HIV-1) Rev protein and Rev-dependent mRNA. Chem. Biol. **4:** 139–147.
4. NISHI, K. *et al.* 1994. Leptomycin B targets a regulatory cascade of crm1, a fission yeast nuclear protein, involved in control of higher order chromosome structure and gene expression. J. Biol. Chem. **269:** 6320–6324.
5. FORNEROD, M. *et al.* 1997. CRM1 is an export receptor for leucine-rich nuclear export signals. Cell **90:** 1051–1060.
6. FUKUDA, M. *et al.* 1997. CRM1 is responsible for intracellular transport mediated by the nuclear export signal. Nature **390:** 308–311.
7. KUDO, N. *et al.* 1997. Molecular cloning and cell cycle-dependent expression of mammalian CRM1, a protein involved in nuclear export of proteins. J. Biol. Chem. **272:** 29742–29751.
8. STADE, K. *et al.* 1997. Exportin 1 (Crm1p) is an essential nuclear export factor. Cell **90:** 1041–1050.
9. KUDO, N. *et al.* 1998. Leptomycin B inhibition of signal-mediated nuclear export by direct binding to CRM1. Exp. Cell Res. **242:** 540–547.
10. TOONE, W. M. *et al.* 1998. Regulation of the fission yeast transcription factor Pap1 by oxidative stress: requirement for the nuclear export factor Crm1 (Exportin) and the stress-activated MAP kinase Sty1/Spc1. Genes Dev. **12:** 1453–1463.
11. TODA, T. *et al.* 1992. Fission yeast pap1-dependent transcription is negatively regulated by an essential nuclear protein, crm1. Mol. Cell. Biol. **12:** 5474–5484.

Melanoma Cell Lines Contain a Proteasome-Sensitive, Nuclear Cytoskeleton-Associated Pool of β-Catenin

P. BONVINI,[a,c] S.-G. HWANG,[a] M. EL-GAMIL,[b] P. ROBBINS,[b] L. NECKERS,[a] AND J. TREPEL[a]

[a]Department of Cell and Cancer Biology, Medicine Branch, National Cancer Institute, National Institutes of Health, Rockville, Maryland 20850 (P.B. & L.N.) and Bethesda, Maryland 20892 (S.-G.H. & J.T.), USA

[b]Surgery Branch, National Cancer Institute, National Institutes of Health, Bethesda, Maryland 20892, USA

Recent studies have shown that colon carcinoma and melanoma cells that contain either deletions of APC or activating mutations in β-catenin contain elevated levels of both cytoplasmic and nuclear β-catenin.[1–4] Similar results were reported following proteasome inhibition of cells containing wild-type β-catenin. Furthermore, in cells containing mutated β-catenin or wild-type β-catenin but no APC, the β-catenin protein has an exceptionally long half-life. These findings led to the hypothesis that lack of APC function or β-catenin mutation result in elevated levels of nuclear β-catenin secondary to elevation of a soluble, proteasome-resistant cytosolic pool of the protein. However, β-catenin exists in several subcellular locations, and little is known of the effect of β-catenin mutations/APC deletions on the response of these pools to proteasome inhibition. To further examine this question, we studied three previously described melanoma cell lines,[3] 1241, which expresses APC but carries a Ser37Æ Phe37 (S37F) β-catenin mutation in the GSK3ß phosphorylation site; 928, which expresses wild-type β-catenin but no detectable APC; and 1011, which contains both wild-type β-catenin and APC.

In this study, the three melanoma cell lines were treated with the proteasome inhibitor ALLnL (100 μM)[5,6] for 6 hours, and the β-catenin steady-state level in several subcellular fractions was compared with that of untreated cells. As predicted from previous studies, soluble β-catenin in 1011 cells was sensitive to proteasome inhibition, but the soluble β-catenin fraction of both 928 and 1241 cells was resistant to proteasome-mediated degradation. A novel finding of this study is that the detergent-insoluble β-catenin fraction from all three cell lines retained proteasome sensitivity. To clarify the nature of this detergent-insoluble fraction, we lysed cells in detergent-free buffer and prepared soluble, microsomal, and pellet fractions, which were analyzed for β-catenin content. As expected, the β-catenin steady-state level in 1011 cells was increased primarily in the soluble fraction after proteasome inhibition. In contrast, in 928 and 1241 cells, β-catenin protein markedly accumulated only

[c]Address for correspondence: Paolo Bonvini, 9610 Medical Center Drive, Suite 300, Rockville, Maryland 20850. Phone, 301/402-3128, ext. 312; fax, 301/402-4422.
e-mail, bonvinip@box-b.nih.gov

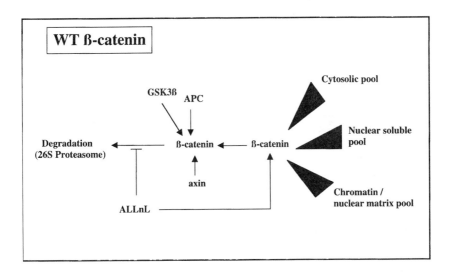

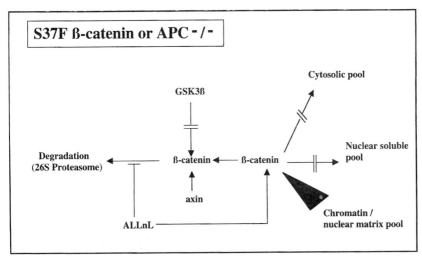

FIGURE 1. Effect of proteasome inhibition on β-catenin subcellular distribution. Wild-type β-catenin was shown to be degraded by the 26S proteasome pathway, by interacting with the APC, axin, and GSKß3 proteins. In 1011 melanoma cells, proteasome inhibition caused an accumulation (▲) of wild-type β-catenin (WT β-catenin) in cytosolic, nuclear detergent-soluble, and nuclear chromatin/nuclear matrix (detergent-insoluble) fractions. However, in 928 (APC −/−) and 1241 (S37F β-catenin) melanoma cells, proteasome inhibition causes accumulation (▲) of β-catenin protein only in the chromatin/nuclear matrix fraction without affecting (⊣⊢►) β-catenin cytosolic and nuclear detergent-soluble fractions.

in the pellet fraction after proteasome inhibition. This fraction is primarily comprised of cytoskeleton/nuclear matrix-associated components. The β-catenin level in the microsomal fraction, which represents membrane-associated β-catenin, remained unaffected by proteasome inhibition in all cell lines. Fluorescence microscopic analysis of cytoskeletal preparations confirmed these observations and demonstrated strong accumulation of nuclear cytoskeleton-associated β-catenin in proteasome-inhibited cells. These results were supported by additional biochemical fractionation studies. We prepared intact nuclei from the three cell lines after proteasome inhibition and analyzed the β-catenin level in soluble and insoluble nuclear fractions. Consistent with our other findings, b-catenin was markedly increased in the insoluble nuclear fraction in 1241 and 928 cell lines following proteasome inhibition. To investigate whether this pool represented transcriptionally active β-catenin, we transiently transfected 928 and 1241 cells with a Tcf-luciferase reporter plasmid, pTOPFLASH,[1] and 24 hours later exposed cells to the proteasome inhibitor ALLnL. Proteasome inhibition resulted in a 3–13-fold increase in Tcf-dependent reporter activity in both 928 and 1241 cells. In agreement with these results, we found that in cells transiently transfected with an HA-LEF expression plasmid,[7] transcriptionally active β-catenin/LEF complexes were localized primarily to the insoluble nuclear fraction both before and after proteasome inhibition.

In summary, even though detergent-soluble, cytoplasmic β-catenin pools lose their sensitivity to the proteasome subsequent to β-catenin mutation or loss of APC, our data demonstrate the existence of a detergent-insoluble nuclear β-catenin pool which remains sensitive to the proteasome, especially in cells harboring β-catenin mutation or loss of APC. This nuclear fractions contains nuclear cytoskeletal elements and chromatin. Preliminary experiments have identified both β-catenin/nuclear filament complexes and β-catenin/chromatin association in this fraction. Finally, the detergent-insoluble nuclear fraction contains proteasome-sensitive β-catenin/LEF complexes, and proteasome inhibition results in a significant elevation of β-catenin-dependent Tcf transactivation. Thus, β-catenin residing in the detergent-insoluble nuclear fraction is transcriptionally active, and this pool remains sensitive to proteasome inhibition even when the detergent-soluble cytosolic β-catenin component from the same cells is resistant. These results argue for differential regulation of β-catenin stability in distinct subcellular compartments.

REFERENCES

1. KORINEK, V., N. BARKER, P.J. MORIN, D. VAN WICHEN, R. DE WEGER, K.W. KINZLER, B. VOLGESTEIN & H. CLEVERS. 1997. Constitutive transcriptional activation by a β-catenin-Tcf complex in APC $^{-/-}$ colon carcinoma. Science 275: 1784–1787.
2. MORIN, P.J., A.B. SPARKS, V. KORINEK, N. BARKER, H. CLEVERS, B. VOLGESTEIN & K.W. KINZLER. 1997. Activation of ß-catenin-Tcf signaling in colon cancer by mutations in ß-catenin or APC. Science 275: 1787–1790.
3. RUBINFELD, B., P. ROBBINS, M. EL-GAMIL, I. ALBERT, E. PORFIRI & P. POLAKIS. 1997. Stabilization of ß-catenin by genetic defects in melanoma cell lines. Science 275: 1790–1792.
4. YOST, C., M. TORRES, J.R. MILLER, E. HUANG, D. KIMELMAN & R.T. MOON. 1996. The axis-inducing activity, stability, and subcellular distribution of ß-catenin is regulated in Xenopus embryos by glycogen synthase kinase 3. Genes Dev.

5. ORLOWSKI, M., C. CARDOZO & C. MICHAUD. 1993. Evidence for the presence of five distinct proteolytic components in the pituitary multicatalytic proteinase complex. Properties of two components cleaving bonds on the carboxyl side of branched chain and small neutral amino acids. Biochemistry **32:** 1563–1572.

6. ROCK, K.L., C. GRAMM, L. ROTHSTEIN, K. CLARK, R. STEIN, L. DICK, D. HWANG & A.L. GOLDBERG 1994. Inhibitors of the proteasome block the degradation of most cell proteins and the generation of peptide presented on MHC Class I molecules. Cell **78:** 761–771.

7. BEHRENS, J., J.P. VON KRIES, M. KUHL, L. BRUHN, D. WEDLICH, R. GROSSCHEDL & W. BIRCHMEIER. 1996. Functional interaction of β-catenin with the transcription factor LEF-1. Nature **382:** 638–642.

Truncated Form of β-Catenin and Reduced Expression of Wild-Type Catenins Feature HepG2 Human Liver Cancer Cells

GIUSEPPE CARRUBA, [a,e] MELCHIORRE CERVELLO,[b] MARIA D. MICELI,[a] ROSARIA FARRUGGIO,[a] MONICA NOTARBARTOLO,[c] LUCREZIA VIRRUSO,[b] LYDIA GIANNITRAPANI,[d] ROBERTO GAMBINO,[b] GIUSEPPE MONTALTO,[d] AND LUIGI CASTAGNETTA[a,c]

[a]Institute of Oncology, and [d]Institute of Internal Medicine, University of Palermo, Palermo, Italy

[b]Institute of Developmental Biology, C.N.R., Palermo, Italy

[c]Experimental Oncology, Palermo Branch of IST-Genoa, c/o M. Ascoli Cancer Hospital Center, Palermo, Italy

The cadherins are a family of calcium-dependent cell to cell adhesion molecules that are primarily involved in both embryonic morphogenesis and structural and functional preservation of adult tissues.[1] Cadherin function is mediated by a group of cytoplasmic proteins, referred to as α-, β- and γ-catenin (plakoglobin). Assembly of the cadherin/catenin complex is accomplished by linkage of E-cadherin to the actin microfilaments of cytoskeleton through both γ- and β-catenin.[2] Therefore, altered expression of the catenin molecules may be responsible for disturbance of the cadherin-mediated adhesion system, eventually leading to the onset of an invasive cell phenotype.[3,4] Reports on the cadherin/catenin system and its regulation in human liver tumor tissues remain sparse and occasionally controversial. In the present work, we compared expression of the various catenins in a human liver cancer cell line (HepG2) with that in a nonneoplastic human hepatocytic cell line (Chang liver) using Western blotting analysis. We also used reverse transcriptase-polymerase chain reaction (RT-PCR) and DNA sequencing analyses to inspect the structure and expression of the β-catenin gene.

MATERIALS AND METHODS

Cell Cultures. Cells were maintained in RPMI 1640 medium supplemented with 10% heat-inactivated fetal calf serum. Both culture medium and cells were periodically tested for mycoplasma contamination. Cells with a narrow range of passage number were used for all experiments.

Gel Electrophoresis and Immunoblotting. Chang liver and HepG2 cells were lysed for 20 minutes in a lysis buffer containing 20 mM TRIS, pH 7.4, 1% Triton, 1%

[e]Address for correspondence: Institute of Oncology, Via Marchese Ugo 56, 90141 Palermo, Italy. Phone +39 091 666-4346; fax, +39 091 666-4352.
e-mail, lucashbl@unipa.it

Nonidet P-40, 10 μg/ml aprotinin, 10 μg/ml leupeptin, and 1 mM phenylmethylsulfonyl fluoride (Sigma, St. Louis, Missouri). Cell lysates were centrifuged at $12,000 \times g$ for 10 minutes at 4°C and the resulting supernatants recovered. Sample protein concentration was determined with a Bio-Rad protein assay kit (Bio-Rad Laboratories SrL, Milan, Italy). Fifty microgram protein aliquots of each supernatant were mixed with reducing 3x Laemmli sample buffer and subjected to SDS-PAGE, as originally described by Laemmli.[5] Proteins were electrophoresed onto a nitrocellulose membrane (Amersham) and membranes probed with a 1:200 to 1:1500 dilution of anti-α, anti-β, or anti-γ-catenin antibody. Hybridization was visualized using an ECL detection kit (Amersham Italia SrL, Milan, Italy), according to the manufacturer's instructions. Relative estimates of hybridized bands were carried out with a GS-670 Bio-Rad Densitometer using the Molecular Analyst/PC image analysis software (version 1.1).

Extraction of Cellular RNA and Reverse-Transcriptase-PCR (RT-PCR). Total RNA was extracted from Chang liver and HepG2 cells by the guanidinium-thiocyanate method according to Chomczynski and Sacchi.[6] Prior to cDNA preparation, all RNA was treated with 5 U of DNAse I (Boehringer). cDNA was made from 5 μg of total RNA using a First-Strand Synthesis Kit (Amersham). PCR was then performed using 1–2 μl of cDNA solution as template. Two pair of primers were designed to examine the entire coding sequence of β-catenin gene into two separate regions. The sequences of the primers used were as follows: S1 (sense), corresponding to nucleotides +192 to +211; A1 (antisense), corresponding to nucleotides +1101 to +1120; S2, corresponding to nucleotides +763 to +782; and A2, corresponding to nucleotides +2590 to +2609. The primers were designed according to the EMBL/GenBank cDNA sequence (accession No. X87838). PCR fragments were analyzed by 1.5% agarose gel electrophoresis.

DNA Sequencing. Primer A888 (corresponding to nucleotides +868 to +888) was designed to amplify a short N-terminal region of β-catenin mRNA. The PCR products obtained using primers S1 and A888 were separated by agarose gel electrophoresis, and the fragment of interest was extracted. Each fragment was cloned using the TOPO-TA cloning kit (Invitrogen). Purified DNA containing β-catenin cDNA was used in a thermocycle sequencing reaction with the Thermo sequenase-radiolabeled terminator cycle sequencing kit (Amersham). All the sequencing reactions were performed using the S1 and A888 primers.

RESULTS

Western blotting experiments revealed expression of normal α-catenin in the two cell lines studied, although HepG2 cells expressed significantly smaller amounts of this 102-kD component with respect to Chang liver cells (FIG. 1A). Analysis of β-catenin expression showed that whereas both cell lines contained a normal 92-kD protein, markedly reduced levels were found in HepG2 cells. In the latter cell line a smaller component of about 75 kD was coexpressed with the wild-type β-catenin protein (FIG. 1B); this resulted in an overall increase of β-catenin expression levels. Greater amounts of γ-catenin were found in Chang liver cells, while again HepG2 cells exhibited a pronounced reduction in γ-catenin expression (FIG. 1C). Relative

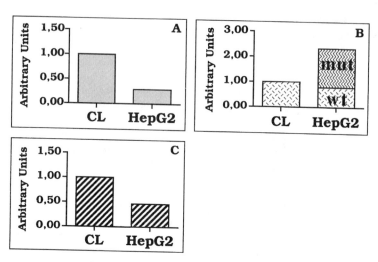

FIGURE 1. Quantification of α-catenin (**A**), β-catenin (**B**), and γ-catenin (**C**) expression in Chang liver and HepG2 cells. Histograms illustrate results obtained by densitometric analysis of Western blotting experiments. mut, mutated form; wt, wild type.

estimates of catenin levels in Chang liver and HepG2 cells revealed a clear increase (2.3-fold) of total β-catenin amounts in HepG2 cells, whereas expression of wild-type α-, β-, and γ-catenins was reduced in this cell line, respectively, being 29%, 78%, and 47% of that seen in Chang liver cells. The potential deletion of β-catenin mRNA in HepG2 cells was investigated by means of RT-PCR. Agarose gel electrophoresis showed that the S1-A1 PCR product from HepG2 cells gave rise to two separate bands, one corresponding to the full-length β-catenin message and one additional band about 350-bases shorter (not shown). Sequencing analysis of the PCR-amplified 5'-terminal S1-A888 fragments from HepG2 revealed a 348-base in-frame deletion from position 287 to 634 of the shorter fragment, resulting in a 116 amino acid deletion (from Trp[25] to Ile[140]) (FIG. 2). As a consequence, the mutated β-catenin molecule consisted of 665 amino acids, with an expected molecular mass of about 73 kD. No sequence mutation was detected in the full-length fragment (not shown).

DISCUSSION

In the present work we report evidence of a truncated form of β-catenin in HepG2 human liver cancer cells, accompanied by a significant decrease in the expression of wild-type α-, β- and γ-catenins. Because both γ- and β-catenins represent an essential requirement for formation of the cadherin/catenin complex, it seems likely that loss of catenin results in alteration of the E-cadherin–mediated cell-cell adhesion system in HepG2 cells. RT-PCR and DNA sequencing analyses showed that HepG2 cells contain a deletion of β-catenin at the NH₂-terminal region of the protein, namely at the potential phosphorylation site of glycogen synthase kinase-3β (GSK-3β).

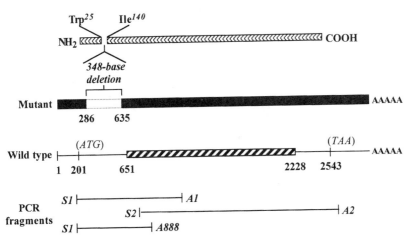

FIGURE 2. Sequencing analysis for mutant β-catenin protein and mRNA in HepG2 cells. The 348-base deletion and resulting 116 amino acid deletion are indicated. Cross hatching, the 13-cycle repeat sequence domain. *ATG*, initiation codon; *TAA*, stop codon. The extension of both sense (S1, S2) and antisense (A1, A2) primers used for RT-PCR as well as that of the primer set (S1, A888) used for DNA sequencing is reported. Numbers indicate the nucleotide positions at boundaries.

This may eventually lead to accumulation of a hypophosphorylated form of β-catenin, because the GSK-3β–induced phosphorylation of β-catenin promotes its turnover.[7] Recently, de La Coste and colleagues detected point mutations or deletions of the β-catenin gene in both human liver tumors and hepatoma cells, leading to accumulation of the β-catenin in the nucleus.[8] All this strongly supports the hypothesis that β-catenin mutations and/or hindrance of its turnover may be involved in human liver carcinogenesis. Further investigation should define the potential biologic role of β-catenin derangements during development of human hepatocellular carcinoma and ascertain whether similar variations are present in both precancerous lesions and primary tumors of the liver.

ACKNOWLEDGMENTS

This study was funded in part by the Italian Association for Cancer Research (AIRC, to L.C.) and by research grants from Italian MURST 60% (to L.C. and G.M.). The authors are grateful to Dr. De Pasqua (Zeneca Pharmaceuticals, Milan, Italy) for financial support of the present study. The authors wish to thank Dr. A. Giallongo (Palermo, Italy) for fruitful discussion and continuous support.

REFERENCES

1. TAKEICHI, M. 1991. Cadherin cell adhesion receptor as a morphogenetic regulator. Science (Washington, DC) **251:** 1451–1455.

2. KEMLER, R. 1993. From cadherins to catenins: Cytoplasmic protein interactions and regulation of cell adhesion. Trends Genet. **9:** 317–321.
3. SHIMOYAMA, Y., A. NAGAFUCHI, S. FUJITA, M. GOTOH, M. TAKEICHI, S. TSUKITA & S. HIROHASHI. 1992. Cadherin dysfunction in a human cancer cell line: Possible involvement of loss of α-catenin expression in reduced cell-cell adhesiveness. Cancer Res. **52:** 5770–5774.
4. NAKANISHI, Y., A. OCHIAI, S. AKIMOTO, H. KATO, H. WATANABE, Y. TACHIMORI, S. YAMAMOTO & S. HIROHASHI. 1997. Expression of E-cadherin, α-catenin, β-catenin and plakoglobin in esophageal carcinomas and its prognostic significance. Oncology **54:** 158–165.
5. LAEMMLI, U.K. 1970. Cleavage of structural proteins during the assembly of the head of bacteriophage T4. Nature **227:** 680–685.
6. CHOMCZYNSKI, P. & N. SACCHI. 1987. Single-step method of RNA isolation by acidic guanidinium thiocyanate-phenol-chloroform extraction. Anal. Biochem. **162:** 156–159.
7. YOST, C., M. TORRES, J.R. MILLER, E. HUANG, D. KIMELMAN & R.T. MOON. 1996. The axis-inducing activity, stability and subcellular distribution of β-catenin is regulated in *Xenopus* embryo by glycogen synthase kinase 3. Genes Dev. **10:** 1443–1454.
8. DE LA COSTE, A., B. ROMAGNOLO, P. BILLUART, C.A. RENARD, M.-A. BUENDIA, O. SOUBRANE, M. FABRE, J. CHELLY, C. BELDIORD, A. KAHN & C. PERRET. 1998. Somatic mutations of the β-catenin gene are frequent in mouse and human hepatocellular carcinoma. Proc. Natl. Acad. Sci. USA **95:** 8847–8851.

Induction of Apoptosis by Gelsolin Truncates

HISAKAZU FUJITA,[a,c] PHILIP G. ALLEN,[b] PAUL A. JANMEY,[b]
TOSHIFUMI AZUMA,[b] DAVID J. KWIATKOWSKI,[b] THOMAS P. STOSSEL,[b]
AND N. KUZUMAKI[a]

[a]Division of Gene Regulation, Cancer Institute, Hokkaido University School of Medicine,
Sapporo 060-8638, Japan

[b]Division of Experimental Medicine, Brigham and Women's Hospital, Harvard Medical
School, Boston, Massachusetts 02115, USA

Gelsolin is an 82-kD protein present in most vertebrate tissue that has been shown to affect the length of actin polymers *in vitro*. Gelsolin severs actin filaments, nucleates actin polymerization, and blocks actin monomer exchange of the fast-growing (barbed) ends of actin filaments.[1] Calcium ions, pH, and polyphosphoinositides regulate these activities *in vitro*.[2] Increased expression of gelsolin in fibroblasts, by stable transfection of the gelsolin cDNA, causes rapid cell movement in tissue culture.[3] Moreover, adult skin fibroblasts from gelsolin null mice move slower and exhibit reduced membrane ruffling compared with wild-type fibroblasts.[4] The amino acid sequence of the gelsolin molecule has six homologous repeats (G1–G6), and extensive studies using proteolytic fragments and recombinant truncates of gelsolin indicate that the various functions of gelsolin involve the cooperative interaction of the domains encoded by repeated sequences. The G1 domain appears to be essential for severing activity, and therefore G1 is regarded as an effector domain for the severing activity of gelsolin. Mutant proteins that lack a functional domain in their normal counterpart can be used to inhibit the activity of the native protein.[5] We previously showed that G2-6 and G2-3, truncates of gelsolin lacking the G1 domain necessary for severing, but not for filament binding or monomer nucleation, function as competitive inhibitors of the actin filament-severing activities of both native forms of gelsolin and cofilin, another family of protein that influences actin filament remodeling.[6] In this study, we transfected the cDNAs encoding gelsolin truncates to examine their effect in the cell.

MATERIALS AND METHODS

Expression Vectors and DNA Transfection

The cDNAs for truncates of gelsolin[6] were subcloned into multicloning sites of LK444 containing the human β-actin promoter. The expression vector was cotransfected with pMiwhph carrying the hygromycin B-resistant (hyg B[r]) gene into B16-BL6 cells by the lipofection method using lipofectin (GIBCO/BRL Life Technolo-

[c]Address for correspondence: Hisakazu Fujita, Division of Gene Regulation, Cancer Institute, Hokkaido University School of Medicine, N15W7, Kita-ku, Sapporo 060-8638, Japan. Phone, +81-11-706-6053; fax, +81-11-06-7869.
e-mail, h_fujita@med.hokudai.ac.jp

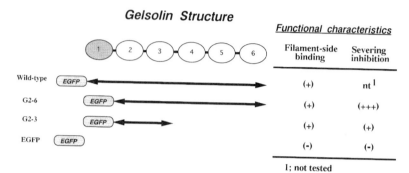

FIGURE 1. Structure and characteristics of gelsolin truncates for transfection.

gies, Inc.). Transfected cells were placed in a selection medium containing hygromycin B (Wako) for 14–20 days, and individual colonies were picked up randomly. For transient expression of EGFP-fused truncate, cDNAs of each truncate were subcloned into multiple cloning sites of pEGFP-C1 or C2 (Clontech).

Cell Death Assays

COS 7 cells were transiently transfected with EGFP fused full-length for each truncate of gelsolin expression plasmid using lipofectAMINE (GIBCO/BRL Life Technologies, Inc.). Two to three days later, the morphology of transfected cells was examined under a fluorescent microscope (TE-300-EF, Nikon Instic, Japan). At least 300 EGFP-positive cells in five to seven separated fields were counted for each transfection ($n = 3$) and identified as apoptotic or nonapoptotic based on morphologic alterations typical of adherent cells undergoing apoptosis including becoming rounded up, becoming condensed, and detaching from the dishes. Apoptotic index was determined by counting the number of apoptotic cells with EGFP signal divided by the total number of EGFP-positive cells.

RESULTS AND DISCUSSION

To examine the effect on cell motility of gelsolin truncates G2-6 or G2-3, which can inhibit the severing activity of gelsolin *in vitro*, we attempted to obtain cells stably expressing these gelsolin truncates. However, no stable transfectant expressing G2-6 or G2-3 was obtained after a number of trials. An *in vitro* transcription-translation experiment with gelsolin truncate cDNAs demonstrated that they were capable of producing the polypeptides of truncates (data not shown). These results suggest that the expression of G2-6 or G2-3 that inhibits the severing activity of gelsolin could be unfavorable for cell growth. Next, we examined the phenotype of COS 7 cells after transient transfection using a vector carrying gelsolin truncate cDNA with an NH_2-terminal EGFP tag under the control of the CMV promoter (FIG. 1). Expression of EGFP-tagged gelsolin truncates as well as cell molphology was monitored by a fluorescence microscope. As shown in FIGURE 2A, cells transfected

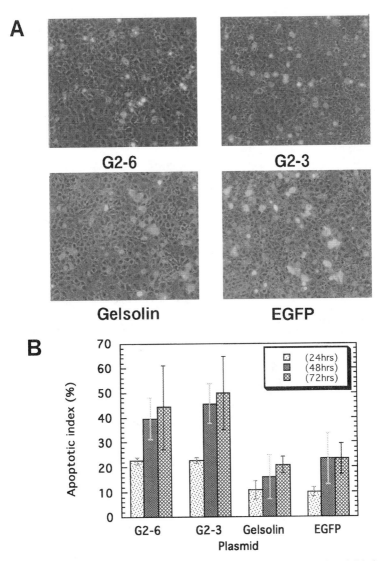

FIGURE 2. (A) Morphologies of COS 7 cells transfected with EGFP-fused G2-6, G2-3, full-length, and EGFP alone at 72 hours after transfection. **(B)** Apoptotic index based on the calculation described in Materials and Methods.

with EGFP-tagged G2-6 or G2-3 appeared to be rounded up, condensed, and finally detached from the dishes at 72 hours after transfection. These morphologic alterations are characteristic of adherent cells undergoing apoptosis. These phenotypes were specific for G2-6 or G2-3, which can inhibit the severing activity of gelsolin, because cells transfected with EGFP-fused full-length gelsolin and EGFP alone were well spread out, and the number of cells showing bright fluorescence signals was increased (FIG. 2A). The morphologic change occurred in a time-dependent manner, and about 50% of transfected cells with EGFP-tagged G2-6 or G2-3 showing a fluorescence signal demonstrated apoptotic cell death (FIG. 2B). These results are consistent with the fact that no stable transfectant expressing G2-6 or G2-3 was obtained. Furthermore, our results indicate that disruption of the actin cytoskeletal reorganization system mediated by a continuous actin polymerization-depolymerization cycle through inhibition of gelsolin's severing activity with truncates eventuates in apoptotic cell death.

REFERENCES

1. YIN, H.L. 1987. Gelsolin: Calcium- and polyphosphoinositide-regulated actin-modulating protein. Bioessays **7:** 176–179.
2. JANMEY, P.A. 1994. Phosphoinositides and calcium as regulators of cellular actin assembly and disassembly. Annu. Rev. Physiol. **56:** 169–191.
3. CUNNINGHAM, C.C., T.P. STOSSEL & D.J. KWIATKOWSKI. 1991. Enhanced motility in NIH 3T3 fibroblasts that overexpress gelsolin. Science **251:** 1233–1236.
4. WITKE, W., A.H. SHARPE, J.H. HARTWIG et al. 1995. Hemostatic, inflammatory, and fibroblast responses are blunted in mice lacking gelsolin. Cell **81:** 41–51.
5. FUJITA, H., P.G. ALLEN, P.A. JANMEY et al. 1997. Characterization of gelsolin truncates that inhibit actin depolymerization by severing activity of gelsolin and cofilin. Eur. J. Biochem. **248:** 834–839.
6. HERSKOWITZ, I. 1987. Functional inactivation of genes by dominant negative mutations. Nature **329:** 219–222.

Reexpression of the Major PKC Substrate, *SSeCKS*, Correlates with the Tumor-Suppressive Effects of SCH51344 on Rat-6/*src* and Rat-6/*ras* Fibroblasts but Not on Rat-6/*raf* Fibroblasts

IRWIN H. GELMAN,[a] QIAORAN XI,[a] AND C. CHANDRA KUMAR[b]

[a]*Department of Microbiology, Mount Sinai School of Medicine, New York, New York 10029, USA*

[b]*Department of Tumor Biology, Schering-Plough Research Institute, Kenilworth, New Jersey, USA*

Oncogenes such as v-*src* and v-*ras* induce oncogenic transformation by activating at least two signaling pathways, a Raf-Mek-Erk pathway controlling proliferation-inducing transcription, and pathways involving Rho-family GTPases that regulate both proliferation and control of cytoskeletal architecture. SCH51344 is a pyrazolo-quinoline derivative that was isolated by its ability to derepress a transformation-sensitive α-actin isoform and was subsequently shown to suppress *ras*-induced oncogenic transformation by inhibiting membrane ruffling controlled by the Rho-family member, Rac.[1–3] Because SCH51344 does not inhibit *ras* activation of either Erk or Jnk, this drug is thought to mediate tumor suppression by reestablishing controls on actin-based cytoskeletal organization rather than by affecting proliferative signaling.

We previously described a new cell cycle-regulated protein kinase C (PKC) substrate, SSeCKS, that interacts with and modulates the organization of the actin-based cytoskeleton.[4–7] SSeCKS expression is downregulated in *src*- and *ras*-, but not in *raf*-transformed rodent fibroblasts,[4] and its reexpression in *src*-transformed fibroblasts or *ras*-transformed prostate cancer epithelial cells suppresses anchorage- and mitogen-independence and reestablishes contact-inhibited growth and cytoskeletal organization.[8] SSeCKS also shares significant similarity with human Gravin, a scaffolder of kinases such as PKC and PKA.[9] Therefore, we surmised that SSeCKS expression might serve as a marker for oncogenes that alter the critical cytoskeletal control pathways involved in transformation. Here we ask if SCH51344 could derepress SSeCKS and if this correlates with a loss of anchorage independence in *src*-, *ras*-, and *raf*-transformed rat-6 fibroblasts.

MATERIALS AND METHODS

Rat-6, rat-6/v-*src*, rat-6/v-*ras*, and rat-6/v-*raf* were cultured in DMEM plus 10% heat-inactivated calf serum (GIBCO-BRL, Gaithersburg, Maryland) as described previously.[4] Proliferation assays and colony formation assays in soft agar were per-

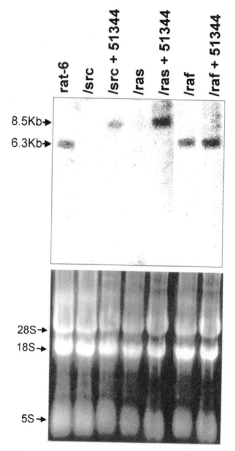

FIGURE 1. SCH51344 derepresses SSeCKS transcript levels in rat-6/*src* and rat-6/*ras* cells, but not in rat-6/*raf* cells. One µg/lane of poly A-selected mRNA from untransformed and transformed rat-6 cells grown for 3 days in DMSO carrier or 40 µM SCH51344 was analyzed by northern blotting using a [^{32}P]-labeled rat SSeCKS cDNA probe. *Bottom panel* shows ethidium bromide staining of the rRNA species of the preselected RNA.

formed as described previously.[8] Northern blotting was performed as described previously using 1 µg per lane of poly A-selected mRNA (Qiagen) from cells grown for 3 days in 40 µM SCH51344 (or DMSO carrier) and probed with [^{32}P]-labeled rat SSeCKS cDNA. Immunoblotting with polyclonal rabbit antibody raised to rat SSeCKS protein was described previously.[5]

RESULTS

FIGURE 1 shows that SSeCKS RNA levels are decreased in *src*- and *ras*-, but not in *raf*-transformed rat-6 cells incubated with DMSO carrier, as we described previ-

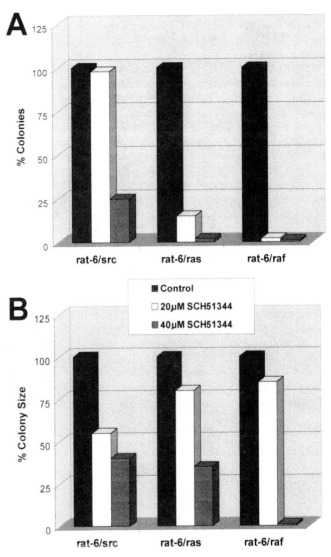

FIGURE 2. Reversal of anchorage-independent growth by SCH51344. *Src*-, *ras*-, or *raf*-transformed rat-6 cells were grown in soft agar medium containing either DMSO carrier or 20 or 40 μM SCH51344 for 2 weeks. **(A)** Percent average colony formation equal to the frequency of colonies formed per 10^5 cells seeded in 6-cm plates (in duplicate) as a percentage of carrier control. **(B)** Average colony size as a percentage of carrier control.

ously.[4] There was a 5–10-fold increase in the accumulation of SSeCKS transcripts in rat-6/*src* and rat-6/*ras* cells treated for 3 days with SCH51344. However, the mRNA induced by SCH51344 was larger than that in untransformed or *raf*-transformed cells

(8.5 vs 6.3 Kb). The steady-state levels of the major SSeCKS protein isoforms, 290 and 280 kD, were also induced by SCH51344 in rat-6/*src* and rat-6/*ras* cells (data not shown), suggesting that the 8.5-Kb transcripts encode these as opposed to novel SSeCKS protein isoforms.

We then determined the effect of the putative Rac inhibitor, SCH51344, on the anchorage-independent growth and proliferation of rat-6/*src*, rat-6/*ras,* and rat-6/*raf.* Colony-forming frequency was defined as the number of colonies formed after a 2-week incubation in soft agar containing drug versus soft agar containing just DMSO carrier. FIGURE 2 shows that 20 μM SCH51344 severely inhibited *ras*- and *raf*-induced colony formation in soft agar, yet had no effect on *src*'s ability to induce colonies. Likewise, 40 μM SCH51344 was more potent at inhibiting *ras*- and *raf*-induced colony formation, although *src*'s colony-forming ability was inhibited 75% at this drug concentration. The average size of colonies formed by all the oncogene-transformed cells was decreased by SCH51344, especially rat-6/*raf* cells, which showed a sharp sensitivity to 40 μM SCH51344. Finally, both concentrations of the drug had little effect on the proliferation rates of all cell types grown in media containing 10% calf serum (data not shown).

CONCLUSION

Our data indicate that SCH51344 suppresses *src*-, *ras*-, and *raf*-induced oncogenic transformation, although the oncogenic growth potentials of rat-6/*ras* and rat-6/*raf* cells are more dependent on pathways blocked by SCH51344 than by rat-6/*src* cells. Reexpression of SSeCKS may contribute to the SCH51344-mediated suppression of *src*- and *ras*-, but not *raf*-induced oncogenesis. Thus, v-*src*, v-*ras,* and v-*raf* require Rac-mediated cytoskeletal reorganization to induce oncogenic transformation, but v-*raf* may activate Rac downstream of SSeCKS.

REFERENCES

1. KUMAR, C.C. *et al.* 1995. Cancer Res. **55:** 5106–5117.
2. HE, H. *et al.* 1998. Mol. Cell Biol. **18:** 3829–3837.
3. COMER, K.A. *et al.* 1998. Oncogene **16:** 1299–1308.
4. LIN, X. *et al.* 1995. Mol. Cell Biol. **15:** 2754–2762.
5. LIN, X. *et al.* 1998. *JBC* **271:** 28,430–28,438.
6. NELSON, P. & I.H. GELMAN. 1997. Molec. Cell. Biochem. **175:** 233–241.
7. GELMAN, I.H. *et al.* 1998. Cell Motil.Cytoskel. **41:** 1–17.
8. LIN, X. & I.H. GELMAN. 1997. Cancer Res. **57:** 2304–2312.
9. NAUERT, J. *et al.* 1997. Curr. Biol. **7:** 52–62.

Subtractive cDNA Cloning and Characterization of Genes Induced by All-Trans Retinoic Acid

YACHI CHEN AND DAVID A. TALMAGE[a]

Institute of Human Nutrition and Department of Pediatrics, Columbia University, New York, New York 10032, USA

Retinoids, a group of natural and synthetic analogs of vitamin A, have proven effective in preventing tumor formation in animal studies and clinical trials[1] (see ref. 2 for reviews). Of all retinoids, all-trans retinoic acid (RA) is the most biologically active vitamin A metabolite. Using an experimental model involving F111/RARα cells (parental F111 rat fibroblasts do not express detectable RARα, β, or γ, whereas F111/RARα cells express RARα and are therefore RA responsive) and polyoma virus middle T antigen as an oncogenic agent, our laboratory has demonstrated that RA, acting via RARα, suppresses mT-induced transformation by blocking transcription of the c-fos gene whose product is a component of the transcription factor AP-1.[3,4] Further study indicated that the observed inhibitory effect of RA on transformation induced by mT resulted from RA preventing mT signaling to the c-fos promoter via the phosphatidylinositol 3-kinase (PI3-kinase)/Rac/Jun N-terminal kinase (JNK) signaling cascade.[5] We think that RA blocks this pathway by inducing expression of some inhibitory proteins that act on the components of this pathway (FIG. 1). Our hypothesis is supported by several observations: (1) activation of RARα, itself a nuclear transcription factor, is required for inhibition of mT-induced transformation; (2) analysis of RA repression of c-fos transcription demonstrated that pretreatment of cells with RA for >6 hours was required and that the observed RA effect on c-fos expression was blocked by the protein synthesis inhibitor cycloheximide; and (3) no RARE has been found in the c-fos promoter and therefore RAR is unlikely to inhibit c-fos expression directly. A full understanding of the mechanism of the anticarcinogenic effect of RA requires identification of these RARα–regulated inhibitory genes.

RESULTS

With the polymerase chain reaction (PCR)-select cDNA subtraction method (Clontech Laboratories, Inc.), seven genes expressed after induction by RA were obtained (TABLE 1). These genes include two novel genes whose sequences do not match with sequences present in the Genbank or EMBL database, and they are designated as M33 and M90. The five known genes are: M61, which is homologous to

[a]Corresponding author: Dr. David A. Talmage, Institute of Human Nutrition, Columbia University, 701 West 168th Street, Hammer Health Science Bldg. Room 5-503, New York, New York 10032. Phone, 212/305-5342; fax, 212/305-3079.
e-mail, dat1@columbia.edu

TABLE 1. Seven RA-induced cDNAs identified

cDNAs	Description
M90	Novel[a]
M33	Novel[a]
M61	• Shares 89% sequence identity at the protein level with hematopoietic lineage switch 2 (HLS2), which is induced during an erythroid to myeloid lineage switch
	• Shares homology with aminopeptidases
Sar1a (M96)	• A GTP-binding protein that functions in vesicular transport between the ER and Golgi
pRbAp46	• Interacts with Rb
	• Inhibits Ras signaling in yeast
	• Found to be associated with histone deacetylases
p190 GAP-associated protein	• Binds to GAP1 (GTPase-activating protein) which negatively regulates Ras signaling
	• Contains two domains, a GTPase domain and a GAP domain that stimulates GTPase activity of Rho, Rac, and Cdc42
	• Acts as a tumor suppressor
	• Overexpression of the p190 GAP domain alone suppresses the c-fos protein expression.
Protein phosphatase 1 (PP1β)	• The β–subunit of the serine/threonine phosphatase, PP1
	• Found bound to the chromatin structure in interphase cells

[a]Novel — sequences submitted do not match with sequences in GenBank or EMBL databases.

hematopoietic lineage switch 2 (HLS2) that is induced during an erythroid to myeloid lineage switch; Sar1a (M96), which functions in vesicular transport between Golgi and ER[6]; pRbAp46, which interacts with Rb and has been shown to inhibit Ras signaling in yeast[7]; p190GAP-associated protein, which acts as a tumor suppressor in a cell culture system[8]; β-type catalytic subunit of the serine/threonine phosphatase protein phosphatase 1,[9] which is bound to the chromatin structure in interphase cells.

We determined the mRNA levels for these seven genes over a time course of 48 hours following RA treatment. Based on the results obtained from the time course study, these genes were induced with three distinct kinetic patterns: (1) rapid, transient: PP1β; (2) rapid, sustained: M90, M61 (HLS-2), and M33; and (3) delayed: 190GAP-AP, Sar1a, and pRbAp46. We found that M33 was expressed at much higher levels in nontransformed than in mT-transformed F111 cells. M33 and Sar1a expression was elevated in RARα-expressing cells. Finally, induction of delayed genes (pRbAp46 and Sar1a), but not the early M61 gene, was inhibited by cycloheximide treatment (2 μg/ml, 15 minutes before RA stimulation).

FUTURE EXPERIMENTS

To biologically characterize isolated RA-induced cDNAs, we plan to test the effects of expression of these genes on c-fos expression and transformation. We have demonstrated that RA inhibits transformation by blocking the PI3-kinase/JNK sig-

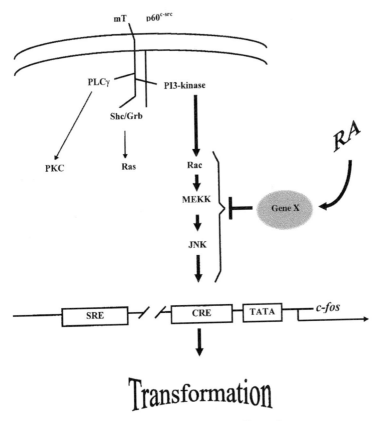

FIGURE 1. Middle T-induced signaling pathways.

naling pathway leading to the c-fos promoter.[5] If RA blocks a specific step in the PI3-kinase signaling pathway to the c-fos promoter by inducing one of the candidate genes, the constitutive expression of the candidate cDNA will inhibit both the activity of the c-fos promoter and any signaling intermediate acting downstream of the targeted step. We will therefore determine the effects of isolated RA-induced cDNAs on the activities of Rac, PAK, MEKK1, SEK, and JNK, which are components of the signaling pathway.

CONCLUSION

We demonstrated that the subtractive cloning procedure is feasible in discovering differentially expressed genes induced by RA, and whether the identified genes indeed mediate RA inhibition of c-fos expression and transformation requires further biological characterization.

REFERENCES

1. HONG, W.K. *et al.* 1990. Prevention of second primary tumors with isotretinoin in squamous-cell carcinoma of the head and neck. N. Engl. J. Med. **323:** 795–801.
2. HILL, D.L. & C.J. GRUBBS. 1992. Retinoids and cancer prevention. Annu. Rev. Nutr. **12:** 111–181.
3. TALMAGE, D.A. & R.S. LACKEY. 1992. Retinoic acid receptor α suppresses polyoma-virus transformation and expression in rat fibroblasts. Oncogene **7:** 1897–1845.
4. TALMAGE, D.A. & M. LISTERUD. 1994. Retinoic acid suppresses polyoma virus transformation by inhibiting transcription of the *c-fos* proto-oncogene. Oncogene **9:** 3557–3562.
5. CHEN, Y. *et al.* 1998. Retinoic acid inhibits transformation by preventing phosphatidylinositol 3-kinase dependent activation of the c-fos promoter. Oncogene **18:** 139–148.
6. KUGE, O. *et al.* 1994. Sar1 promotes vesicle budding from the endoplasmic reticulum but not Golgi compartments. J. Cell Biol. **125:** 51–65.
7. QIAN, Y.-W. & E. Y.-H. P. LEE. 1995. Dual retinoblastoma-binding proteins with properties related to a negative regulator of ras in yeast. J. Biol. Chem. **270:** 25507–25513.
8. WANG, D.Z.M. *et al.* 1997. The GTPase and Rho GAP domains of p190, a tumor suppressor protein that binds the M_r 120,000 Ras GAP, independently function as anti-ras tumor suppressors. Cancer Res. **57:** 2478–2484.
9. DA CRUZ E SILVA, E.F. *et al.* 1995. Differential expression of protein phosphatase1 isoforms in mammalian brain. J. Neurosci. **15:** 3375–3389.

Purification and Functional Characterization of a Novel Protein Encoded by a Retinoic Acid-Induced Gene, RA28

ZHIHUA LIU,[a] AIPING LUO, GUANGHU WANG, XIUQIN WANG, AND MIN WU

National Laboratory of Molecular Oncology, Department of Cell Biology, Cancer Institute, Chinese Academy of Medical Sciences and Peking Union Medical College, Beijing 100021, P.R. China

Retinoic acid (RA), a derivative of vitamin A, is a key molecule in controlling differentiation and development.[1] RA has been used in the treatment of leukemia, severe cystic acne, and other chronic skin diseases; however, the successful use of retinoic acid in the treatment of leukemia and the prevention of solid tumors in experimental animals and human populations has made it an effective reagent in tumor differentiation treatment. All-trans retinoic acid (ATRA) was used in this laboratory to induce differentiation of human lung adenocarcinoma cell line GLC-82 *in vitro*, and several novel genes were isolated using a subtraction strategy. In this report, one of the retinoic acid-induced genes, RA28, and its encoded protein were studied.

MATERIALS AND METHODS

All-trans retinoic acid was purchased from Sigma. *Cell culture*: Human lung adenocarcinoma cell line GLC-82 was kindly provided by Prof. Mingda Liang from Kunming Medical College, China. The cells were grown in DMEM supplemented with 15% fetal calf serum and treated with 1×10^{-5}M ATRA after seeding to allow for cell adhesion. Culture medium with or without ATRA was replaced every 24 hours.

Gene isolation: Subtractive hybridization was carried out between the cells treated with or without ATRA, and many of the genes were obtained. Among them, RA28 was selected for further study.

Gene localization on chromosome: Radiation hybrid (RH) technology was used to localize RA28 on chromosome. The presence or absence of each marker in the GeneBridge 4 radiation hybrid panel (Research Genetics Inc.) was determined by polymerase chain reaction (PCR). Data of the PCR results were sent to Whitehead Institute, MIT, for further analysis.

Protein expression and purification: The predicted open reading frame sequence of RA28 (nucleotide 260-595) was subcloned into the expression vector pET-22b(+) (Novagen Inc.) and transformed into the BL21(DE3) strain of *Escherichia coli*. The RA28/His fusion protein was produced in the BL21(DE3) strain of *E. coli* in the

[a]To whom correspondence should be addressed. Phone, +86-10-67723789; fax, +86-10-67715058.
e-mail, liuzh@pubem.cicams.ac.cn

1   2   3   4   5   6   7

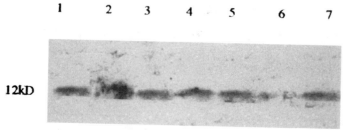

12kD

FIGURE 1. Western blot analysis showing RA28 protein expression in different human tumor cell lines. (1) Colon HR8348; (2) hepatic 7402; (3) lung adenocarcinoma LTEP-a2; (4,5) prostate TSUp21 and DU145; (6) lung adenocarcinoma GLC-82; (7) esophageal EC8712.

presence of 0.4 mM IPTG, cells were harvested and broken by sonication, and the fusion protein was purified by 6X His affinity tag immobilized metal affinity chromatography (IMAC, Clotech) according to the manufacturer's directions. The purified protein was analyzed by 15% SDS-PAGE using the Tris-Tricine buffer system.

Antibody production and purification: Polyclonal antisera against RA28 protein were raised by a synthesized peptide (NDLEDKNSPFYYDWHQ, which is amino acid 21-36) coupled to KLH and purified by the caprylic acid method as well as by BSA-coupled RA28 peptide linked to the affinity gel method. Western blot and northern blot analyses were performed according to standard protocol.

Microscopic analysis of cells expressing green fluorescent fusion protein (GFP): Green fluorescent protein has emerged as a unique tool for examining intracellular phenomena in living cells. Expression vectors encoding the pEGFP-RA28 fusion protein were transfected into GLC-82 cells using lipofectamine-mediated gene transfer following manufacturer's instructions (Life Technologies, Inc.); after 36–48 hours' incubation at 37°C in 5% CO_2, the living cells were examined under fluorescence microscopy.

RESULTS

1. RA28 (GenBank accession No. U28249) is a cDNA of 1475 bp with a polyadenylation signal and a polyA tail at the 3' end; a 330-bp open reading frame is predicted from nucleotide 260-595. Sequence analysis showed that it shared high homology with Mat-8 (mammary tumor 8 kD[2]), a phospholemman-like protein expressed in human breast tumor; however, it is distinctly different from Mat-8 because it contains an additional 26 amino acids. Computational analysis revealed one casein kinase II phosphorylation site and four *N*-myristoylation sites within the RA28 sequence.

2. Gene RA28 was localized to the chromosome 19q13.1 region by linkage analysis (Lod>15); the gene locus lies in close proximity to marker D19S224 (Distance = 7.36 cR). More precisely, the gene was localized between D19S425 and D19S421. The genetic distance between markers was estimated to be about 3.3 cm.

3. The recombinant protein was expressed and purified from the BL21(DE3) strain of *E. coli*; almost 20% of the supernatant protein was RA28/His. The SDS-

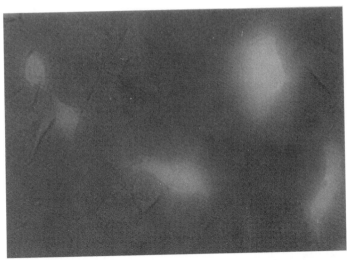

FIGURE 2. Microscopic analysis of cells expressing GFP/RA28 fusion protein showing that RA28 protein is a membrane protein. (The original figure was in color.)

PAGE/IEF showed that RA28 (ORF) had a molecular weight of 12 kD with a neutral PI of 7.0.

4. Western blot analysis showed that RA28 protein was detected in all the tissues we examined (lung, brain, and esophageal tissue) and in all the cell lines we checked (colon, liver, lung, prostate, and esophageal cancer cell lines) with a molecular weight of 12 kD, coinciding with the ORF we predicted, which indicates that the ORF we predict is correct. Furthermore, RA28 does not exhibit a distinct tissue-specific pattern of protein expression.

5. Microscopic analysis of cells expressing GFP/RA28 fusion protein showed that RA28 protein is a membrane protein, which coincides with the computational analysis that RA28 is a membrane protein with a single membrane-spanning domain.

6. Preliminary functional studies showed that RA28 could induce carcinoma cells to differentiation and apoptosis to some extent.

DISCUSSION

RA28 was obtained from a human lung cancer cell line, whereas Mat-8 was first obtained from murine breast tumor and then from human breast tumor as well. It was believed that Mat-8 is a marker of a cell type preferentially transformed by Neu or Ras oncoproteins.[2] Given the homology between RA28 and Mat-8, we hypothesized that RA28, like Mat-8, might be involved in certain classes of oncogenic events.

A universal feature of the communication is that the external signal must in some way be able to penetrate the lipid bilayer surrounding the cell; however, studies over the last decade have demonstrated additional pathways for directing proteins to cells that co- or posttranslationally modify protein by specific lipids. The particularly exciting thing is that *N*-myristoylation protein plays a critical role in cell growth and development, transmembrane signaling, oncogenesis, virus replication and assembly, and the like.[3] Motif analysis showed that RA28 has four *N*-myristoylation sites with a transmembrane domain, so we presumed that RA28 might participate in the signaling processes and closely relate with classes of oncogenic events. However, this hypothesis needs further investigation.

ACKNOWLEDGMENTS

This work was supported by the National Natural Science Foundation of China (39700168) and the National Climbing Project (18).

REFERENCES

1. GUDAS, L.J. *et al.* 1994. Cellular biology and biochemistry of the retinoids. *In* The Retinoids. M.B. Sporn *et al.,* Eds. :443–520. Raven Press. New York.
2. MORRISON, B.W. *et al.* 1996. Mat-8, a novel phospholemman-like protein expressed in human breast tumors, induces a choride conductance in *Xenopus oocytes*. J. Biol. Chem. **270**: 2176–2182.
3. CASEY, P.J. *et al.* 1995. Protein lipidation in cell signaling. Science **268:** 221–225.

Augmented Inhibition of Tumor Cell Proliferation in Combined Use of Electroporation with a Plant Toxin, Saporin

H. MASHIBA,[a] Y. OZAKI, AND K. MATSUNAGA

Division of Immunology, National Kyushu Cancer Center, 3-1-1 Notame, Minami-ku, Fukuoka 811-1347, Japan

Electroporation (EP) utilizing high voltage electric pulses has been employed to introduce vectors, antitumor drugs, and other agents into cytoplasm. EP has been widely used in *in vitro* and *in vivo* experiments in the field of gene therapy[1] and chemotherapy.[2] Electrochemotherapy using local EP in combination with bleomycin has been applied clinically in the treatment of metastatic nodules of head and neck squamous cell carcinoma and breast carcinoma, melanoma and other cutaneous malignancies.[3,4]

In the present studies utilizing EP, we have attempted to introduce intracellularly a plant toxin, saporin (MW, 30 kD), which is a single polypeptide chain (A chain) that inactivates ribosomes. Saporins are relatively nontoxic to cells, because they lack the binding chain (B chain), but one molecule of saporin is considered sufficient to kill a target cell once it has been introduced into cytoplasm. Various human cancer cell lines and a murine fibrosarcoma cell line (MethA) were used as target cells. By changing voltage, length of electric pulses, and the number of pulses, we examined the EP condition in which a strong antiproliferative effect on target cells could be induced. The antitumor effect of combination therapy with local EP and saporin injected intralesionally on established MethA tumors was also studied.

MATERIALS AND METHODS

In Vitro *Experiments*. Cancer cells derived from human cancer cell lines ASPC-1 (pancreatic cancer), HeLa (uterine cervical cancer), HOC (ovarian cancer), PC9 (lung cancer), or MethA tumor cells were electroporated in serum-free medium in the presence or absence of various concentrations of saporin (10^{-3} to 10^3 ng/ml) using disposable cuvette electrodes (2 mm gap), BTX 620, and the Electro Cell Manipulator ECM 2001 (BTX Inc., USA). Treated or nontreated cells were transferred to 24-well culture plates, and the concentrations of saporin were adjusted to equal those in the group that had been electroporated in the presence of saporin. After 72 hours' incubation, viable cells were counted by the trypan blue dye exclusion method after trypsinization of adhering cells. The degree of inhibition of cell proliferation

---

[a]Address of corresponding author: Division of Immunology, National Kyushu Cancer Center, 3-1-1 Notame, Minami-ku, Fukuoka 811-1347, Japan. Phone, 81-92-541-3231, Ext. 2435 or 2436; fax, 81-92-551-4585.
e-mail: hmashiba@nk-cc.go.jp

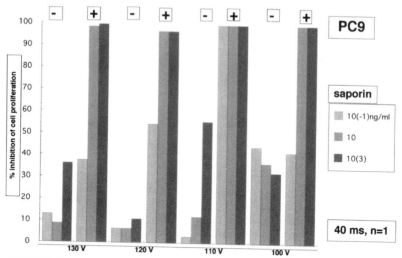

FIGURE 1. PC9 cells (human lung cancer cell line) were electroporated in the presence (+) or absence (−) of saporin. After 72 hours' incubation, the degree of proliferation inhibition was determined by comparing the viable cell number with that of each medium control group.

was determined by comparing the viable cell number in the experimental group with that of medium control in each voltage group taken as 0%.

In Vivo *Experiments.* MethA tumor cells were inoculated sc into Balb/c mice (2×10^6 cells/mouse). After 8 days in which the diameter of the tumor reached approximately 7 mm, the tumor was electroporated twice in crisscross fashion using needle-type electrodes 3 minutes after intratumoral injection of saporin (1 μg) or phosphate- buffered saline solution (PBS). Thereafter, tumor growth was observed by measuring the diameter of the tumors.

RESULTS AND CONCLUSION

Attempts to cause temporary pore formation of the cancer cell membrane and to introduce intracellularly a plant toxin, saporin, which is relatively nontoxic because it lacks membrane-binding sites, were made utilizing high-voltage electric pulses. Human cancer cell lines ASPC-1, HeLa, HOC, and PC9 and a murine tumor cell line, MethA tumor cell line, were electroporated in the presence or the absence of saporin. Nontoxic concentrations to nontreated target cells were used in each cell line (10^{-1} to 10^3 ng/ml in human cancer cell line and 10^{-3} to 10 ng/ml in MethA tumor cell line). Almost complete inhibition of target cell proliferation was observed in all cell lines when the cells were electroporated (100–140 V, 40 ms, $n = 1$) in the presence of saporin; however, a low or moderate inhibitory effect was caused by the addition of saporin after electroporation (EP) (FIG. 1). Similar marked inhibition of cell proliferation was obtained with the other condition of EP (70–90 V, 10 ms, $n = 8$).

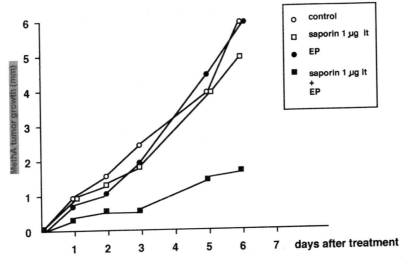

FIGURE 2. MethA tumor cells (2×10^6 cells/mouse) were inoculated subcutaneously into Balb/c mice. After 8 days in which the diameter of the tumors reached approximately 7 mm, tumors were treated with electroporation (EP) 3 minutes after intralesional injection of phosphate-buffered saline solution (1 μg/mouse). Thereafter, the increase in tumor size was measured and plotted.

As marked inhibition of cell proliferation was obtained with the combined use of EP with saporin *in vitro*, the antitumor effect was examined using established MethA tumors in syngeneic Balb/c mice. The tumors, which reached approximately 7 mm in diameter, were electroporated (200 V/cm, 10 ms, $n = 8$) twice 3 minutes after the intratumoral injection of saporin (1 mg/mouse). Tumor necrosis was observed 24–48 hours after the combination therapy, and marked inhibition of tumor growth was obtained; however, saporin or EP alone was ineffective in inhibiting tumor growth (FIG. 2). Combination therapy utilizing EP and saporin seems to promising in cancer therapy in the future.

REFERENCES

1. CHAVANY, C., Y. CONNELL & L. NECKERS. 1995. Contribution of sequence and phosphorothioate content to inhibition of cell growth and adhesion caused by c-myc antisense oligomers. Molec. Pharmacol. **48:** 738–746.
2. MASHIBA, H., Y. OZAKI, Y. ICHINOSE & K. MATSUNAGA. 1997. Augmentation of cytostatic effect on cultured tumor cell lines in combination of electroporation with actinomycin D. 20th Int. Cog. Chemother. Programme & Book of Abstracts, p. 58. Int. Soc. of Chemotherapy. Sydney, Australia.
3. DOMENGE, C., S. ORIOWSKI, J. BELEHHADEK, JR., T. DE BAERE, G. SCHWAAB, B. LUBOINSKI & L. M. MIR. 1995. Phase I-II treatment of large permeation nodules of head and neck squamous cell carcinoma (HNSCC) and breast adenocarcinoma (BA) by electrochemotherapy. Proc. Annu. Meet. Am. Assoc. Cancer Res. **36:** A1476.
4. GLASS, L.F., N.A. FENSKE, M. JAROSZESKI, R. PERROTT, D.T. HARVEY, D.S. REINTGEN & R. HELLER. 1996. Bleomycin-mediated electrochemotherapy of basal cell carcinoma. J. Am. Acad. Dermatol. **34:** 82–86.

Expression of Matrix Metalloproteinases and Their Inhibitors in Human Brain Tumors

RICHARD BÉLIVEAU,[a,d] LOUIS DELBECCHI, [a] EDITH BEAULIEU,[a] NATHALIE MOUSSEAU,[a] ZARIN KACHRA,[a] FRANCE BERTHELET,[b] ROBERT MOUMDJIAN,[b] AND ROLANDO DEL MAESTRO[c]

[a]Laboratoire de médecine moléculaire, centre de cancérologie Charles-Bruneau, Hôpital Ste-Justine-UQAM, Montreal, Quebec, Canada

[b]Hôpital Notre-Dame, Montréal, Québec, Canada

[c]The Brain Tumor Tissue Bank, London, Ontario, Canada

Brain tumors are among the most vascularized solid tumors in which the degree of angiogenesis is important in discriminating between low grade and high grade tumors.[1] Both angiogenesis and tumor invasion require controlled degradation of the extracellular matrix (ECM) components to allow cell migration and tissue formation.[2] Matrix metalloproteinases (MMPs) are zinc-dependent endopeptidases that play a fundamental role in these processes.[3] To date, 14 human MMPs are known and are classified into four groups based on their protein domain structure.[4] The smallest subgroup consists of matrilysin (MMP-7), whereas the second group is comprised of collagenases (MMP-1, MMP-8, and MMP-13), stromelysins (MMP-3, MMP-10, and MMP-11), and metalloelastase (MMP-12). The third group contains 72- and 92-kD gelatinases (MMP-2 and MMP-9, respectively), and the fourth group consists of membrane-type MMPs (MT-MMPs: MMP-14 or MT1-MMP, MMP-15, MMP-16, and MMP-17). MMP activity is regulated by tissue inhibitors of metalloproteinases (TIMPs), which inhibit active forms of MMPs and thus prevent degradation of ECM components. Four TIMPs (TIMP-1, TIMP-2, TIMP-3, and TIMP-4) have been identified to date.[5] In this study we present data on MMP and TIMP expression in human brain tumors ranging from grade I to IV.

MATERIAL AND METHODS

Tumors. Tumor tissues obtained from The Brain Tumor Tissue Bank (London, Ontario, Canada) were homogenized in 5 volumes of medium containing 250 mM sucrose, 10 mM Hepes/Tris pH 7.5, and the samples were frozen at -80°C until use.

Zymography. In a sample buffer, 50 µg of protein samples/well were denatured in a sample buffer without β-mercaptoethanol, and zymography was carried out on 7.5% polyacrylamide gels containing 0.1% gelatin, as described previously.[6]

[d]Address for correspondence: Laboratoire de médecine moléculaire et centre de cancérologie Charles Bruneau, hôpital Ste-Justine-UQAM, C.P. 8888, succursale Centre-ville, Montréal (Québec), Canada, H3C 3P8. Phone, 514/987-3000 (8551); fax, 514/987-0246.
e-mail, beliveau.richard@uquam.ca

Fluorometric Assays. Assays were performed using EnzChek Collagenase/Gelatinase and Enz/Chek Elastase Assay kits from Molecular Probes (Eugene, Oregon). Tumor protein 25 μg was mixed with fluorescein-conjugated gelatin or elastin-labeled with BODIPY FL,[7] and the rate of proteolysis was determined using a Fluoroskan II fluorometer.

RESULTS

MMP Expression by Western Blotting. MMP-2 is detected in almost every sample, but in modest amount. MMP-9 is present in most tumors, but it is expressed in

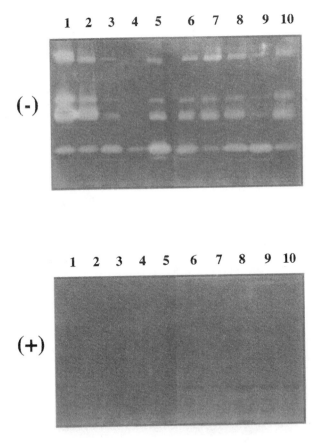

FIGURE 1. Zymographic analysis of MMP activity in meningioma. Tumor samples (50 μg/well) were denatured in a sample buffer without β-mercaptoethanol and subjected to SDS-PAGE on 7.5% polyacrylamide gels containing 0.1% gelatin. Zymograms were developed in the presence (+) or absence (−) of 0.5 mM 1,10 phenanthroline.

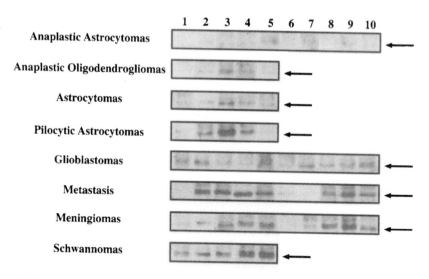

FIGURE 2. Western blot analysis of TIMP-2 expression. Tumor samples (25 μg) were subjected to SDS-PAGE using 12.5% polyacrylamide gel, Western blotting, and ECL detection. In the metastasis group, *lanes 1–5* correspond to melanoma metastases and *lanes 6–10* to lung metastases.

low amounts in schwannomas, meningiomas, and metastasis, and MMP-12 is expressed at moderate-to-high levels in most tumors but it is not detectable in anaplastic oligodendrogliomas, metastasis, meningiomas, and schwannomas. Statistical analysis of the data did not reveal any correlation between tumor grades and the expression levels of four MMPs examined.

MMP Expression by Zymography. A common pattern of gelatinolysis is observed with two bands of 72 kD (MMP-2) and 92 kD (MMP-9) in most tumors. A representative zymogram showing gelatinolytic activity of MMP-2 and MMP-9 in meningioma is shown in FIGURE 1. A good correlation is observed between zymographic data and Western blotting analysis.

MMP Activity by Fluorometric Assay. Low levels of proteolytic activities are observed in tumor samples by fluorometric assay than by zymography. This may be explained by the presence of TIMPs in the tumors that are dissociated from MMPs in SDS gel electrophoresis during zymography. The variability of our results and the lack of correlation between MMPs and tumor grades may be due to: (1) the small number of the sample population examined, (2) interpatient variablity in a given group of tumors, and (3) the amount of normal tissue present in surgically removed tumors.

TIMP Expression by Western Blotting. TIMP's expression levels are significantly higher in schwannomas but lower in anaplastic astrocytomas, anaplastic oligodendrogliomas, and astrocytomas. TIMP-2 levels of expression among tumors examined are shown in FIGURE 2.

CONCLUSION

High expressions of TIMP-1 and TIMP-2 are found in low grade tumors and low levels are seen in high grade tumors, suggesting that TIMPs may be a valuable marker for tumor malignancy. MMPs and TIMPs may have an important role in the progression and development of human brain tumors.

SUMMARY

Sixty human brain tumors, including grade I meningiomas, schwannomas, and pilocytic astrocytomas, grade II astrocytomas, grade III anaplastic astrocytomas and oligodendrogliomas, and grade IV glioblastomas and lung and melanoma metastases were analyzed for expression of four matrix metalloproteinases (MMPs), two tissue inhibitors of MMPs (TIMPs), and MMP activity. No marked correlation was found between MMP expression and the degree of malignancy. Western blotting analysis revealed a more uniform pattern of distribution of MMP-2 (gelatinase A) than of MMP-9 (gelatinase B) and MMP-12 (metalloelastase) among tumors. All 60 tumors showed a similar pattern of activity in zymography, MMP-2 being the major species detected. Interestingly, TIMP-1 and TIMP-2 expression levels were low in tumors of grade III but significantly higher in tumors of grade I, particularly schwannomas. Altogether, these data suggest that: (1) the balance between MMP-2 and TIMP-2 is important in human brain tumors; and (2) TIMP expression may be a valuable marker for tumor malignancy.

ACKNOWLEDGMENT

This work was supported by the Natural Sciences and Engineering Research Council of Canada and Fondation Charles Bruneau.

REFERENCES

1. ASSIMAKOPOULOU, M. 1997. Microvessel density in brain tumors. Anticancer Res. **17:** 4747–4754.
2. MIGNATTI, P. & D.B. RIFKIN. 1996. Plasminogen activators and matrix metalloproteinases in angiogenesis. Enzyme Protein **49:** 117–137.
3. RAY, J.M. AND W.G. STETLER-STEVENSON. 1994. The role of matrix metalloproteinases and their inhibitors in tumor invasion, metastasis and angiogenesis. Eur. Respir. J. **7:** 2062–2072.
4. POWELL, W.C. & L.M. MATRISIAN. 1996. Complex roles of matrix metalloproteinases in tumor progression. Curr. Top. Microbiol. Immunol. **213:** 1-21.
5. GREENE J. *et al.* 1996. Molecular cloning and characterization of human tissue inhibitor of metalloproteinase 4. J. Biol. Chem. **271:** 30375–30380.
6. KLEINER, D.E. & W.G. STETLER-STEVENSON. 1994. Quantitative zymography: Detection of picogram quantities of gelatinases. Anal. Biochem. **218:** 325–329.
7. JONES, L.J. *et al.* 1997. Quenched BODYPI dye-labeled casein substrates for the assay of protease activity by direct fluorescence measurement. Anal. Biochem. **251:** 144–152.

Plasmin-Depletion Therapy

A New Approach to Overcoming Tumor Cell Drug Resistance

MYUNG CHUN[a,c] AND MICHAEL K. HOFFMANN[b]

[a]Bioeast, 200 East End Avenue, New York, New York 10128, USA

[b]New York Medical College, Valhalla, New York, New York 10595, USA

Most anticancer agents destroy cancer cells by activating the apoptosis pathway.[1] We have shown that plasmin can render cancer cells resistant to apoptosis-inducing drugs and may alter their growth pattern.[2,3]

The adverse effect of plasmin on the growth of cancer has been recognized. The precursor of plasmin is plasminogen. Cancer cells often express the protease urokinase, which converts plasminogen to plasmin. Urokinase has been detected in breast cancer, colorectal cancer, lung cancer, melanoma, prostate cancer, stomach cancer, and ovarian cancer.[4–6] Plasmin generation by urokinase in tumor tissues is known to correlate with a poor prognosis.[4–6] In the last decade, extensive but unsuccessful attempts have been made to inhibit the generation of plasmin on cancer cells by blocking tumor cell urokinase.[4–6]

We have taken a different approach. We blocked plasmin generation on cancer cells by eliminating the urokinase substrate plasminogen rather than by inhibiting the enzyme itself. This therapeutic approach is referred to as plasmin-depletion therapy. The plasmin-depletion therapy principle is illustrated in FIGURE 1.

Plasmin-depletion therapy induces systemic conversion of the patient's plasminogen to plasmin. On conversion, plasmin is rapidly inactivated by decay. As it takes approximately 2 days for the body to regenerate plasminogen, plasmin-depletion therapy provides a plasminogen-free state in patients and deprives cancer cells of the plasmin precursor plasminogen. During this period, cancer cells are unable to block the apoptosis process and remain sensitive to apoptosis-inducing drugs (FIG. 1).

Preclinical data show that plasmin-depletion therapy enhances the efficacy of anticancer agents and of the host's anticancer defense. Tissue culture studies were performed with several apoptosis-inducing anticancer agents and a variety of human breast and colon cancer cell lines. The following are examples of *in vivo* experiments. Immunodeficient nu/nu mice were inoculated intradermally with HT29 human colon cancer cells. One day later, the animals received saline as control, PDT, a suboptimal dose of doxorubicin, or doxorubicin plus PDT. Tumor volumes were assessed at 21 days. The volume of the tumors in the group treated with doxorubicin plus PDT was less than half that in the group treated with either doxorubicin or PDT alone. Tumor volume in the latter two groups was approximately 85% that of the control group. In immunotherapies, similar results were obtained. Fourteen days af-

[c]For correspondence: phone, 212/360-6631; fax, 212/360-6631.
e-mail, chun01@sprynet.com

UNTREATED

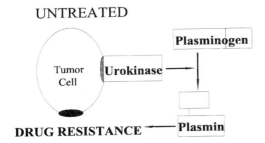

TREATED

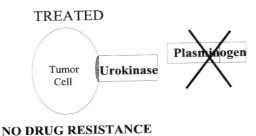

NO DRUG RESISTANCE

FIGURE 1. Plasmin-depletion therapy principle. *Untreated:* Plasmin generated from patient's plasminogen by urokinase induces drug resistance. *PDT treated:* Plasmin-depletion therapy depletes patient's plasminogen, the source of plasmin generated by cancer cells, and thus suppresses drug resistance.

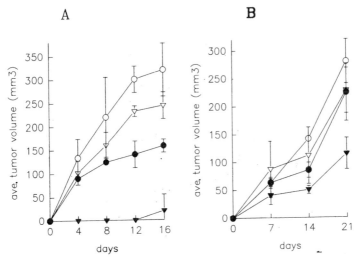

FIGURE 2. Plasmin-depletion therapy increases the efficacy of chemotherapeutic and immunotherapeutic drugs *in vivo*. **(A)** Balb/C athymic nude mice were injected intraperitoneally with either 0.2 ml saline (○,●) or plasmin-depletion therapy (PDT, 150 units urokinase in 0.2 ml saline) (△,▲). Thirty minutes later, mice were injected with saline solution or PDT twice more at 10-minute intervals. Two hours after the first injection, 2 million HT29 cells were inoculated intradermally into the abdomen. Mice were treated twice, 24 and 48 hours after tumor inoculation, with 0.2 ml saline (○,△) or 100 μg/ml M79 antibody in

ter treatment, tumor volume in the group treated with monoclonal tumor-reactive antibody was 50% that of the control group. Tumor volume in the animals receiving PDT alone was 80% of control. In animals treated with monoclonal antibody plus PDT, tumors were not detected (FIG. 2).

In conclusion, these observations indicate that plasmin-depletion therapy, by overcoming a key form of drug resistance, provides a means to increase the efficacy of systemic therapies.

REFERENCES

1. da SILVA C.P., C.R. DE OLIVEIRA, M. DA CONCICAO & P. DE LIMA. 1996. Apoptosis as a mechanism of cell death induced by different chemotherapeutic drugs in human leukemic T- lymphocytes. Biochem Pharmacol. **51:**1331–1340.
2. CHUN, M. 1997. Plasmin induces the formation of multicellular spheroids of breast cancer cells. Cancer Lett. **117:** 51–56.
3. CHUN, M. & M.K.HOFFMANN. 1997. Patent application. PCT/US97/14231. Date of Application: August 13, 1997.
4. BACHMANN, F. 1994. Basic Principles and Clinical Practice. Lippincott. Co. Philadelphia, PA.
5. FAZIOLI, F. & F. BLASI. 1994. Urokinase-type plasminogen activator and its receptor: New targets for anti-metastatic therapy? Trends Pharmacol. Sci **15:** 25–29.
6. ANDREASEN, P.A., L. KJOLLER, L. CHRISTENSEN & M.J. DUFFY. 1997. The urokinase-type plasminogen activator system in cancer metastases: A review. Int. J. Cancer **72:** 1–22.

FIGURE 2 (*continued from previous page*)
0.2 ml saline (●,▲). On the days indicated, the formation of tumors as well as the volume of tumors was assessed. Tumor volume = the length × the width × the height. (**B**) One million HT29 cells were inoculated into the abdomen of nude mice. Twenty hours later, animals were treated with either plasmin-depletion therapy (i.e., 150 units urokinase) (△,▲) or saline (○,●) twice at 30-minute intervals. After 24 hours, animals were treated with either 0.2 ml saline (○,△) or 50 μg doxorubicin in 0.2 ml saline (●,▲) intravenously twice at 4-hour intervals. Tumors were measured as described in **A** on the days indicated.

Polysulfated Heparinoids Selectively Inactivate Heparin-Binding Angiogenesis Factors

G. ZUGMAIER,[a,e] R. FAVONI,[b] R. JAEGER,[a] N. ROSEN,[c] AND C. KNABBE[d]

[a]Department of Hematology/Oncology, Philipps-University, D-35033 Marburg, Germany

[b]Istituto Nazionale per la Ricerca sul Cancer, Viale Benedetto XV, 10, 16132 Genoa, Italy

[c]Department of Medicine, Memorial-Sloan Kettering Cancer Center, New York, New York 10021, USA

[d]Department of Clinical Pathology, Robert-Bosch Krankenhaus, D-70376 Stuttgart, Germany

Angiogenesis, the process of forming new blood vessels, is an essential part of reproduction, development, and wound repair.[1] Under these conditions, angiogenesis is a process controlled according to the physiologic requirements of the organism.[1]

Many diseases, however, are driven by persistent unregulated angiogenesis as a pathophysiologic process.[1] Pathologic angiogenesis plays an important role in the growth and metastasis of malignant tumors.[1] Since 1983, several factors responsible for angiogenesis have been identified. It gradually has become clear that polysaccharides, such as heparin and heparan sulfate, play a key role through their affinity for certain polypeptide growth factors.[1] These heparin-binding growth factors are capable of inducing angiogenesis.[1] The family of heparin-binding growth factors, which had initially been purified by Gospodarovic et al.[2] consist of structurally related polypeptides. Two members, heparan-binding growth factor 1 (HBGF1) and HBGF2, have been studied under many different names.[2] Most commonly they are known as acidic and basic fibroblast growth factor (FGF) because of their influence on the proliferation of mesoderm- and neuroectoderm-derived cells.[2] The interactions of the FGFs with heparin have important physiologic implications.[2] Heparin increases the biologic activity of acidic FGF and protects acidic and basic FGF from degradation by heat, acid, and proteases.[2] The binding of FGFs to heparan sulfate is essential for the binding of FGFs to their receptor on the cell surface.[2]

Because FGFs play such an important role in angiogenesis,[2] their inactivation might become an important step towards cancer therapy by blocking angiogensis. The present study investigates the selective inactivation of FGFs by heparin-like polysaccharides.

RESULTS

Soft agar cloning assays were used as an experimental model to study the inactivation of heparin-binding and nonheparin-binding growth factors. SW13 cells,

---

[e]To whom correspondence should be addressed.

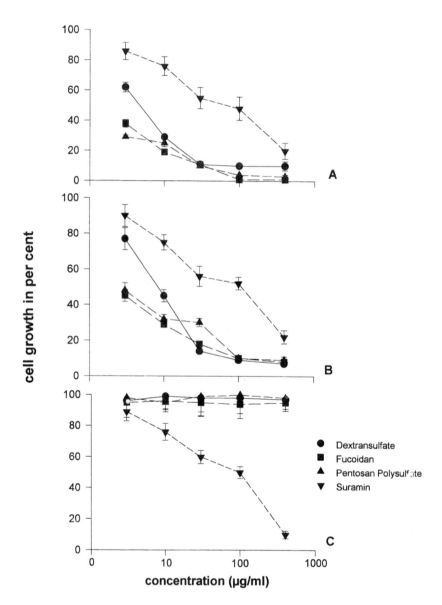

FIGURE 1. Soft agar cloning assays. Cell line SW 13, derived from carcinoma of the adrenal cortex, was stimulated with 10 ng/ml basic FGF (**A**) or 10 ng/ml acidic FGF (**B**). Estrogen-receptor–positive breast cancer cell line MCF7 was stimulated under serum-free conditions with 100 ng/ml IGF1 (**C**). Polyanions were added at increasing concentrations. Dishes were incubated 7–9 days at 37°C in a 5% CO_2 atmosphere. Colonies larger than 40 μm were counted.

whose anchorage-independent growth depends on the presence of fibroblast growth factor (FGF), were incubated with 10 ng/ml acidic or basic FGF (FIG. 1A and B). Cells were treated with the polyanions dextransulfate, fucoidan, pentosan polysulfate, and suramin at concentrations ranging from 1–400 μg/ml.

In the assays with basic FGF, the half-maximal inhibitory concentrations (IC_{50}s) were 1 μg/ml for pentosan polysulfate and fucoidan, 5 μg/ml for dextransulfate, and 100 μg/ml for suramin (FIG. 1A). In the assays with acidic FGF, the IC_{50}s were 3 μg/ml for pentosan polysulfate, and for fucoidan, 10 μg/ml for dextran sulfate and 100 μg/ml for suramin (FIG. 1B).

Anchorage-independent growth of breast cancer cell line MCF7, stimulated by 100 ng/ml insulin-like growth factor 1 (IGF1), was applied as an experimental model for inactivation of nonheparin-binding growth factors (FIG. 1C). Cells were incubated with the polyanions dextran sulfate, fucoidan, pentosan polysulfate, and suramin at concentrations ranging from 1–400 μg/ml. The IC_{50} for suramin was 100 μg/ml; the heparinoids dextran sulfate, fucoidan, and pentosan polysulfate had no effect (FIG. 1C).

Competitive binding assays were used to study the effects of polyanions on receptor binding of heparin-binding and nonheparin-binding growth factors (FIG. 2). Cells were incubated with labeled growth factors at concentrations similar to the respective K_d. Nonspecific binding was excluded by adding excess amounts of nonradioactive ligand. The polyanionic compounds dextransulfate, fucoidan, pentosan polysulfate, and suramin were added at concentrations ranging from 1–1,000 μg/ml.

The IC_{50}s for the binding of basic FGF to its receptor were 1 μg/ml for pentosan polysulfate, 5 μg/ml for fucoidan, 1 μg/ml for dextran sulfate, and 100 μg/ml for suramin (FIG. 2A). The IC_{50}s for binding of acidic FGF to its receptor were 3 μg/ml for pentosan polysulfate and for fucoidan, 50 μg/ml for dextransulfate, and 100 μg/ml for suramin (FIG. 2B).

The polysulfated heparinoids had no effect on binding of IGF1 to its receptor. The IC_{50} for binding of IGF1 to its receptor was 100 μg/ml for suramin (FIG. 2C).

DISCUSSION

We have shown that polysulfated heparinoids selectively inactivate heparin-binding angiogenesis factors basic FGF and acidic FGF. The effects of heparinoids are more potent on basic FGF than on acidic FGF. Basic FGF exhibits a higher affinity for heparin (1.5 MNaCl) than does acidic FGF (1.0 MNaCl). In addition, we demonstrated that heparinoids can also inactive heparin-binding growth factors, which do not belong to the FGF family, such as heregulin or pleiotrophin (data not shown). Heparinoids exert no effect on nonheparin-binding growth factors, as demonstrated for IGF1 (FIG. 1C and 2C), EGF, and TGF$_\alpha$ (not shown). Suramin inactives heparin-binding and nonheparin-binding growth factors. The concentrations of suramin necessary for inactivation of heparin-binding growth factors are 100 times higher than the necessary concentrations of heparinoids. Suramin, a polyanion, has been shown to inhibit cancer growth in various clinical trials. However, nonselective binding to proteins induces toxic side effects.[4]

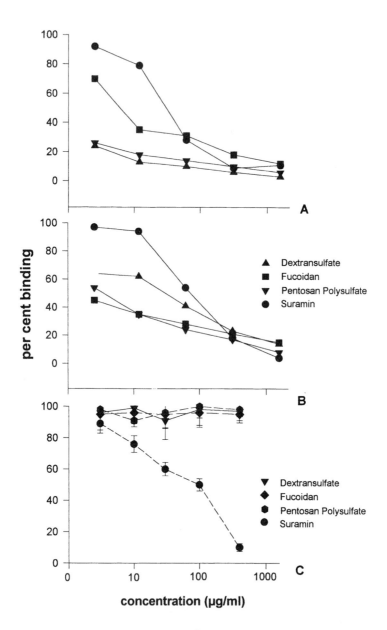

FIGURE 2. Radioreceptor assay: 3×10^5 SW 13 cells (**A,B**) or MCF7 cells (**C**) were plated in 24-well plates. After the cells had been washed and incubated with binding buffer for 1 hour, 30,000 c/m of iodinated basic FGF (**A**), acidic FGF (**B**), or IGF1 (**C**) were added. Nonspecific binding was excluded by the addition of the non-radioactive growth factors at an excess concentration of 100 ng/ml. Polyanions were added at increasing concentrations. Radioactivity was measured by a γ-counter, and specific binding was calculated. Standard deviations < 10% are not shown (**A,B**).

The angiogenetic capacities of basic and acidic FGF have been demonstrated in several publications.[1-3] High expression of FGF has been associated with progressive growth of fibrosarcomas,[3] astrocytomas,[5] glioblastomas,[6] pancreatic carcinomas,[7] renal carcinomas,[8] colon carcinoma,[9] and head and neck tumors.[10] Elevated levels of basic FGF have been detected in the urine of patients with a wide spectrum of cancers.[11]

Our data indicate that the affinity of FGFs for heparin can be used for selective inactivation of these and other growth factors that bind to heparin. The mechanism of inactivation of heparin-binding growth factors by heparinoids has not yet been clarified. Studies of the fucoidan-binding properties with various proteins have demonstrated that the number and disposition of sulfate groups are important for the interaction of the heparinoid with basic amino acids such as arginine, lysine, or histidine.[12,13] Our experiments (data not shown) have demonstrated that the binding sites of heparin and the heparinoid pentosan polysulfate on FGF are not identical. Similar results have been obtained from binding studies of heparin and pentosan polysulfate to antithrombin.[14]

We therefore may speculate that polysulfated heparinoids inactivate the FGFs by preventing their binding to heparin in a noncompetitive way, and through this mechanism prevent the binding of FGF to its receptor. It has been shown that FGF binding to the receptor is dependent on heparin.[15]

In conclusion, our data show that polysulfated heparinoids exert a selective inhibitory effect on heparin-binding angiogenesis factors. In contrast, suramin inhibits growth factors in a nonselective way. However, the concentrations of suramin, necessary to block heparin-binding growth factors, are 100 times higher than the concentrations of polysulfated heparinoids. Various studies have demonstrated that polysulfated heparinoids can inhibit tumor growth *in vivo*.[16-19]

The present study might provide some insight into the mechanism of action through which polysulfated heparinoids exert their growth inhibitory effects on tumor cells. The application of polysulfated heparinoids might block metastatic tumour growth by inhibiting angiogenesis factors.

SUMMARY

Angiogenesis is a prerequisite for tumor expansion and metastasis. The angiogenic potential of the heparin-binding growth factors acidic fibroblast growth factor (FGF) and basic FGF has been demonstrated in various publications. We studied the inhibitory effects of suramin and the polysulfated heparinoids pentosan polysulfate, dextran sulfate, and fucoidan on the action of FGF. As an experimental model, we used the adrenal cancer cell line SW 13, whose anchorage-independent growth depends on the presence of FGF. The polysulfated heparinoids inhibited FGF-induced growth and binding to the receptor at an IC_{50} of 0.5–3 µg/ml. Suramin inhibited FGF at an IC_{50} of 100 µg/ml. The polysulfated heparinoids exerted no effect on IGF-1 or TGFα–related growth. Suramin inhibited the anchorage-independent growth induced by IGF-1 or TGFα only at an IC_{50} of 100 µg/ml. Our results indicate that suramin inhibits growth factors in a nonselective way. By contrast, polysulfated heparinoids exert a selective inhibitory effect on heparin binding angiogenesis factors at an IC_{50}, which is 100 times below the IC_{50} of suramin. Therefore, the administration of polysulfated heparinoids might become a novel approach to tumor therapy based on blocking angiogenesis.

REFERENCES

1. FOLKMAN, J. & Y. SHING. 1992. Angiogenesis. J. Biol. Chem. **267:** 10931–10934.
2. BURGESS, W.H. & T. MACIAG. 1989. The heparin-binding (fibroblast) growth factor family of proteins. Annu. Rev. **58:** 575–606.
3. KANDEL, J. *et al.* 1991, Neovascularization is associated with a switch to the export of the bFGF in the multistep development of fibrosarcoma. Cell **66:** 1095–1104.
4. STEIN, C.A. 1993. Suramin: A novel antineoplastic agent with multiple potential mechanisms of action. Cancer Res. **53:** 2239–2248.
5. MAXWELL, M. *et al.* 1991. Expression of angiogenic growth factor genes in primary human astrocytomas may contribute to their growth and progression. Cancer Res. **51:** 1345–1351.
6. STEFANIK, D.F. *et al.* 1991. Acidic and basic fibroblast growth factors are present in glioblastoma multiforme. Cancer Res. **51:** 5760–5765.
7. YAMANAKA, Y. *et al.* 1993. Overexpression of acidic and basic fibroblast growth factors in human pancreatic cancer correlates with advanced tumor stage. Cancer Res. **53:** 5289–5296.
8. NANUS, D.M. *et al.* 1993. Expression of basic fibroblast growth factor in primary human renal tumors: Correlation with poor survival. J. Natl. Cancer Inst. **85:** 1597.
9. DIRIX, L.Y. *et al.* 1996. Serum basic fibroblast growth factor and vascular endothelial growth factor and tumour growth kinetics in advanced colorectal cancer. Ann. Oncol. **7:** 843–848.
10. DELLACONO, F.R. *et al.* 1997. Expression of basic fibroblast growth factor and its receptors by head and neck squamos carcinoma tumor and vascular endothelial cells. Am. J. Surg. **174:** 540–544.
11. NGUYEN, M. *et al.* 1993. Elevated levels of an angiogenic peptide, basic fibroblast growth factor, in the urine of patients with a wide spectrum of cancers. J. Natl. Cancer Inst. **86:** 356–361.
12. JONES, R. 1990. Unusual, fucoidin-binding properties of chymotryspinogen and trypsinogen. Biochim. Biophys. Acta **1037:** 227–232.
13. DEANGELIS, P. & C.G. GLABE. 1988. Role of basic amino acids in the interaction of binding with sulfated fucans. Biochemistry **27:** 8189–8194.
14. SUN, X. & J. CHANG. 1989. The heparin and pentosan polysulfate binding sites of human antithrombin overlap but are not identical. Biochemistry **185:** 225–230.
15. ORNITZ, D.M. & P. LEDER. 1992. Ligand specificity and heparin dependence of fibroblast growth factor receptors 1 and 3. J. Biol. Chem. **267:** 16305–16311.
16. COOMBE, D.R. 1987. Analysis of the inhibition of tumour metastasis by sulphated polysaccharides. Int. J. Cancer **39:** 82–88.
17. NGUYEN,, N.M., J.E. LEHR & K.J. PIENTA. 1993. Pentosan inhibits angiogenesis in vitro and suppresses prostate tumor growth in vivo. Anticancer Res. **13:** 2143–2147.
18. WELLSTEIN, A., G. ZUGMAIER *et al.* 1991. Tumor growth dependent on Kaposi's sarcoma-derived fibroblast growth factor inhibited by pentosan polysulfate. J. Natl. Cancer Inst. **83:** 716.
19. ZUGMAIER, G., M.E. LIPPMANN & A. WELLSTEIN. 1992. Inhibition by pentosan polysulfate (PPS) of heparin-binding growth factors released from tumor cells and blockage by PPS of tumor growth in animals. Int. Cancer Inst. **84:** 1716–1724.

RPR 130401, a Nonpeptidomimetic Farnesyltransferase Inhibitor with *in Vivo* Activity

P. VRIGNAUD,[a] M.C. BISSERY, P. MAILLIET, AND F. LAVELLE

Rhône-Poulenc Rorer S.A., Centre de recherche de Vitry-Alfortville, 13 quai Jules Guesde, B.P. 14, 94403 Vitry sur Seine, France

A nonpeptidomimetic farnesyltransferase inhibitor (FTI) was identified through an enzymatic Ras screening, leading to the synthesis of benzo[f]perhydroisoindole derivatives, a new class of competitive inhibitors with the farnesyl pyrophosphate substrate.[1] One compound of this family, exhibiting enzymatic and cellular activities at a micromolar level, was evaluated *in vivo*, but was found inactive.[2] Thereafter, new chemical modifications were performed. RPR 130401 was selected for its cytostatic *in vitro* activity in a colony formation assay against human Ki-Ras carcinoma cells, inhibiting concentration 50% (IC_{50}) ranging from 0.045 to 0.48 µM. The goal of the work presented herein was to evaluate its *in vivo* activity.

According to the chemotherapy methods previously described,[3] the *in vivo* antitumor efficacy of RPR 130401 was evaluated against human Ki-Ras carcinomas obtained from the American Type Culture Collection and xenografted in Swiss nude mice: two colons (HCT 116 and SW620), one pancreas (MIA PaCa-2), and one lung (H460). Swiss nude mice were grafted sc with tumor implants on day 0. Tumors were measured with a caliper 2–3 times a week, and tumor weight was evaluated using the following formula: tumor weight (mg) = length (mm) × width^2 (mm^2)/2. RPR 130401 was suspended in water containing 0.5–1% polysorbate 80 and 0.5% methyl cellulose. It was administered orally twice a day for 19 consecutive days to mice bearing palpable sc tumors at dosages of 248, 400, and 645 mg/kg/administration. A dosage producing 20% body weight loss or drug-related death was declared toxic. The end points were tumor growth delay (T-C = difference in median times required for treatment and control groups to reach a predetermined size) and $\log_{10}$ cell kill net (lck net = tumor growth delay – treatment duration/3.32 × tumor doubling time). Cytostatic activity was obtained for a tumor growth delay corresponding at least to the treatment duration. A negative lck net indicated that tumor grew under treatment.

Pharmacokinetics of RPR 130401 was determined following a single administration of 250 mg/kg in nontumor-bearing B6D2F$_1$ mice (FIG. 1). The area under the curve (AUC_{0-24h}) was 820.3 h.µg/ml, with a 2.8-hour half-life of elimination. Peak plasma concentration was 142.1 µg/ml 2 hours postdose, a concentration 100 times greater than the *in vitro* IC_{50} (~0.091 µg/ml in HCT 116 colony formation assay), and 19.9 µg/ml 8 hours postdose. Therefore, for efficacy studies, this compound was administered orally twice a day, 7 hours apart, for 3 consecutive weeks.

[a]Phone, 33 1 55 71 36 29; fax, 33 1 55 71 34 71.
e-mail, Patricia.VRIGNAUD@RP-RORER.FR

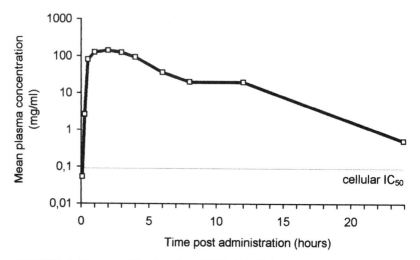

FIGURE 1. Pharmacokinetics of oral RPR 130401. RPR 130401 was suspended in water containing 0.5% polysorbate 80 and 0.5% methyl cellulose and administered to B6D2F$_1$ female mice at 250 mg/kg. Plasma was collected at 5, 15, and 30 minutes and 1, 2, 3, 4, 6, 8, 12, and 24 hours postdose. Plasma levels were determined by HPLC with UV detection (LC-MS/MS, limit of quantification was 0.05 µg/ml).

Against the most *in vitro* sensitive tumor, colon HCT 116, tumor size at the start of therapy ranged between 80 and 180 mg in the various treatment and control groups. The highest dosage administered was well tolerated with no body weight loss and no adverse effects. Cytostatic activity was achieved with a tumor growth delay of 22.8 days and an 0.3 lck net (FIG. 2). There was a clear dose response effect in the tumor growth delays at the two dosages below 400 and 248 mg/kg/administration with a transient cytostatic effect. Tumor growth delays were 17.3 and 11.7 days, respectively, with a negative lck net.

In mice bearing colon carcinoma SW620 with a 0–179 mg tumor weight at the start of therapy, the highest dosage tested of 645 mg/kg/administration was well tolerated and produced a tumor growth delay of 15.7 days for a treatment duration of 19 days and a negative lck net (−0.3). This indicates that no cytostatic activity was obtained. The two lowest doses of 400 and 248 mg/kg/administration were also inactive.

At the highest dose tested, 645 mg/kg/dam, RPR 130401 was toxic in lung H460-bearing mice, with two of eight drug-related deaths associated with excessive body weight loss. Tumor size at the start of therapy ranged between 100 and 200 mg. The optimal dosage of 400 mg/kg/administration produced no cytostatic activity with a tumor growth delay of 15.2 days for a treatment duration of 19 days and a negative lck net (−0.4). The lowest dosage was also inactive.

In the same way, three of eight drug-related deaths occurred at the highest dosage tested of 645 mg/kg/administration in mice bearing pancreas MIA PaCa-2, with tumor size at the start of therapy ranging from 80–170 mg. Although we observed a slow down in tumor growth in mice treated at the optimal dosage of 400 mg/kg/ad-

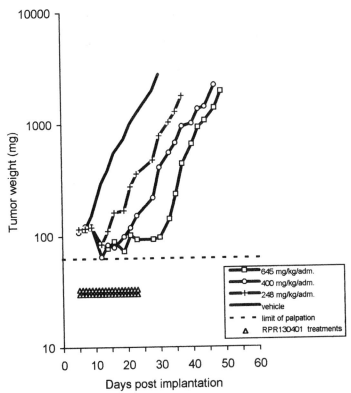

FIGURE 2. RPR 130401 *in vivo* **efficacy against human colon carcinoma HCT116.**
RPR 130401 was administered orally twice daily for 19 consecutive days at dosages of 248
(+), 400 (O), and 645 mg/kg/administration (□) to Swiss nu/nu mice bearing measurable
human colon HCT116 (80–180 mg). Each curve represents the median tumor growth of each
group. Cytostatic activity = (tumor growth delay ≥ treatment duration), corresponding to a
positive $\log_{10}$ cell kill net.

ministration, RPR 130401 did not produce any cytostatic activity (T – C = 10.6 days;
–0.7 lck net).

In conclusion, RPR 130401 was bioavailable by the oral route and produced cytostatic activity against one Ki-Ras activated carcinoma, colon HCT 116, xenografted in nude mice. Further *in vivo* evaluation of RPR 130401 will be performed in
human and murine tumors exhibiting no Ki-Ras mutations, the main point being to
evaluate this type of compound in combination with chemotherapy.

REFERENCES

1. MAILLIET, P. *et al.* 1997. Proc. Am. Assoc. Cancer Res. **39:** 2347.
2. VRIGNAUD, P. *et al.* 1997. Proc. Am. Assoc. Cancer Res. **39:** 2348.
3. SCHABEL, F.M., JR. *et al.* 1977. Quantitative evaluation of anticancer agents in experimental animals. Pharmacol. Ther. Part A **1:** 411–435.

Cellular Effects of a New Farnesyltransferase Inhibitor, RPR-115135, in a Human Isogenic Colon Cancer Cell Line Model System HCT-116

P. RUSSO,[a,d,f] C. OTTOBONI,[a,d] C. FALUGI,[b] W. REINHOLD,[a] J.F. RIOU,[c] S. PARODI,[d] AND P.M. O'CONNOR[a,e]

[a]Laboratory of Molecular Pharmacology, Division of Basic Sciences, National Cancer Institute, National Institutes of Health, Bethesda, Maryland 20892, USA

[b]Department of Developing Biology, University of Genoa, Genoa, Italy

[c]Anticancer Research Program, Centre de Recherche Rhone-Poulenc Rorer, Vitry F-94403, France

[d]Laboratory of Experimental Oncology, National Cancer Institute and Department of Clinical and Experimental Oncology, University of Genoa, Genoa I-16132, Italy

This work focused on the cellular effects of a new nonpeptidomimetic farnesyltransferase (FTase) inhibitor, namely, RPR-115135, tested in a human colon cancer HCT-116 isogenic cell line model system. HCT-116 line, which harbors a K-Ras mutation,[1] was transfected with an empty control pCMV vector or with a dominant-negative mutated p53 transgene (248R/W) to disrupt p53 function, as previously described.[2]

Of the many signal transduction mechanisms that are emerging as potential targets for drug hunting in cancer, prenylation of Ras family proteins, such as Ras, RhoB, and Rab (virtually all members of the Ras superfamily of proteins), is receiving particular attention from both pharmaceutical companies and academic groups.[3–9] Interest in protein prenylation has escalated because of the importance of this modification in the function of Ras proteins, GTP-binding proteins[10] that, when mutated, contribute to the development of different types of cancers.[11–13]

RPR-115135 is a new and selective inhibitor of FTase in vitro (farnesylation of lamin-B, H-Ras, or K-Ras), unaffecting the closely related enzyme geranyl-geranyltransferase I.[14] Kinetic experiments showed that this compound inhibits FTase in an FPP-competitive way (Y. Lelievre, personal communication).

We found that relative to control transfectants [two different clones: CMV-2 (IC_{50} = 2.81 ± 0.42 μM) and CMV-4 (5.75 ± 3.10 μM)], there was a tendency for mutated-p53 transfectant HCT-116 clones [Mu-p53-2 (0.55 ± 0.37 μM) and Mu-p53-4 (0.77 ± 0.28 μM)] to be more sensitive to RPR-115135 (≥ 5-fold difference at the IC_{50} value)

[e]Present address: Oncology Research Division, Agouron Pharmaceuticals, Inc., San Diego, CA 92121, USA

[f]To whom correspondence should be addressed: Department of Experimental Oncology, National Cancer Institute, Largo Rosanna Benzi 10, I-16132 Genoa, Italy. Phone, +39 010 5600212; fax, +39 010 5600210.

e-mail, patrusso@hp380.ist.unige.it.

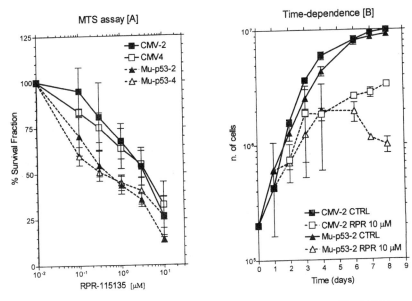

FIGURE 1. (**A**) Cell growth inhibition induced by RPR-115135 in HCT-116 human isogenic colon cancer cell line system. Each point represents the mean ± SD of at least three independent experiments performed in sextuplicate. MTS assay was performed after 6 days of continous exposure. (**B**) Time-course sensitivity to RPR-115135 over 6 days of exposure in CMV-2 and Mu-p53-2 clones. Each point represents the mean ± SD of at least three independent experiments performed in sextuplicate.

(FIG. 1A). In addition, the two Mu-p53 clones were slightly more resistant to 5-FU (data not shown) than were the two CMV clones and the parental one.

Time-course experiments conducted over 6 days with continual exposure to 10 μM RPR-115135 (IC$_{75-85}$) revealed that HCT-116 cells were still able to grow up to 72 hours following drug administration, but thereafter, clear growth inhibition was observed (FIG. 1B). Growth inhibition could not easily be accounted for on the basis of a specific cell cycle arrest phenotype, as assayed by flow cytometry (data not shown). Thus, the effect on the composition of the cell cycle was apparently similar in untreated control cells and treated cells when corrected for the same number of viable cells.

Apoptotic events were infrequently observed in 10 μM RPR-115135–treated cells (less than 1–5%), but other morphologic alterations were present 48–72 hours after treatment and might explain the observed growth inhibition. In treated cell lines, high percentages of hypertrophic and vacuolated cells were found. This phenomenon was evident already at the second incubation day (FIG. 2) in the Mu-p53-2 clone, whereas in CMV-2 cells a relevant presence of this "giant" cell type was observed from the third incubation day. Six days after the beginning of treatment with 10 μM RPR-115135, practically 100% of treated cells presented the altered morphology just described. In the course of a 6-day treatment the frequency of cells with a "giant" size increased progressively, whereas the cells tended to clump together, forming big rounded clusters of

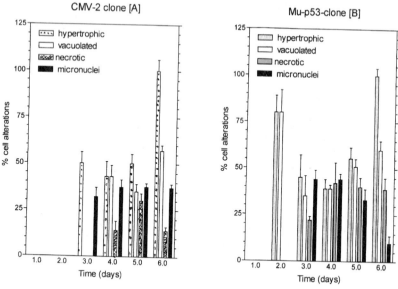

FIGURE 2. Percentage of cell morphology alterations (toluidine staining) and micronuclei induction (DAPI staining) over a 6-day treatment period with 10 µM RPR-115135. **(A)** CMV-2 cells; **(B)** Mu-p53-2 cells. At least 500 cells were counted for each slide; experiments were performed in duplicate for three different times. Mean ± SD of at least three independent experiments.

cells with huge nuclei, sometimes in the form of polykarions, and large cytoplasms (about 4–5 times ∅ the control cell size).

In treated Mu-p53-2 cells, a tendency towards necrosis was observed, whereas apoptotic figures were poorly represented (≅ in the same % as in controls) (FIG. 2).

Three days after the beginning of treatment, exposure to 10 µM RPR-115135 produced a large number of micronuclei (FIG. 2). In CMV-2 cells, a maximum number of micronuclei was reached after 4 days of treatment. They remained at a plateau level throughout the subsequent days of treatment (FIG. 2). In Mu-p53-2 cells there was a tendency to form a greater amount of micronuclei after 3 or 4 days of treatment. After 5 or 6 days of treatment, counting micronuclei became technically difficult because of the tendency of treated cells to form small compact cell clusters, with nuclei with highly condensed chromatin. In control cells the number of micronuclei was always less than 3%. An important observation was that an unusually large amount (> 30%) of micronuclei were found in treated cells (FIG. 2). As an example, ethylmethanesulfonate (EMS, an alkylating genotoxic agent) at very high concentrations (60 mM) in V79 cells induces about 10% of micronuclei,[15] and usually the frequency of micronuclei is expressed per 1,000 nuclei. In our experiments the frequency was expressed per 100 nuclei. It is well known that both clastogens (i.e., EMS or X-rays) and aneugens (i.e., podophyllotoxins, colchicine, nocodazole, and vinblastine) can induce micronuclei in V79 cells, so this assay is considered generally valid for aneuploidy detection.[15] Our results showed that for the first time a farnesyltransferase inhibitor could induce important cell morphologic alterations, and the high percentage of induced micronuclei suggests a potential ability for RPR-115135 to be an aneuploidy-inducing agent. More detailed analyses to discriminate between aneuploidy due to chromosome nondisjunction or chromosome loss are ongoing. Preliminary results suggest a possible role for RPR-115135 as an aneugen agent (in preparation).

In conclusion, RPR-115135 can induce cell growth inhibition independently from the status of p53. Its growth-inhibiting effect cannot be ascribed to the induction of classic programmed cell death, but rather to large alterations in cell morphology. In addition, RPR-115135 could be an aneuplody-inducing agent.

ACKNOWLEDGMENTS

This work was partially supported by AIRC (Associazione Italiana per la Ricerca sul Cancro) 1997, Milan, Italy (grant to P.R.), Progetto Finalizzato Ministero Sanità, 1997, Rome, Italy, and Progetto Interuniversitario: Terapie antineoplastiche innovative, MURST 1997, Rome, Italy (grant to S.P.). Dr. Patrizia Russo received a fellowship (Martha Galle-Sacerdote Momigliano, 1997) and Dr. Cristina Ottoboni received a second fellowship, both awarded by FIRC (Fondazione Italiana per la Ricerca sul Cancro), Milan, Italy.

REFERENCES

1. KOO, H.-M. *et al.* 1996. Enhanced sensitivity to 1-β-D-arabinofuranosylcytosine and topoisomerase II inhibitors in tumor cell lines harboring activated ras oncogens. Cancer Res. **56:** 5211–5216.
2. FAN, S. *et al.* 1997. Cell lacking CIP1/WAF1 genes exhibits preferential sensitivity to cisplatin and nitrogen mustard. Oncogene **14:** 2127–2136.
3. GIBBS, J.B & A. OLIFF. 1997. The potential of farnesyltransferase inhibitors as cancer chemotherapeutics. Ann. Rev. Pharmacol. Toxicol. **37:** 143–166.
4. LEONARD, D.M. 1997. Ras farnesyltransferase. A new therapeutic target. Med. Chem. **40:** 2971–2990.
5. LERNER, E.C. *et al.* 1997. Inhibition of Ras prenylation: A signaling target for novel anti-cancer drug design. Anti-Cancer Drug Design **12:** 229–238.
6. MAILLET, P. *et al.* 1997. Synthesis and in vitro structure-activity relationship of a new promising series of non peptidic protein-farnesyl-transferase inhibitors. Proc. Am. Assoc. Cancer Res. **8:** 350.
7. OMERCH, A. *et al.* 1997. Farnesylproteintransferase inhibitors as agents to inhibit tumor growth. BioFactors **6:** 359–366.
8. QIAN, Y. *et al.* 1997. Farnesyltransferase as a target for anticancer drug design. Biopolymer **43:** 25–41.
9. SEBTI, S.M. & A.D. HAMILTON. 1997. Inhibition of Ras prenylation: A novel approach to cancer chemotherapy. Pharmacol. Ther. **74:** 103–114.
10. KATZ, M.E. & F. MCCORMICK. 1997. Signal transduction from multiple Ras effectors. Curr. Opin. Gen. Dev. **7:** 75–79.
11. KHOSRAVI-FAR, R. *et al.* 1996. Oncogenic Ras activation of Raf/mitogen-activated protein kinase independent pathways is sufficient to cause tumorigenic transformation. Mol. Cell. Biol. **16:** 3923–3933.
12. ZACHOS, G. & D.A. SPANDIDOS. 1997. Expression of ras proto-oncogenes: Regulation and implications in the development of human tumors. Crit. Rev. Oncol. Hematol. **26:** 65–75.

13. WHITE, A.M. *et al.* 1995. Multiple Ras functions can contribute to mammalian cell transformation. Cell **80:** 533–541.
14. CLERC, F.F. *et al.* 1995. Constrained analogs of KCVFM with improved inhibitory properties against farnesyl transferase. Bioorg. Med. Chem. Lett. **5:** 1779–1784.
15. Genetic Toxicology and Environmental Mutagenesis. Special Issue: 1997. The CB in vitro micronucleus assay in human lymphocytes. Mut. Res. **392:** 1–280.

The Farnesyltransferase Inhibitor L-744,832 Inhibits the Growth of Astrocytomas through a Combination of Antiproliferative, Antiangiogenic, and Proapoptotic Activities

MATTHIAS M. FELDKAMP, NELSON LAU, AND ABHIJIT GUHA[a]

Samuel Lunenfeld Research Institute, Mount Sinai Hospital, and Division of Neurosurgery, The Toronto Hospital and University of Toronto, Toronto, Ontario, Canada

The 21-kD cellular protein Ras is known to play a critical role in a wide range of cellular events, including proliferation, cytoskeletal rearrangement, development, and apoptosis. Activated Ras is bound to GTP, whereas Ras•GDP represents the inactive protein. Up to 30% of human malignancies express a mutant form of this protein in which Ras is constitutively present in its activated GTP-bound form. Such oncogenic mutations have not been identified in glioblastoma multiforme (GBM). We have however demonstrated that Ras activation is critical in the proliferation of these tumors[1] as well as important in the secretion of the angiogenic factor vascular endothelial growth factor (VEGF[2]), with Ras activation occurring secondary to overexpression of the receptor tyrosine kinases platelet derived growth factor receptor (PDGF-R) and epidermal growth factor receptor (EGF-R).[1] As farnesyltransferase inhibitors (FTIs) inhibit the posttranslational modification of Ras, preventing the association of Ras with its upstream activators at the cell surface, we hypothesized that astrocytoma cells would be growth inhibited by such agents.

The FTI L-744,832 was provided by Allen Oliff (Merck Research Laboratories, West Point, Pennsylvania). Six astrocytoma cell lines were evaluated, including five established lines (U87, U118, U138, U343, and U373). In addition, U118:EGFRvIII cells were evaluated, which express the constitutively activated truncated receptor EGFRvIII, expressed in a large subset of GBMs. We previously showed that U118:EGFRvIII cells constitutively express higher levels of activated Ras•GTP. Cells were treated with L-744,832 at doses ranging from 10 nM to 100 μM, and the concentration of vehicle was kept constant in all wells (0.1% methanol). Cells were grown in 96-well plates, and proliferation was measured using the tetrazolium compound MTS, which is bioreduced by viable cells into a colored formazan product. Dose-response curves (Hill plots) were constructed by modeling a log normal dose-response relationship. Logistic regression (probit analysis) was used to estimate the LD_{50} for each cell line as the dose at which proliferation was reduced to 50% of control wells. All astrocytoma cell lines were growth inhibited by L-744,832, with IC_{50} ranging from 5.3 to 17.4 μM. Cells expressing EGFRvIII were more sensitive to L-

[a]Address correspondence to: Abhijit Guha, MD, Division of Neurosurgery, Toronto Western Hospital, 399 Bathurst St., Toronto, Ontario, Canada, M5T 2S8. Phone, 416/603-5740; fax, 416/603-5298.

e-mail, ab.guha@utoronto.ca

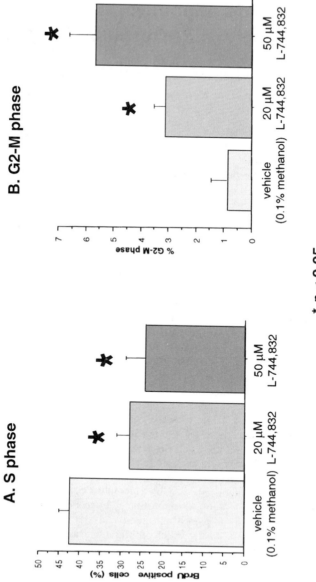

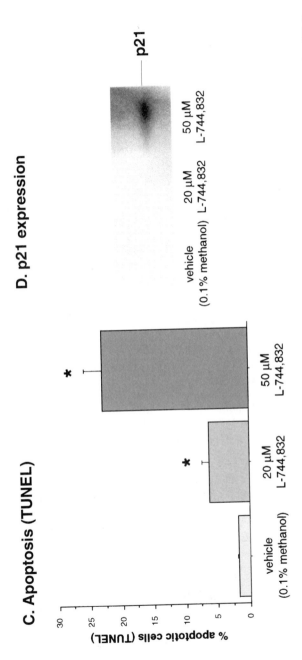

FIGURE 1. Effect of L-744,832 on U373 cells. Entry into the S phase of the cell cycle was measured using BrdU incorporation (**A**). Progression through the G2-M checkpoint of the cell cycle was determined using FACS (**B**). L-744,832 induced a dose-dependent induction of cellular apoptosis, as measured using a TUNEL assay (Boehringer Mannheim; **C**). These effects on cell cycle progression and apoptosis may be mediated through p21, which is upregulated by L-744,832 in U373 cells (anti-p21, PharMingen; **D**). *Statistical significance by factorial ANOVA, with $p < 0.05$.

744,832 (4.36 vs. 11.21 μM). L-744,832 demonstrated both cytostatic as well as cytotoxic activity, depending on the dose. At doses near the IC_{50} (20 μM), the agent demonstrated primarily a reversible cytostatic effect. At higher doses (50 μM), however, L-744,832 demonstrated a cytotoxic effect towards astrocytoma cells; this cytotoxic effect was not reversible on discontinuation of drug treatment. The dose-dependent effects demonstrated by this agent are consistent with progressive inhibition of Ras processing and membrane localization on S-100/P-100 fractionation experiments, and we also demonstrated a modest inhibition of MAPK activity (as determined by a radioactive myelin basic protein kinase assay).

The mechanism for the antiproliferative effects of L-744,832 on astrocytoma cells was evaluated in two cell lines: U87 cells are wild-type for p53, whereas U373 cells express mutant p53. Results were similar for both cell lines, suggesting a p53-independent mechanism. L-744,832 20 μM significantly reduced incorporation of bromodeoxyuridine (BrdU) in both cell lines, consistent with inhibition of cell cycle progression through the G1-S checkpoint (FIG. 1A). In addition, FACS analysis revealed a significant dose-dependent increase in the G2-M fraction of the cycle, further suggesting inhibition of cell cycle progression through the G2-M checkpoint (FIG. 1B). Our results thus imply a dual effect of L-744,832 on the cell cycle, with inhibition at both the G1-S and G2-M checkpoints. We propose that such a dual effect may be mediated through increased p21 expression, as demonstrated for U373 cells (FIG. 1D).

Consistent with its predominantly cytostatic effect at low doses, L-744,832 20 μM induced only a small increase in apoptosis, as detected using a TUNEL assay (FIG. 1C). Vehicle-treated U373 cells demonstrated an apoptosis rate of $1.7 \pm 0.1\%$, whereas L-744,832 20 μM increased this to $6.3 \pm 1.1\%$. Consistent with its strong cytotoxic effect at higher doses, 50 μM L-744,832 further increased the rate of apoptosis in U373 cells to $22.9 \pm 2.9\%$ for U373 cells ($p < 0.0001$). Similar results were obtained in U87 cells.

Finally, previous evidence from our laboratory and others has implicated a role for Ras in regulating expression of the potent angiogenic factor VEGF.[2] In the current paper, we have demonstrated that L-744,832 exerts a potent dose-dependent inhibitory effect on VEGF secretion from astrocytoma cells under both normoxic and hypoxic conditions.

Our experiments thus provide further evidence supporting the relevance of Ras-mediated signaling in the molecular pathogenesis of GBMs. The FTI L-744,832 potently inhibits the proliferation of astrocytoma cells in culture, through a combination of antiproliferative and proapoptotic events. Furthermore, we predict that this agent may have substantially greater effect *in vivo* by combining these effects with its antiangiogenic effect of reducing VEGF secretion. FTIs may thus prove to be promising agents in the management of these presently terminal human brain tumors.

REFERENCES

1. GUHA, A., M.M. FELDKAMP, N. LAU, G. BOSS & T. PAWSON. 1997. Proliferation of human malignant astrocytomas is dependent on Ras activation. Oncogene **15:** 2755–2766.
2. FELDKAMP, M.M., N. LAU, J. RAK, R.S. KERBEL & A. GUHA. 1999. Astrocytoma cell lines express high levels of Vascular Endothelial Growth Factor (VEGF), which is reduced by inhibition of the Ras signaling pathway. Int. J. Cancer. **81:** 118–124.

Isolation of Farnesyltransferase Inhibitors from Herbal Medicines

BYOUNG-MOG KWON,[a] SEUNG-HO LEE, MI-JEONG KIM, HYAE-KYEONG KIM, AND HWAN MOOK KIM

Korea Research Institute of Bioscience and Biotechnology (KRIBB), P.O Box 115, Yusung, Taejon 305-600, Republic of Korea

Ras proteins (H, K, and N) are small guanine nucleotide binding proteins that undergo a series of posttranslational modifications including farnesylation onto cysteine 186 at C-terminal of Ras by farnesyl protein transferase (FPTase). This is a mandatory process before Ras anchoring to plasma membrane, which is critical for its biologic activity, such as cell proliferation and tumorigenesis. Evidence now exists that specific inhibitors of FPTase will have an antitumorigenic effect. Many research teams are working on the isolation of natural inhibitors to give chemical leads to develop effective therapeutic agents for the treatment of cancers.[1,2]

In the course of our screening for potent inhibitors of FPTase from herbal medicines, we isolated 2-hydroxycinnamaldehyde, rhombenone, and arteminolide as inhibitors of FPTase.

MATERIALS AND METHODS

Isolation and Purification

The chloroform extract of the dried materials was fractionated by silica gel flash chromatography eluting with 5–10% MeOH in chloroform. Active fractions were further purified by C-18 column chromatography and gel filtration (Sephadex LH-20). Finally, the purified compounds were obtained by preparative reverse phase HPLC (YMC J'sphere ODS-H80, 250×20 mm ID column).

Structure Determination

The isolated compounds were determined by interpretation of NMR, IR, and mass spectral data. Analysis of HRFABMS and ^{13}C NMR spectra of 2-hydroxycinnamaldehyde, rhombenone, and arteminolide led to the molecular formulas $C_9H_9O_2$, $C_{29}H_{46}O_4$, and $C_{35}H_{42}O_8$, respectively. The ^{13}C NMR, HMQC experiment, and DEPT spectra served to identify the protons attached to a specific carbon. The ^1H-^1H COSY spectra and HMBC correlations between nonprotonated carbons and neighboring protons gave the key informations for the determination of structures. The relative stereochemistry of the compounds was determined by analysis of NOESY experiments.

[a]Phone, 82-42-860-4557; fax, 82-42-861-2675.
e-mail, kwonbm@kribb4680.kribb.re.kr

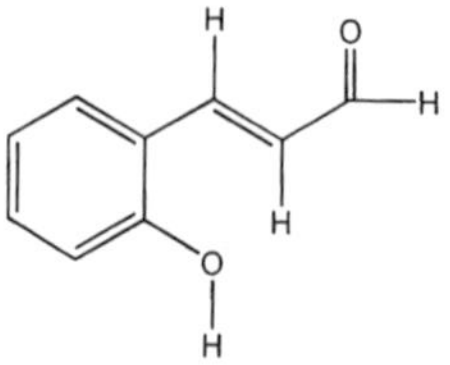

Compound   (1)

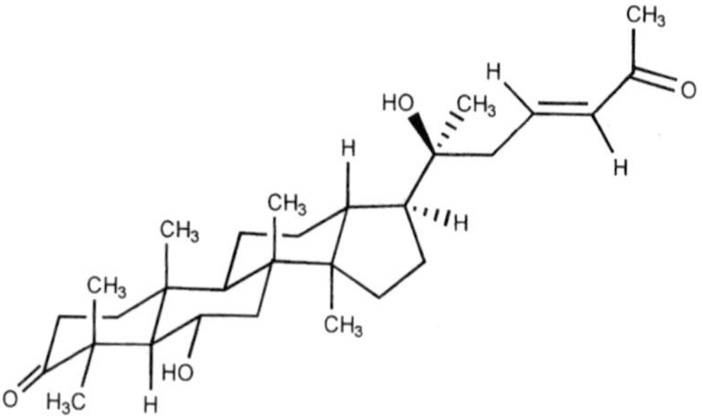

Compound (2)

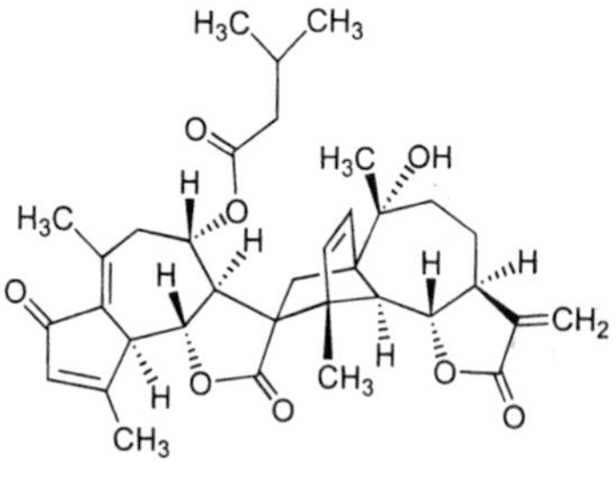

Compound (3)

FIGURE 1. Structure of FPTase inhibitors.

In Vivo Antitumor Activity of Cinnamaldehyde

SW-620 human colon adenocarcinoma cells (1×10^7 cells/ml) were implanted into the right flank of nude mice. Compound was dissolved in 0.5% tween 80 and was intraperitoneally administered at concentrations of 30 and 100 mg/kg. Adriamycin was used as a reference compound.

Tumor Weight of SW620 (Day 19)

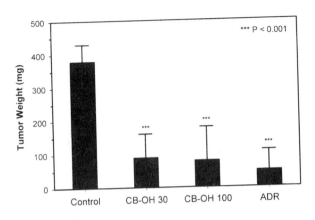

Body weight changes of nude mice
xenografted with SW620

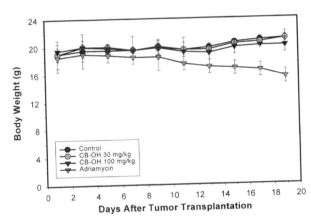

FIGURE 2. *In vivo* growth of SW-620 human tumor xenograft.

RESULTS

2-Hydroxycinnamaldehyde. 2-Hydroxycinnamaldehyde was isolated from the stem bark of *Cinnamomum cassia* Blume (Lauracea). It was the first time that we isolated it from natural sources. Extract of the bark of *C. cassia* has been used in China and Korea as a therapeutic agent for various diseases including hypertension and indigestion.

The compound also inhibited angiogenesis in a chick embryo chorioallantoic membrane (CAM).[3,4]

Rhombenone. We isolated rhombenone from the leaves of *Hedera rhombea* Bean (Araliaceae). Extract of the leaves of *H. rhombea* has been used as a therapeutic agent for various diseases including hemorrhage, chronic catarrh, jaundice, lithiasis, and convulsion. Rhombenone inhibited a recombinant rat FPTase with an IC_{50} of 2.3 μM.

Arteminolide. Arteminolide was isolated from the leaves of *Artemisia sylvatica* Maxim. (Compositae). Members of the *Artemisia* genus are important medicinal plants found throughout the world. Artemisinin, which was isolated from *Artemisia annua* L, is well known as an antimalarial agent.[5] Isolated arteminolide is a sesquiterpene lactone that exhibits a wide range of biologic activities. Arteminolide inhibited recombinant rat FPTase with an IC_{50} of 360 nM and appeared to be selective for FPTase. It did not inhibit rat squalene synthase ($IC_{50} \gg 200$ M) and recombinant rat geranyl-geranyl protein transferase I ($IC_{50} \gg 200$ M).

REMARKS

Although the FPTase inhibitors, isolated from Korean herbal medicines, mildly inhibit FPTase in comparison with the synthetic compounds,[6] they have different structures. Therefore, the compounds might be useful lead compounds for the development of antitumor drugs through the control of Ras-mediated signal transduction.

REFERENCES

1. GIBBS, J.B. *et al.* 1994. Farnesyltransferase inhibitors: Ras research yields a potential cancer therapeutic. Cell **77:** 175–178.
2. QIAN, Y. *et al.* 1998. Farnesyltransferase as a target for anticancer drug design. Biopoly. **43:** 25–41.
3. WEBB, C.P. *et al.* 1998. Signaling pathways in Ras-mediated tumorigenicity and metastasis. Proc. Natl. Acad. Sci. USA **95:** 8773–8778.
4. ARBISER, J.L. 1997. Oncogenic H-ras stimulates tumor angiogenesis by two distinct pathways. Proc. Natl. Acad. Sci. USA **94:** 861–866.
5. PICMAN, A.K. 1986. Biological activities of sesquiterpene lactones. Biochem. System. Ecol. **14:** 255–281.
6. SEBTI, S.M. & A.D. HAMILTON. 1998. New approaches to anticancer drug design based on the inhibition of farnesyltransferase. DDT **3:** 26–33.

Farnesyltransferase Inhibitor-Induced Regression of Mammary Tumors in TGFα and TGFα/*neu* Transgenic Mice Correlates with Inhibition of Map Kinase and p70s6 Kinase Phosphorylation

PETER NØRGAARD,[a–c] BRIAN K. LAW,[a] HANS S. PLOVISSON,[b] AND HAROLD L. MOSES[a]

[a]*Vanderbilt Cancer Center, Vanderbilt University, Nashville, Tennessee 37232, USA*

[b]*Section for Radiation Biology, The Finsen Center Rigshospitalet, Copenhagen, DK-2100, Denmark*

Recent research has provided us with detailed knowledge of the biochemical characteristics by which cancer cells differ from their normal progenitor cells. This has led to a conceptual shift in anticancer drug development, and compounds have been developed that selectively target these specific biochemical processes. One such target is the protooncoprotein p21-Ras, which plays a central role as signal transducer in mitogenic signaling pathways "downstream" of receptor-protein-tyrosine kinases (RTK) such as epidermal growth factor (EGF) receptor. Ras is mutationally activated in a wide range of human cancers and as such is presumed to play a significant role in the malignant phenotype of these cancers. Farnesyltransferase inhibitors (FTI) inhibit the posttranslational processing of Ras, and treatment of MMTV-H-*ras* transgenic mice with mammary and salivary tumors with the FTI L-744,832 resulted in dramatic regression of the tumors due to induction of apoptosis and/or G1 cell cycle arrest depending on the presence and nature of additional genetic alterations.[1,2]

In breast cancer, Ras is rarely mutated; however, it is presumed to play a significant role as transducer of mitogenic signals from tyrosine-kinase receptors (e.g., EGF receptor), which are activated because of mutation, gene amplification, or overexpression of ligands for the receptors (e.g., TGFα).

FARNESYLTRANSFERASE INHIBITOR-INDUCED REGRESSION OF MAMMARY TUMORS

To examine the sensitivity to FTI of tumors in which mitogenic activation emerged upstream of wild-type Ras, we measured the effect of L-744,832 on the growth of mammary tumors in MMTV-TGFα mice, in which tumor latency time was reduced by either of three different approaches, multiparicity, DMBA treatment, or

[c]Corresponding author: Peter Nørgaard, Institute of Pathological Anatomy, Glostrup University Hospital, DK-2600 Glostrup, Denmark. Phone, +45-4323 2555; fax, +45 4323 3944.
e-mail, norgaard@forum.dk

TABLE 1. Mammary tumor regression *in vivo* by farnesyltransferase inhibitor L-744,832 (FTI)

	FTI mean MGR[a] (mm³/day)	Vehicle mean MGR[a] (mm³/day)		
All MMTV-TGFα and -TGFα/*neu*	−7.4 +/−1.6	19.0 +/−3.4	$p = 0.0001$	
MMTV-TGFα-multiparous	−8.4 +/−2.2	10.6 +/−2.7		
MMTV-TGFα-DMBA-treated	−3.1 +/−3.6	31.7 +/−13.4		
MMTV-TGFα/*neu*	−4.5 +/−2.4	23.4 +/−7.3		
MMTV–H-*ras*	−5.4 +/−1.9	16.7 +/−3.5	$p < 0.001$	(1)
MMTV–*ras/myc*	−10.2 +/−5.0	43.6 +/−12.7	$p < 0.005$	(2)
MMTV–H-*ras*/p53 +/+	−7.7 +/−1.1	11.8 +/−1.6	$p < 0.005$	(2)
MMTV–H-*ras*/p53 −/−	−12.3 +/−1.9	26.3 +/−4.9	$p < 0.001$	(2)

[a]MGR = Mean growth rate for a particular tumor was calculated from the tumor growth curve (tumor volume plotted as a function of treatment time in days) with the following formula: MGR = $[(\text{sumAUC}_n) - (\text{vol}_1 \times (\text{day}_1))]/(\text{day}_n - \text{day}_1)^2$, where AUC = area under the tumor growth curve was calculated with the formula; AUC = $[(\text{vol}_1 + \text{vol}_2)/2] \times (\text{day}_2 - \text{day}_1)$.

concomitant expression of an MMTV-*neu* transgene. The mice were treated with daily, subcutaneous injections of 40 mg/kg L-744,832 or an isosmotic vehicle for 5 weeks, after which half of the mice were crossed over to the opposite treatment. L-744,832 induced reversible regression of the tumors of an order of magnitude (mean growth rate = MGR) comparable to those previously observed with Ras transgenic mice (TABLE 1). The incidence of carcinomas relative to "benign" tumors (hyperproliferative lesions and adenomas) was higher in DMBA-treated and TGFα/*neu* mice than in multiparous mice, as were the growth rates. However, no statistical differences were noted between the responses to L-744,832 among tumors in these three groups of mice. Also, benign tumors responded to FTI the same as did carcinomas. In addition to tumor volume, we monitored treatment response by serum level of TGFα encoded by the transgene, which was closely correlated with tumor volume. Serum TGFα decreased in mice with regressing tumors and increased in mice with growing tumors. This effect was probably secondary to tumor regression, because a direct effect on TGFα expression would stem from FTI affecting the MMTV promoter, which we found unlikely.

TUMOR REGRESSION BY FTI WAS PARALLELED BY INDUCTION OF APOPTOSIS AND G1 CELL CYCLE ARREST

Histologic examination demonstrated a decreased number of mitotic figures and an increased number of apoptotic bodies in FTI-treated compared to vehicle-treated tumors. For a more detailed analysis, we compared biopsy specimens obtained from tumors in individual mice before and during treatment with L-744,832. By TUNEL-staining we found that tumor regression was paralleled by an increased apoptotic index (TABLE 2). In addition, FACS analysis demonstrated an increased fraction of cells in G1 cell cycle phase in response to FTI treatment in all cases examined (TABLE 2).

TABLE 2. Effects of farnesyltransferase inhibitor L-744,832

In vivo Mammary tumors in MMTV-TGFα and -TGFα/*neu* mice	*In vitro* EGF treated BALB-MK cells
Tumor volume ↓	
Serum h-TGFα ↓	
Apoptosis index ↑	
G1 cell cycle fraction ↑	Protein synthesis ↓[b]
DNA synthesis ↓[a]	DNA synthesis ↓[c]
MAP kinase phosphorylation ↓	p70s6 kinase phosphorylation ↓
MAP kinase activity ↓	p70s6 kinase activity ↓
p70s6 kinase phosphorylation ↓	PHAS-1 phosphorylation ↓

[a]Brdu incorporation.
[b]^{35}S-methionine incorporation.
[c]^{3}H-thymidine incorporation.

INHIBITION OF MAP KINASE AND P70S6 KINASE BY FTI

Mitogenic signals emerging from receptor tyrosine kinases such as the EGF receptor are transduced through different signaling pathways such as the Ras/Map kinase (Mapk) and the Ras/PI3 kinase (PI3k) pathways, the latter involving p70s6 kinase (p70s6k), which was recently shown to regulate the translation of a subset of transcripts containing polypyrimidine tracts at their 5' ends.[3] To identify the signaling pathways that FTI inhibited *in vivo*, we analyzed protein extracts from pre- and posttreatment tumor biopsy specimens. Immunoblotting with an antibody recognizing the active (dually phosphorylated) Mapk demonstrated a reduction in Mapk phosphorylation in the tumors in response to FTI treatment (TABLE 2). This reduction in activity was confirmed by direct measurement of Mapk activity in the protein extracts. Immunoblotting with an anti-p70s6k antibody demonstrated a reduction inp70s6k phosphorylation in the posttreatment tumor biopsy specimens relative to pretreatment levels.

To further investigate these findings *in vitro*, we studied protein extracts from EGF-stimulated mouse keratinocytes (BALB-MK cells). These cells responded to L-744,832 treatment with an inhibition of DNA and protein synthesis (TABLE 2). This was paralleled by a dose-dependent inhibition in p70s6k phosphorylation and a reduction in p70s6k activity towards s6 substrate peptide. Phosphorylation of PHAS-1, another PI3k-dependent regulator of protein synthesis, was also inhibited by FTI, whereas we observed little or no inhibition of Mapk activation under these experimental conditions. Expression of a dominant negative Ras inhibited both Mapk and p70s6k activation by EGF, indicating a requirement for Ras activity during Mapk and p70s6k activation.

In Ras-overexpressing MK cells we demonstrated inhibition of farnesylation of Ras by L-744,832. However, in neither wild-type MK cells nor mouse tumors could endogenous Ras be detected with the methods employed.

ANNALS NEW YORK ACADEMY OF SCIENCES

CONCLUSION

Together these results showed that L-744,832 induced regression of mouse mammary tumors in which oncogenic activation emerged upstream of wild-type Ras. The data suggested that this effect was due in part to a G1 arrest and increased apoptosis, which were in turn paralleled by inhibition of mitogenic signal transducers Mapk and p70s6k. These findings were supported by *in vitro* data demonstrating that Ras is required for mitogenic activation of Mapk and p70s6k and that FTI inhibited DNA and protein synthesis at a point upstream of Mapk as well as p70s6k and PHAS-1.

These results suggest that the potential clinical use of FTI could be expanded to include cancers harboring activated receptor tyrosine kinases as well as those containing activated Ras.

REFERENCES

1. KOHL, N.E., C.A. OMER, M.W. CONNER, N.J. ANTHONY, J.P. DAVIDE, S.J. DESOLMS, E.A. GIULIANI, R.P. GOMEZ, S.L. GRAHAM, K. HAMILTON, L.K. HANDT, G.D. HARTMAN, K.S. KOBLAN, A.M. KRAL, P.J. MILLER, S.D. MOSSER, T.J. O'NEILL, E. RANDS, M.D. SCHABER, J.B. GIBBS & A. OLIFF. 1995. Inhibition of farnesyltransferase induces regression of mammary and salivary carcinomas in *ras* transgenic mice. Nature Med. **1:** 792–797.
2. BARRINGTON, R.E., M.A. SUBLER, E. RANDS, C.A. OMER, P.J. MILLER, J.E. HUNDLEY, S.K. KOESTER, D.A. TROYER, D.J. BEARS, M.W. CONNER, J.B. GIBBS, K. HAMILTON, K.S. KOBLAN, S.D. MOSSER, T.J. O'NEILL, M.D. SCHABER, E.T. SENDERAK, J.J. WINDLE, A. OLIFF & N.E. KOHL. 1998. A farnesyltranferase inhibitor induces tumor regression in transgenic mice harboring multible oncogenic mutations by mediating alterations in both cell cycle control and apoptosis. Mol. Cell. Biol. **18:** 85–92.
3. KAWASOME, H., P. PAPST, S. WEBB, G. KELLER, G. JOHNSON, E. GELFAND & N. TERADA. 1998. Targeted disruption of p70(s6k) defines its role in protein synthesis and rapamycin sensitivity. Proc. Natl. Acad. Sci. USA **95:** 5033–5038.

Inhibition of Protein Tyrosine Kinase Activity by 1a-Docosahexaenoyl Mitomycin C

MAYUMI SHIKANO,[a,b] KENJIRO ONIMURA,[b] HIDESUKE FUKAZAWA,[a] SATOSHI MIZUNO,[a] KAZUNAGA YAZAWA,[b] AND YOSHIMASA UEHARA[a,c]

[a]Department of Bioactive Molecules, National Institute of Infectious Diseases, 1-23-1 Toyama, Shinjuku-ku, Tokyo 162-8640, Japan

[b]Sagami Chemical Research Center, 4-4-1 Nishi-Ohnuma, Sagamihara, Kanagawa 229-0012, Japan

Protein kinases play an important role in many signal transduction pathways, and unregulated acceleration of protein kinase activities is often responsible for serious diseases including malignant tumors. Therefore, attempts have been made to develop protein kinase blockers to be applied in antiproliferative therapeutics and as probes to elucidate the role of these enzymes in cellular signal transduction. We synthesized a series of mitomycin C derivatives (TABLE 1) conjugated with various fatty acids at position 1a through amide bond and examined their effect on protein kinase A (PKA), protein kinase C (PKC), calmodulin-dependent protein kinase III (CaMK), and protein tyrosine kinase (PTK) of v-src-transformed NIH 3T3 cells, as described previously.[1,2]

Among these compounds, 1a-docosahexaenoyl mitomycin C (DMMC) alone inhibited PTK activity in a dose-dependent manner, and its inhibitory activity was almost the same as that of herbimycin A (FIG. 1A, TABLE 1). DMMC hardly affected PKC and inhibited PKA and CaMK only at the highest concentration, 100 μg/ml (FIG. 1A, TABLE 1). On the other hand, 1a-arachidonyl mitomycin C attenuated PTK activity faintly although it inhibited CaMK effectively (TABLE 1). Other mitomycin C derivatives showed no effect on any kinase activities (TABLE 1). The results suggested that there is a critical fatty acid selectivity of mitomycin C derivative for PTK inhibition.

The effect of docosahexaenoic acid and/or mitomycin C, both of which are the component of DMMC, on protein kinase activities was also evaluated. As was already reported for unsaturated fatty acids,[3,4] complete inhibition of PKC but not other kinases was observed with 50 μg/ml of docosahexaenoic acid (FIG. 1B). Mitomycin C did not affect any protein kinase activity at a concentration of 50 μg/ml, and coexistence of the two compounds reflected only the effect of docosahexaenoic acid (FIG. 1B). Thus, covalent binding of this fatty acid to position 1a of mitomycin C resulted in the acquisition of a new property that neither of the components originally possessed. It could be postulated that the addition of mitomycin C, to docosahexaenoic acid molecule altered its specificity in kinase inhibition. This

[c]Address for correspondence: Department of Bioactive Molecules, National Institute of Infectious Diseases, 1-23-1 Toyama, Shinjuku-ku, Tokyo 162-8640, Japan. Phone, 81-5285-1111; fax, 81-5285-1272.

e-mail, yuehara@nih.go.jp

TABLE 1. Structure of 1a-acly mitomycin C derivatives and their effects on protein kinase activities

R		Inhibition			
		PTK	PKC	PKA	CaMK
Palmityl		−	−	−	−
α-Linolenyl		−	−	−	−
γ-Linolenyl		−	−	−	−
Arachidonyl		±	−	−	++
Eicosapentaenoyl		−	−	−	−
Docosahexaenoyl		+++	−	−	+

SYMBOLS: −, no effect at 100 μg/ml; +, inhibitory at 100 μg/ml; ++, inhibitory at 30 μg/ml; +++, inhibitory at 10 μg/ml.

hypothesis might be supported by the fact that arachidonic acid, which had the same effect as docosahexaenoic acid on PKC (data not shown), inhibits CaMK when conjugated with mitomycin C (TABLE 1).

DMMC also inhibited autophosphorylation of immunoprecipitated p60[v-src] and p210[bcr-abl] of human leukemia cell line K562, whereas it showed no effect on kinase activity of EGF receptor at all (data not shown). The reduced phosphorylation of p60[v-src] did not recover by extensive washing of DMMC-treated immune complex prior to the phosphorylation assay, indicating that inhibition of PTK activity by DMMC is irreversible. In the presence of 2-mercaptoethanol or dithiothreitol, DMMC only slightly inhibited p60[v-src] kinase activity (data not shown). It is supposed that DMMC might form an adduct with some thiol moiety of p60[v-src] protein.

A

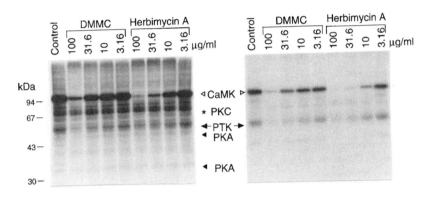

B

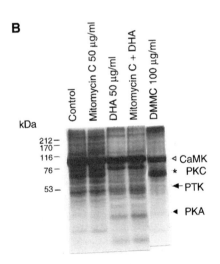

FIGURE 1. Effect of DMMC and its components on protein kinase activities in post-nuclear fraction of v-*src*–transformed NIH 3T3 cells. **(A)** The indicated concentration of DMMC or herbimycin A or DMSO (control) was added to the postnuclear fraction, and the kinase reaction was carried out as described before.[1,2] Autoradiography of the gel before (*left*) and after (*right*) the alkali treatment is indicated. *Open arrowheads, asterisks, arrows,* and *closed arrowheads* represent the positions of protein bands phosphorylated by CaMK, PKC, PTK, and PKA, respectively. **(B)** Docosahexaenoic acid (DHA) and/or mitomycin C (MMC), 50 µg/ml each, were added to the postnuclear fraction before the kinase reaction.

It is reported that reductive activation of mitomycin C to semiquinone is required as the initial step, followed by cleavage of the aziridine ring to produce two sites of attack by nucleophils, C-1 and C-10[5,6] by which the molecules bind DNA. Our results indicate that these sites in DMMC might react with thiol moiety of p60[v-src] protein, consequently making DHA, which possesses kinase-inhibitory ability, accessible to PTK. Yet, another possibility cannot be excluded: the addition of a reducing agent to DMMC might create conditions favorable to maintenance of the unstable semiquinone radical, which attacks the double bond in DHA and degenerates the molecule.

All results just described were obtained in experiments in a cell-free system. We treated v-src–transformed NIH 3T3 cells with DMMC, but no change in PTK activity of p60[v-src] (data not shown) was observed. We synthesized radiolabeled DMMC from [1-^{14}C]docosahexaenoic acid and examined the metabolism of the compound in these cells. TLC analyses of recovered radioactivity from the cells revealed that the amount of DMMC incorporated into the cells increased for up to 3 hours, but after longer incubation most radioactivity was found in the phospholipid fraction (data not shown). This implies the release of docosahexaenoic acid from DMMC and acylation into phospholipid. If DMMC were able to interact with the PTK molecule within the first 3 hours, distinct inhibition of PTK activity would be observed; it is therefore assumed that DMMC might be localized in some part of the cells where it cannot interact with the PTK molecule. It is likely that DMMC might anchor in the plasma membrane with the hydrophobic fatty acyl chain, leaving the hydrophilic mitomycin C part out of the cell. In this case, DMMC would be unable to interact with PTK which is thought to localize in the intracellular side of the plasma membrane or cytosol. Modification of the structure of DMMC so as to penetrate the plasma membrane and inhibit PTK activity would be beneficial. Such a compound is expected to be a promising candidate for novel antiproliferative therapeutics.

REFERENCES

1. FUKAZAWA, H. et al. 1993. Methods for simultaneous detection of protein kinase A, protein kinase C, protein tyrosine kinase, and calmodulin-dependent protein kinase activities. Anal. Biochem. 212: 106–110.
2. LI, P.-M. et al. 1993. Evaluation of protein kinase inhibitors in an assay system containing multiple protein kinase activities. Anticancer Res. 13: 1957–1964.
3. MAY, C.L. et al. 1993. Inhibition of lymphocyte protein kinase C by unsaturated fatty acids. Biochem. Biophys. Res. Commun. 195: 823–828.
4. TAPPIA, P.S. et al. 1995. Influence of unsaturated fatty acids on the production of tumour necrosis factor and interleukin-6 by rat peritoneal macrophages. Mol. Cell. Biochem. 143: 89–98.
5. TOMASZ, et al. 1974. The mode of interaction of mitomycin C with desoxyribonucleic acid and other polynucleotides in vitro. Biochemistry 13: 4878–4887.
6. EGBERTSON, M. & S.J. DANISHEFSKY. 1987. Modeling of the electrophilic activation of mitomycins: Chemical evidence for the intermediacy of mitosene semiquinone as the active electrophile. J. Am. Chem. Soc. 109: 1833–1840.

Activation of a 36-kD MBP Kinase, an Active Proteolytic Fragment of MST/Krs Proteins, during Anticancer Drug-Induced Apoptosis

HIDEAKI KAKEYA, RIE ONOSE, AND HIROYUKI OSADA[a]

Antibiotics Laboratory, The Institute of Physical and Chemical Research (RIKEN), 2-1 Hirosawa, Wako-shi, Saitama 351-0198, Japan

Apoptosis is a systematic suicide of cells within an organism during normal morphogenesis, tissue remodeling, and in response to viral infections or other irreparable cell damage.[1,2] In addition, failure in an apoptosis program often leads to an imbalance in cell number, and some of those abnormalities might lead to tumorigenesis. Based on this concept, control of apoptosis has emerged as an important strategy in cancer chemotherapy.

We recently isolated a novel anticancer drug, cytotrienin A (FIG.1), that induces apoptosis in human promyelocytic leukemia HL-60 cells.[3,4] Cytotrienin A induced marked morphologic changes in the cell, including membrane blebbing, cell shrinkage, chromatin condensation, internucleosomal degradation of chromosomal DNA, and fragmentation of the cell into apoptotic bodies. To gain insight into the mode of action of cytotrienin A-induced apoptosis, we performed an in-gel kinase assay using myelin basic protein (MBP) as a substrate and found activation of a kinase with an apparent molecular mass of 36 kD (termed p36 MBP kinase). The dose of cytotrienin A required to activate the p36 MBP kinase was consistent with that required to induce apoptotic DNA fragmentation in HL-60 cells. This p36 MBP kinase was activated with kinetics distinct from the activation of JNK (c-Jun N-terminal kinase)/SAPK (stress-activated protein kinase) and p38 MAPK. By contrast, p36 MBP kinase activation and apoptotic DNA fragmentation were inhibited by antioxidants such as N-acetylcysteine and reduced-form glutathione. The p36 MBP kinase activation was also observed during hydrogen peroxide (H_2O_2)-induced apoptosis. These results suggest that reactive oxygen species (ROS) including H_2O_2 play a key role in the activation of p36 MBP kinase and the subsequent apoptotic pathway induced by cytotrienin A.

In addition, a broad specificity inhibitor of caspases (Z-Asp-CH_2-DCB) blocked the activation of p36 MBP kinase induced by cytotrienin A, but it did not inhibit the activation of JNK/SAPK and p38 MAPK, indicating that the p36 MBP kinase activation is the downstream of the activation of Z-Asp-CH_2-DCB–sensitive caspase(s) and plays an important role in the apoptotic signaling pathway for DNA fragmentation. Moreover, we revealed that p36 MBP kinase is an active proteolytic product of MST1/Krs2 and MST2/Krs1 based on Western blotting analysis using antibodies against MST/Krs proteins. On cytotrienin A treatment, the amount of full-length

[a]To whom correspondence should be addressed. Phone, +81-48-467-9541; fax, +81-48-462-4669.
e-mail, antibiot@postman.riken.go.jp

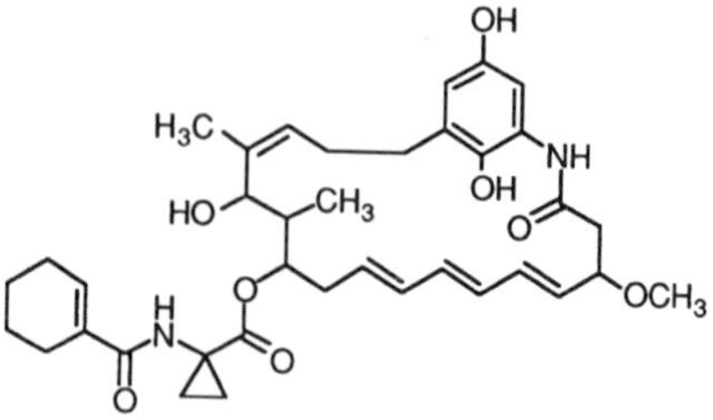

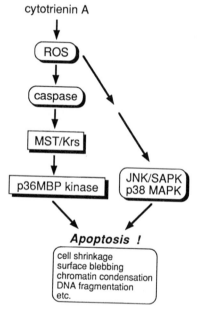

FIGURE 1. Structure of cytotrienin A.

FIGURE 2. A proposed model for cytotrienin A-induced signaling pathways.

MST1/Krs2 and MST2/Krs1 bands diminished in parallel with the appearance of p36 MBP kinase activity, whereas pretreatment of Z-Asp-CH$_2$-DCB or N-acetylcysteine blocked the caspase-mediated proteolysis of MST1/Krs2 and MST2/Krs1 in response to cytotrienin A treatment. MST/Krs proteins are Ste20-related serine/threonine kinases and consist of two family members, MST1/Krs2 and MST2/Krs1. The proteolytic cleavage sites of MST1/Krs2 and MST2/Krs 1 are ^{323}DEMD^{326}S and ^{319}DELD^{322}S, respectively, which is optimal to caspase-3. The C-terminal truncation of MST1/Krs2 gave about 10 times the activation compared with the full-length molecule in *in vitro* experiments.[5–7] Furthermore, MT-21 (3-acetyl-4,5-dimethyl-5-octyloxy-3-pyrrolin-2-one), our synthetic apoptosis inducer, also generated these proteolytic active MST/Krs proteins, p36 MBP kinase, mediated by caspase-3 during apoptosis.[8,9] In addition, this 36 MBP kinase was activated in response to anticancer drugs including camptothecin and etoposide as well as cytotrienin A. Recently, two other groups reported that MST/Krs proteins are cleaved to generate a 36-kD active fragment by caspase-3–like activity during apoptosis induced by Fas (CD95/APO-1),[10,11] which is consistent with our data showing the significance of the p36 MBP kinase pathway during anticancer drug-induced apoptosis.[12] A hypothetical model of our proposed signaling pathways in cytotrienin A-induced apoptosis is shown in FIGURE 2.

Thus, p36 MBP kinase, which is an active proteolytic fragment of MST/Krs proteins mediated by caspase(s), might be a common component of the diverse signaling pathways leading to apoptosis, and controlling this p36 MBP kinase pathway might be a novel strategy in cancer chemotherapy.

REFERENCES

1. NAGATA, S. 1997. Apoptosis by death factor. Cell **88:** 355–365.
2. NICHOLSON, D.W. *et al.* 1997. Caspases: Killer proteases. Trends Biochem. Sci. **22:** 299–306.
3. KAKEYA, H. *et al.* 1997. Cytotrienin A, a novel apoptosis inducer in human leukemia HL-60 cells. J. Antibiot. **50:** 370–372.
4. ZHANG, H.-P. *et al.* 1997. Novel Triene-ansamycins, cytotrienins A and B inducing apoptosis on human leukaemia HL-60 Cells. Tetrahedron Lett. **38:** 1789–1792.
5. CREASY, C.L. *et al.* 1995. Cloning and characterization of a human protein kinase with homology to Ste20. J. Biol. Chem. **270:** 21695–21700.
6. CREASY, C.L. *et al.* 1996. The Ste20-like protein kinase, Mst1, dimerizes and contains an inhibitory domain. J. Biol. Chem. **271:** 21049–21053.
7. TAYLOR, L.K. *et al.* 1996. Newly identified stress-responsive protein kinases, Krs-1 and Krs-2. Proc. Natl. Acad. Sci. USA **93:** 10099–10104.
8. KAKEYA, H. *et al.* 1997. Neuritogenic effect of epolactaene derivatives on human neuroblastoma cells which lack high-affinity nerve growth factors. J. Med. Chem. **40:** 391–394.
9. WATABE, M. *et al.* 1999. Requirement of protein kinase (Krs/MST) activation for MT-21-induced apoptosis. Oncogene **18:** 5211–5220.
10. GRAVES, J. D. *et al.* 1998. Caspase-mediated activation and identification of apoptosis by the mammalian Ste20-like kinase Mst1. EMBO J. **17:** 2224–2234.
11. LEE, K.-K. *et al.* 1998. Proteolytic activation of MST/Krs, STE-20-related protein kinase, by caspase during apoptosis. Oncogene **16:** 3029–3037.
12. KAKEYA, H. *et al.* 1998. Caspase-mediated activation of a p36 myelin basic protein kinase during anticancer drug-induced apoptosis. Cancer Res. **58:** 4888–4894.

Peptides Mimicking Sialyl-Lewis A Isolated from a Random Peptide Library and Peptide Array

INSUG O, THOMAS KIEBER-EMMONS,[a] LASZLO OTVOS, JR., AND
MAGDALENA BLASZCZYK-THURIN[b]

*The Wistar Institute and [a]University of Pennsylvania, Philadelphia,
Pennslvania 19104, USA*

Cell surface carbohydrate structures are an important class of tumor antigens. SA-Le[a] and its structural isomer SA-LeX have been identified as carbohydrate determinants expressed on many carcinomas,[1] and both have been shown to represent functional ligands of selectins. The crucial role of selectin-dependent neutrophil adhesion in their recruitment process and metastasis was confirmed by *in vivo* blockage of E-selectin–dependent interaction.[2] These data imply that analogous molecular mechanisms do indeed underlie inflammation and metastasis and that similar therapeutic approaches can be used to intervene with both processes. Highly diverse peptide libraries offer many distinct advantages over difficult chemical or enzymatic synthesis of complex carbohydrates, providing notably inexpensive and rapid identification and optimization of novel ligands. The peptides described here provide excellent leads for the development of potent antagonists of carbohydrate-protein interaction and in particular antimetastatic and antiinflammatory therapeutic agents.

MATERIALS AND METHODS

Monoclonal antibody (mAb) NS19-9 was generated at the Wistar Institute.[3] Peptides were synthesized at Research Genetics, Inc. (Huntsville, Alabama). SA-Le[a] was obtained from Glycotech, Inc. (Rockville, Maryland). The 12-mer peptide library for these studies was obtained from Invitrogen Inc. (Carlsbad, California).[4] The ability of peptides to block mAb recognition of SA-Le[a] carbohydrate was determined in competition ELISA, using various peptide concentrations. IC_{50} values were calculated by nonlinear least-squares regression of a four-parameter logistic equation. An array of 163 synthetic 12-mer peptides was synthesized by standard Fmoc chemistry on polyethylene glycol modified cellulose membrane at the Wistar Institute and tested for binding of mAb NS19-9.[5]

[b]Address for correspondence: Dr. M. Blaszczyk-Thurin, The Wistar Institute, 3601 Spruce Street, Philadelphia, PA 19104. Phone, 215/898-3829; fax, 215/898-3868.
e-mail, mthurin@wistar.upenn.edu

TABLE 1. Peptide sequence families mimicking SA-Le^a carbohydrate structure

I	#2:	VGIWSVVSEGSR	II	#1:	RCSVGVPFTMES
	#3	QDGVWEHVLEGG		#4:	DLWDWVVGKPAG
	#15:	VELSGRGGLCTW		#12:	VIGAASHDEDVD
	#18:	TIEPVLAEMFMG		#14:	DKETFELGLFDR
				#15:	FSGVRGVYESRT
				#19:	PDDAPMHSTRVE

RESULTS

Random Peptide Library Screening. Several bacterial clones that bind the SA-Le^a–specific NS19-9 mAb were isolated and sequenced. Clones isolated with the carbohydrate-specific mAb in the final selection cycle were tested for protein expression using SDS-PAGE and identified after probing by Western blot with the mAb. Peptide library screening yielded families of peptides with unique consensus sequences. Two distinct consensus sequences, GXWXXVLEG and VVGXP, were identified in families of peptides isolated with mAb NS19-9 (TABLE 1). This may indicate that peptides based on two different motifs isolated with the same mAb can mimic different structural topographies of SA-Le^a carbohydrate, and these subsets of peptides may very likely represent nonoverlapping surfaces of cognate antigen.

Identification of Sequences Critical for mAb Binding Using Peptide Array. To identify the residues critical for mAb binding and to analyze amino acid substitutions that might improve peptide-mAb interaction, we generated an array of 163 peptides based on the sequence of peptide #4 isolated from family II and probed with mAb NS19-9 (FIG. 1). Results suggest that most substitutions at the very N-terminus (residues 1 and 2) were well tolerated and did not influence mAb binding, whereas critical residues were clearly identified at positions 3 to 5. The most important single amino acid for mAb binding was Trp at position 3, because most of the amino acid substitutions at this position blocked mAb recognition. Replacement of Trp3 with H, Y, A, D, and S completely abolish mAb binding, whereas M significantly decreased it. Similarly, substitutions of W at position 5 with H, A, R, and K abolished mAb binding. Several of the substitutions within the identified consensus sequence, in particular VVGK, were not tolerated by the mAb, whereas others allowed for mAb binding. No preference for amino acids was evident from the substituted peptides within positions 10 to 12 of the C-terminus. By contrast, several amino acid replacements resulted in increased binding of the peptides for mAb. The most favorable amino acid with respect to mAb binding was substitution of Trp at position 5 with Phe resulting in the sequence DLWDFVVGKPAG (A#44) that displayed increased binding affinity as compared to the original peptide. Amino acid substitutions within the consensus sequence, at positions 6 to 10 mainly with K, R, and E, also resulted in higher binding of mAb as compared with the original peptide. These data demonstrate that peptides with higher binding properties for the anticarbohydrate mAb were selected using the peptide array approach. These results further confirm that ar-

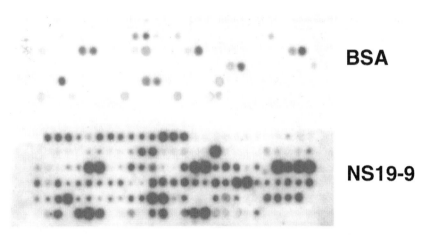

FIGURE 1. Reactivity of mAb NS19-9 with a series of solid-phase single amino acid substituted dodecapeptides based on peptide #4. (*Lower panel*) Background binding to the membrane, using BSA instead of primary antibody (*upper panel*).

omatic amino acids may play an important role in mimicking carbohydrate structures.

Synthetic Peptides Mimic the Carbohydrate Antigen Detected with mAb NS 19-9. To test whether peptide #4 and peptide A#44 are true mimics of SA-Le^a and to determine the concentration of peptides required for blocking of 50% of mAb binding to native carbohydrate antigen, competition ELISA was carried out. Both peptides blocked the binding of NS19-9 to a fixed amount of carbohydrate antigen in a dose-dependent manner. The IC$_{50}$ for peptide #4 blocking of mAb–SA-Le^a binding was 700 μM. Peptide A#44 showed more prominent inhibition of the mAb-SA-Le^a binding as compared to peptide #4, as demonstrated with the IC$_{50}$ value of 70 μM. This suggests that substitution of Phe within the original amino acid sequence generated a peptide with higher affinity for the mAb better mimicking topography for SA-Le^a. Overall, our data demonstrate that the peptides sterically interfere with mAb binding to carbohydrate antigen, implying that the sequences DLWDWVVGKPAG and DL-WDFVVGKPAG represent solvent-accessible epitopes and that the peptides represent cognate determinants for the antibody.

Secondary Structure of Peptides Mimicking Carbohydrate. Both peptides #4 and A#44 highlight the functional role played by the aromatic-X-aromatic motif within the peptide. Secondary structure analysis indicates some propensity for extended and helix structures centered on the W/FVVG region using a neutral net analysis. It is possible that these structure types might be realized within the antibody-combining site. This is consistent with modeling and crystal structure analysis of this motif type which suggested their ability to adopt type I and type II turns within the antibody-combining site. The increased binding of peptide with substitution of Phe for Trp would suggest that the hydrophobic stacking interactions are important for increased antibody binding and consequently antigenic mimicry.

COMMENTS

Functional equivalence of chemically dissimilar molecules such as carbohydrates and proteins sharing common surface topology has been identified previously as a naturally occurring phenomenon. Combinatorial technologies available in recent years have provided an avenue to dissect the molecular basis for such mimicry. Using a combinatorial library screening approach we isolated families of mimics of tumor-associated antigen and E-selectin ligand. We chose one sequence as a lead peptide to delineate the specific residues that may contribute to the mimicry of carbohydrate structures by re-screening of a peptide array. The mAb could tolerate a variety of amino acid substitutions within the lead peptide sequence, still retaining functional specificity. Furthermore, cross-reactive peptides of higher affinity were identified. This suggests that different amino acids can improve structural mimicry within identified peptide. The peptides with various consensus sequences that were identified with the same mAb suggest that indeed different residues act as structural mimics. Alternatively, distinct consensus sequences mimic nonoverlapping topographies of a carbohydrate epitope recognized by the antibody. The prospect of finding mimicking peptides of carbohydrate tumor antigens that competitively inhibit carbohydrate-specific receptor interaction will allow for the design of antagonists of E-selectin and other endolectins with enhanced therapeutic potential to prevent metastasis.

REFERENCES

1. BECHTEL, B., A.J. WAND, K. WROBLEWSKI, H. KOPROWSKI & J. THURIN. 1990. Conformational analysis of the tumor-associated carbohydrate antigen 19-9 and its Lea blood group antigen component as related to the specificity of monoclonal antibody CO19-9. J. Biol. Chem. **265**: 2028–2037.
2. BRODT, P., L. FALLAVOLLITA, R.S. BRESALIER, S. METERISSIAN, C.R. NORTON & B.A. WOLITZKY. 1997. Liver endothelial E-selectin mediates carcinoma cell adhesion and promotes liver metastasis. Int. J. Cancer **71**: 612–619.
3. MAGNANI, J.L., M. BROCKHAUS, D.F. SMITH, V. GINSBURG, M. BLASZCZYK, K.F. MITCHELL, Z. STEPLEWSKI & H. KOPROWSKI. 1981. A monosialoganglioside is a monoclonal antibody defined antigen of colon carcinoma. Science **212**: 55–56.
4. LAVALLIE, E.R., E.A. DIBLASIO, S. KOVACIC, K.L. GRANT, P.F. SCHENDEL & J.M. MCCOY. 1993. A thioredoxin gene fusion expression system that circumvents inclusion body formation in the *E. coli* cytoplasm. Bio/Technology **11**: 187–193.
5. RUDIGER, S., L. GERMEROTH, J. SCHNEIDER-MERGENER & B. BUKAU. 1997. The substrate specificity of the DnaK chaperone determined by screening cellulose-bound peptide libraries. EMBO J. **16**: 1501–1507.

B4112, a Novel Tetramethylpiperidine-Substituted Phenazine That Inhibits the Proliferation of Multidrug-Resistant Cancer Cell Lines

C.E.J. VAN RENSBURG,[a] G. JOONÉ, E. VAN NIEKERK, AND R. ANDERSON

Medical Research Council Unit for Inflammation and Immunity, Department of Immunology, University of Pretoria, Pretoria, South Africa

Overcoming the ominous threat posed by multidrug resistance (MDR), be it pre-existing (intrinsic) or acquired during the course of chemotherapy, is currently perceived to be the most daunting challenge confronting those involved in the development of anticancer pharmacologic agents.

Riminophenazines are a novel class of anticancer agents that have the potential to subvert both intrinsic and acquired MDR.[1] Clofazimine, the prototype riminophenazine, is currently used as a component of the multidrug antimicrobial chemotherapy of leprosy and has been shown by us (1) to be active against all cancer cell lines tested *in vitro*, including those with intrinsic MDR,[2] (2) to neutralize P-glycoprotein (Pgp)-mediated acquired MDR *in vitro*,[3] and (3) to have an unusual site (the outer membrane) and mechanism of anticancer action, which is achieved indirectly by inhibition of Na[+], K[+]-ATPase.[3] Moreover, clofazimine is reported to possess therapeutic activity in murine models of experimental oncology[4,5] as well as in humans with unresectable, and in some cases metastatic, primary hepatocellular carcinoma.[6]

A recently completed intensive screening program was undertaken by us with the primary objective of identifying novel riminophenazines with more potent Pgp-neutralizing and cytotoxic properties. This has resulted in the development of a novel subgroup of riminophenazines, the tetramethylpiperidine(TMP)-substituted phenazines, of which B4112 (FIG. 1) is one of the most promising.

The effects of B4112 (0.01–1 µg/ml) alone and in the presence of a fixed, noncytotoxic concentration (3 ng/ml) of the conventional anticancer agent vinblastine, on the proliferation of a Pgp-expressing erythroleukemic cell line (K562/MMB)[1,3] are shown in FIGURE 1. Proliferation of the cancer cell line was measured using a colorimetric procedure based on the metabolism of MTT by viable cells[3] following incubation for 3 days at 37°C in an atmosphere of 5% CO_2 in tissue culture medium RPMI supplemented with 10% fetal calf serum. At a concentration of 8 ng/ml, B4112 caused 50% restoration of chemosensitivity of this cancer cell line to vinblastine, while the corresponding concentration of B4112, which caused 50% direct cytotoxicity, was 200 ng/ml.

[a]Address for correspondence: Dr. C.E.J. van Rensburg, PO Box 2034, Pretoria 0001, South Africa. Phone, +27-12-319 2622; fax, +27-12-323 0732.
e-mail, cmedlen@medic.up.ac.za

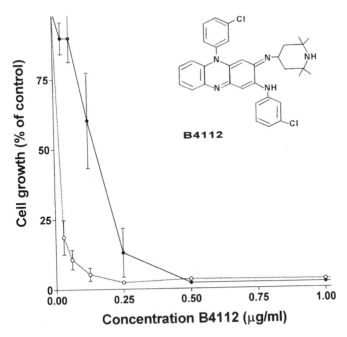

FIGURE 1. Effects of B4112 alone (●—●) and in combination with a fixed, non-cytotoxic concentration (3 ng/ml) of vinblastine (○—○) on the proliferation of a Pgp-expressing erythroleukemic cancer cell line (K562/MMB). Results of three experiments are expressed as the mean percentage growth of the drug-free control systems ± standard error of the mean.

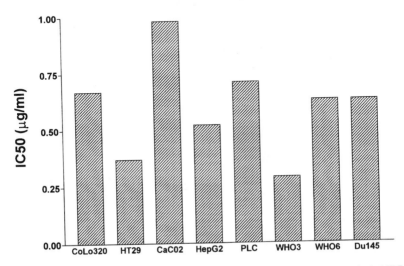

FIGURE 2. Effects of B4112 only on the proliferation of a range of mostly intrinsic MDR, colon, liver, esophageal, and prostate cancer cell lines. Results of four experiments are expressed as the mean concentration of B4112 required to cause 50% inhibition of cell growth (IC_{50}).

The direct cytotoxic effects of B4112 for a range of reference colon (CoLo 320 DM, HT29, $Caco_2$), liver (Hep G2, PLC), and esophageal (WHO3, WHO4) cancer cell lines with varying patterns of intrinsic MDR, as well as a drug-sensitive prostate carcinoma cell line (DU145) are shown in FIGURE 2. The cell lines, which were exposed to B4112 for 3–4 days, were all sensitive to this TMP-phenazine with IC_{50} values that ranged from 0.29–0.98 µg/ml.

These results clearly demonstrate that B4112 is a particularly potent antagonist of Pgp, being active in the low nanogram range. Although neutralization of Pgp is a potentially useful property of anticancer agents, it is noteworthy that this is only one of many mechanisms used by cancer cells to resist the cytotoxic effects of conventional chemotherapeutic agents. Of potentially greater significance, therefore, is the observation that B4112 is broadly active against a range of cancer cell lines, each with a different profile of MDR. These findings suggest that B4112 may subvert all types of MDR, including that which is mediated by Pgp.

REFERENCES

1. VAN RENSBURG, C.E.J., R. ANDERSON & J.F. O'SULLIVAN. 1997. Riminophenazine compounds: Pharmacology and anti-neoplastic potential. Crit. Rev. Oncol. Hematol. 25: 55–67.
2. VAN RENSBURG, C.E.J., A.M. VAN STADEN & R. ANDERSON. 1993. The riminophenazine agents clofazimine and B669 inhibit the proliferation of cancer cell lines *in vitro* by phospholipase A_2-mediated oxidative and non-oxidative mechanisms. Cancer Res. 53: 318–323.
3. VAN RENSBURG, C.E.J., R. ANDERSON, M.S. MYER *et al.* 1994. The riminophenazine agents clofazimine and B669 reverse acquired multidrug resistance in a human lung cancer cell line. Cancer Lett. 85: 59–63.
4. VAN RENSBURG, C.E.J., C. DURANDT, P.J. GARLINSKI *et al.* 1993. Evaluation of the antineoplastic activities of the riminophenazine agents clofazimine and B669 in tumor-bearing rats and mice. Int. J. Oncol. 3: 1011–1013.
5. SRI-PATHMANATHAN, R.M., J.A. PLUMB & K.C.H. FEARON. 1994. Clofazimine alters the energy metabolism and inhibits the growth rate of a human lung-cancer cell line *in vitro* and *in vivo*. Int. J. Cancer 56: 900–905.
6. RUFF, P., M.R. CHASEN, J.E.H. LONG *et al.* 1998. A phase II study of oral clofazimine in unresectable and metastatic hepatocellular carcinoma. Ann. Oncol. 9: 217–219.

The Anti-RAS Cancer Drug MKT-077 Is an F-Actin Cross-Linker

HIROSHI MARUTA,[a,c] ANJALI TIKOO,[a] RUSHDI SHAKRI,[a] AND TADAO SHISHIDO[b]

[a]Ludwig Institute for Cancer Research, Melbourne, Australia 3050

[b]Ashigara Research Labs., Fuji Photo Film Co., Kanagawa 250-0193, Japan

A rhodacyanine dye called MKT-077 has shown highly selective toxicity towards several distinct human malignant cell lines and has been subjected to clinical trials for cancer therapy.[1] However, both the specific oncogenes responsible for its selective toxicity towards cancer cells and its target proteins in these cancer cells still remain to be determined. In this paper, using NIH 3T3 fibroblasts, we demonstrate that oncogenic Ras mutants, such as v-Ha-Ras, are responsible for its selective toxicity. Furthermore, using an MKT-077 derivative, called "compound 1,"[2] as a specific ligand, we have affinity-purified and identified the major target protein of 45 kD (p45) that binds MKT-077 in v-Ha-Ras–transformed cells, but not in the parental normal cells. p45 is actin. Like a few cytoskeletal tumor-suppressive proteins such as HS1, alpha-actinin, and vinculin,[3–5] MKT-077 bundles actin filaments by cross-linking.[6] These findings suggest that specific F-actin cross-linkers are potentially useful in the chemotherapy of Ras-associated cancers.

RESULTS AND DISCUSSION

Ras is responsible for selective toxicity of MKT-077 towards malignant cells. To determine the possible contribution of oncogenic Ras mutants, such as v-Ha-Ras, to the selective toxicity of MKT-077 towards malignant cells, we compared the effects of this drug on the growth of normal and v-Ha-Ras transformed NIH 3T3 fibroblasts (2 x 10^4 cells). MKT-077 1.5 µM inhibits the growth of Ras transformants by 60%, but it causes no effect on normal cell growth. Furthermore, it inhibits almost completely the focus formation of Ras transformants at their confluence. Since the parental normal cells form no focus, MKT-077-treated Ras transformants behave like the parental normal cells. These results seem to be compatible with the previous observation that malignant cells, such as human EJ bladder carcinoma cells, are around 100 times more sensitive to this drug than are normal cells such as CV-1 (African green monkey kidney cell line).[1] Interestingly, EJ cells also carry an oncogenic c-Ha-Ras mutant. These observations clearly indicate that (1) oncogenic Ras mutations are responsible, at least in part, for the selective cytostatic effect of this drug towards malignant cells, and (2) MKT-077 reverses Ras-induced malignant phenotype.

[c]Corresponding author. Fax, 613/9341-3104.
e-mail, hiroshi.maruta@ludwig.edu.au

Actin is the major target protein of MKT-077. To identify and affinity-purify the major target proteins of Ras transformants, we generated an immobilized derivative of MKT-077 by conjugating compound 1, a carboxyl derivative of MKT-077, with sepharose beads, as described previously.[2] This conjugate is called "ligand beads" here. Using the ligand beads, we identified a 45-kD protein (p45) as its major target. MKT-077 binds p45 in Ras transformants, but not in the parental normal cells. p45 comigrates with actin in SDS-PAGE, and in fact MKT-77 binds directly purified actin in both monomeric (G) and filamentous (F) forms.

MKT-077 is an F-actin cross-linker. To further characterize the biochemical nature of MKT-077 /actin complex, we examined the superprecipitation of actin filaments (3 µM) with a series of MKT-077 concentrations under the conditions in which actin filaments alone are hardly precipitated. Like many F-actin cross-linkers/bundlers,[3] MKT-077 (300 µM) is sufficient to superprecipitate most of the actin filaments. These observations suggest that MKT-077 causes the formation of either actin meshworks or bundles by cross-linking actin filaments loosely or tightly, respectively.

To distinguish between meshworks and bundles of actin filaments, we compared the high-shear viscosity of MKT-077–treated F-actin solution with the control actin. If actin filaments form meshworks, viscosity is increased. However, if they form bundles, it is reduced. The specific viscosity of control F-actin (10 µM) is around 0.28, whereas that of the MKT-treated one is around 0.13, strongly supporting the notion that MKT-077 is an F-actin bundler. Electron microscopy has indeed confirmed the actin bundle formation by this drug.

REFERENCES

1. KOYA, K., Y. LI, H. WANG, T. UKAI, N. TATSUTA, M. KAWAKAMI, T. SHISHIDO & L.B. CHEN. 1996. MKT-077, a novel rhodacyanine dye in clinical trials, exhibits anticarcinoma activity in preclinical studies based on selective mitochondrial accumulation. Cancer Res. **56:** 538–543.
2. KAWAKAMI, M., N. SUZUKI, Y. SUDO, T. SHISHIDO & M. MAEDA. 1998. Development of an enzyme-linked immunosorbent assay (ELISA) for antitumor agent MKT-077. Anal. Chim. Acta **362:** 177–186.
3. HE, H., T. WATANABE, X. ZHAN, C. HUANG, E. SCHUURING, K. FUKAMI, T. TAKENAWA, C.C. KUMAR, S.J. SIMPSON & H. MARUTA. 1998. Role of PIP2 in Ras/Rac-induced disruption of the cortactin-actomyosin II complex and malignant transformation. Mol. Cell Biol. **18:** 3829–3837.
4. FERNANDEZ, J.L.R., B. GEIGER, D. SALOMON, I. SABANAY, M. ZOELLER & A. BEN-ZE'EV. 1992. Suppression of tumorigenicity in SV40-transformed cells after transfection with vinculin cDNA. J. Cell Biol. **119:** 427–438.
5. GLUECK, U., D. KWIATKOWSKI & A. BEN-ZE'EV. 1993. Suppression of tumorigenicity in SV40-transformed 3T3 cells transfected with alpha-actinin cDNA. Proc. Natl. Acad. Sci. USA **90:** 383–387.
6. MARUTA, H., A. TIKOO, R. SHAKRI, L. ZUGARO, Y. HIROKAWA, T. SHISHIDO, B. BOWERS, L.H. YE, K. KOHAMA & R. SIMPSON. 1999. The anti-cancer drug MKT-077 cross-links actin filaments and binds HSC70 chaperone ATPase in v-Ha-Ras transformants. Cancer Res. **59.** In press.

Construction of a Cell-Permeable CDC42 Binding Fragment of ACK That Inhibits v-Ha-Ras Transformation

M.S.A. NUR-E-KAMAL,[a,c,d] M.M. QURESHI,[a] J.M. KAMAL,[a,d] W. MONTAGUE,[a] AND H. MARUTA[b]

[a]Department of Biochemistry, Faculty of Medicine and Health Sciences, UAE University, Al Ain, G.P.O. Box 17666, United Arab Emirates

[b]Ludwig Institute for Cancer Research, P.O. Royal Melbourne Hospital, Victoria 3050, Australia

Oncogenic Ras mutants, such as v-Ha-Ras, cause malignant transformation by activating several distinct effectors such as Raf and PI-3 kinase. We showed previously that v-Ha-Ras transformation is suppressed by overexpressing minimal Ras-binding fragments of neurofibromin and Raf-1. It has been suggested that Ras transformation requires Rho family GTPases including Rho, Rac, and CDC42 that control rearrangement of actin cytoskeleton. At least Rac is known to be activated by an end product of PI-3 kinase that is activated by Ras directly. We found that overexpression of a 42 amino acid fragment (ACK42) of the kinase ACK, which binds only CDC42 in the GTP-bound form, suppresses Ras transformation. A cell-permeable peptide vector of 16 amino acids called penetratin or its derivative WR has been used to deliver polypeptides of less than 100 amino acids into target cells. Thus, we have constructed a cell-permeable ACK42 derivative by conjugating WR with ACK42 and hemagglutinin (HA) tag, called WR-HA-ACK42. A thrombin-cleavable GST fusion protein of WR-HA-ACK42 was affinity purified from *Escherichia coli* and then cleaved by thrombin. We found that WR-HA-ACK42 penetrates v-Ha-Ras–transformed cells and inhibits growth.

Rho family GTPases (Rho, Rac, and CDC42) play an important role in the regulation of rearrangement of cytoskeleton.[1] Rho is required for the formation of stress fibers, focal adhesion, and contractile ring. Rac is essential for membrane ruffling. CDC42 is required for microspike/filopodium formation.[2] Ras is involved in the activation of some of these Rho family members. For instance, Rac is activated by a Rac GDS called vav that is activated by tyrosine kinase, Lck, and an end product of PI-3 kinase, the later kinase being activated by Ras.[3] CDC42 is activated through bradykinin B2 receptor (BB2R), and the BB2R gene is induced by Ras through an as yet uncharacterized signaling pathway. These findings suggest that Ras is involved in the activation of CDC42. In fact, CDC42 and Rac were shown to be essential for Ras-induced malignant transformation of fibroblasts.[4] In addition, Rho GTPase was also shown to be needed for Ras transformation. It was recently sug-

[c]Corresponding author. Phone, 732/235-4082; fax, 732/235-4073.
e-mail, nurekasa@umdnj.edu
[d]Present address: Department of Pharmacology, R.W. Johnson Medical School, University of Medicine & Dentistry of New Jersey, 675 Hoes Lane, Piscataway, NJ 08854-5636, USA.

TABLE 1. Effect of WR-HA-ACK42 on the growth of v-Ras transformed NIH 3T3 cells[a]

WR-HA-ACK42		Thrombin	
μg/ml	Cell number (10^3)	μg/ml	Cell number (10^3)
0	50	0	55
0.5	30	0.5	53
1.0	25	1.0	55
2.0	26	2.0	55

[a]About 20,000 cells were seeded in 2 ml RPMI containing 1% fetal calf serum. After overnight incubation, cells were treated with various amounts of penetratin, WR-HA-ACK42, and incubated for another 48 hours under standard conditions. Cells were then trypsinized, collected, and counted under a microscope. Results shown below are the average value of three independent experiments with a standard deviation of less than 5%.

gested that Rho is activated by Ras through the SH3 domain of a Ras GAP of 120 kD.[5]

A nonreceptor tyrosine kinase, ACK, was recently cloned and a small domain of it (42 amino acids in length, named ACK42) was found to bind specifically to CDC42 GTPase.[6] We found that overexpression of ACK42 inhibits v-Ras–induced malignant transformation of NIH 3T3 cells.[7] It raises the potential of ACK42 to inhibit Ras-induced transformation if it could be delivered to target cells. A 16 amino acid peptide (or its derivative, penetratin) corresponding to the third helix of the homeodomain (Antennapedia) protein can translocate across membrane. Fusion protein between penetratin and any foreign polypeptide was reported to be able to act as an internalization vector of polypeptides of about 100 amino acids. Such chemically synthesized conjugated polypeptides were found to block various signaling processes in the cell.[8] We constructed recombinant DNA (plasmid) that encodes fusion protein between penetratin and ACK42. The fusion protein was overexpressed in *E. coli* as GST-bound form and affinity purified. Penetratin-ACK42 chimeric protein was cleaved from GST by thrombin (FIG. 1).

Thrombin-cleaved penetratin (WR-HA-ACK42) was tested for its ability to enter into NIH 3T3 and v-Ras–transformed NIH 3T3 cells. By immunostaining with an antibody against HA tag, penetratin was found to translocate into both types of cells (data not shown). A constitutively active form of Ras was found to be associated with transformation of mammalian cells, and Rho GTPases are involved in such a transformation. It was also shown that the CDC42-binding fragment (ACK42) of kinase ACK inhibits v-Ras-induced transformation.[7] Therefore, we tested if ACK42-containing penetratin could block Ras transformation. v-Ras–transformed cells were treated with various amounts of penetratin. Our penetratin construct inhibited the growth of v-Ras–transformed cells at or above the concentration of 0.5 μg/ml (TABLE 1). We generated restriction sites at either side of DNA encoding ACK42. Therefore, it would be possible to replace the ACK42 part of plasmid DNA by any foreign gene or gene fragment, resulting in construction of a variety of penetratin. Such cell-permeable penetratin constructs would be useful tools in studying the cell signaling process.

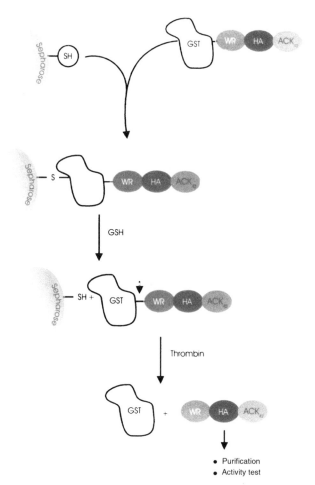

FIGURE 1. Construction of recombinant plasmid and overexpression of GST-WR-HA-ACK42 chimeric protein. A template DNA for WR-HA was generated by end filling re-action using primers, BHRS (5''G GAA GGA TCC AGG AGA TGG AGA AGG TGG TGG AGG AGA TGG TGG AGA AGG 3') and RHA (5' TAC TTC TTG CCT TTG TAC TCT CCT CCA CCT TCT GGA CCA TCT CCT 3'). Part of the ACK gene that encodes ACK42 was amplified by PCR using primers HAS (5' ATG AAG AAC GGA AAC ATG GGC CTG TCG GCC CAG G 3') and EAA (5' TT GAA TTC CTA GTT TCC CAG ATA CAG T 3'). Templates from end filling and PCR reactions were separated by agarose gel electrophoresis followed by purification using "Sephaglass Band Prep Kit, Pharmacia" according to the manufacturer's instructions. Both of these pieces of DNA were ligated and amplified by PCR using primers BHRS and EAA. The PCR product was digested with *Bam*HI and *Eco*RI and cloned into the *Bam*HI and *Eco*RI sites of pGEX-2TH vector. *E. coli* cells were trans-formed with subclone, and ampicillin-resistant colonies were screened for the presence of insert GST-WR-HA-ACK42 plasmid containing *E. coli* cells were grown in LB medium. IPTG was added to a final concentration of 20 μM when cell density reached 1.0 at 600 nm and incubated for 7 hours. Cells were harvested and lysate was prepared. GST fusion protein was purified on a GSH-agarose affinity column. Penetratin was cleaved off GST by treating GST-WR-HA-ACK42 with thrombin (Sigma).

REFERENCES

1. HALL, A. 1998. Rho GTPase and actin cytoskeleton. Science **279:** 509–514.
2. CRESPO, P., K.E. SCHUEBEL, A.A. OSTROM, J.S. GUTKIND AND X.R. 1997. Phosphotyrosine-dependent activation of Rac1 GDP/GTP exchange by the Vav. Nature **385:** 169–172.
3. HAN, J., K. LUBY-PHELPS, B. DAS *et al.* 1998. Role of substrates and products of PI-3 kinase in regulating activation of Rac by Vav. Science **279:** 558–560.
4. Qui, R.G., A. Abo, F. McCormick & M. Symons. 1997. CDC42 regulates anchorage-independent growth and is necessary for Ras transformation. Mol. Cell. Biol. **17:** 3449–3458.
5. LEBLANC, V., B. TOCQUE & I. DELUMEAU. 1998. Ras GAP controls Rho-mediated cytoskeletal rearrangement through its SH3 domain. Mol. Cell. Biol. **18:** 5567–5578.
6. MANSER, E., T. LEUNG, H. SALIHUDDIN, L. TAN & L. LIM. 1993. A non-receptor tyrosine kinase that inhibits the GTPase activity of p21^{CDC42}. Nature **363:** 364–367.
7. NUR-E-KAMAL, M.S.A., J.M. KAMAL, M.M. QURESHI & H. MARUTA. 1999. The CDC42-specific inhibitor derived from ACK-1 blocks v-Ha-Ras–induced transformation. Oncogene **18:** in press.
8. WILLIAMS E.J., D.J. DUNICAN, P.J. GREEN, F.V. HOWELL, D. DEROSSI, F.S. WALSH & P. DOHERTY. 1997. Selective inhibition of growth factor-stimulated mitogenesis by a cell permeable Grb2-binding peptide. J. Biol. Chem. **272:** 22349–22354.

Rational Development of Cell-Penetrating High Affinity SH3 Domain Binding Peptides That Selectively Disrupt the Signal Transduction of Crk Family Adapters

CHRISTIAN KARDINAL,[a] GUIDO POSERN,[a] JIE ZHENG,[b]
BEATRICE S. KNUDSEN,[c] AMGEN PEPTIDE TECHNOLOGY GROUP,[d]
ISMAIL MOAREFI,[e] AND STEPHAN M. FELLER[a,f]

[a]Laboratory of Molecular Oncolology, MSZ, University of Würzburg, Würzburg, Germany

[b]Department of Structural Biology, St. Jude Childrens Hospital, Memphis, Tennessee

[c]Department of Pathology, New York Hospital, New York, New York

[d]Boulder, Colorado

[e]Max Planck Institute for Biochemistry, Martinsried, Germany

The Crk family of adapter proteins selectively binds to specific tyrosine-phosphorylated epitopes on various receptors and their substrate proteins via the Src homology 2 (SH2) domains (FIG. 1, reviewed in ref. 1). By contrast, SH3 domains are molecular adhesives that mediate intracellular signaling events by binding to specific proline-rich epitopes on signal-transducing proteins downstream of the adapters.[1] With the Crk and Crk-like (CRKL) proteins, these include guanine nucleotide release factors that regulate small GTPases such as Ras and Rap1 as well as Abl family tyrosine kinases and PAK-superfamily serine/threonine kinases.[1] Based on previous biophysical and ultrastructural studies,[2,3] short motifs that bind to the SH3(1) domain of Crk/CRKL were defined. These were subsequently selectively mutagenized to generate Crk/CRKL SH3-binding peptides of high affinity and selectivity (HACBPs). Affinities were increased up to 20-fold compared to the best wild-type sequence, whereas selectivity was not only retained, but also sometimes increased.[4] A GST-HACBP fusion protein precipitated Crk/CRKL proteins out of ^{35}S-labeled cell lysates. Very little binding of other cellular proteins to HACBP was detectable, indicating a great preference of HACBPs for Crk/CRKL when compared to other endogenous cellular proteins.[4] Antennapedia (Antp) and integrin-derived shuttle sequences that allow the penetration of peptides through membranes of living cells[5] were subsequently attached to the HACBPs and analyzed for interference with SH3 binding in vitro. Antp-tagged peptides were then selected for further testing in vivo.

[f]Address for correspondence: Stephan Feller, PhD, Laboratory of Molecular Oncology, MSZ-Medical Institute for Radiation & Cell Research, Versbacherstr. 5, D-97078 Wuerzburg, Germany. Phone, + 49-(0)931-201-3840; fax, + 49-(0)931-201-3835.
e-mail, stephan.feller@mail.uni-wuerzburg.de

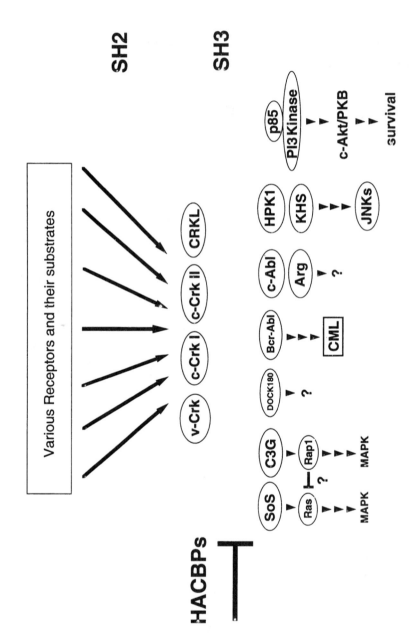

FIGURE 1. SH3 domain-interacting proteins and signal transduction pathways downstream of Crk family adapter proteins.

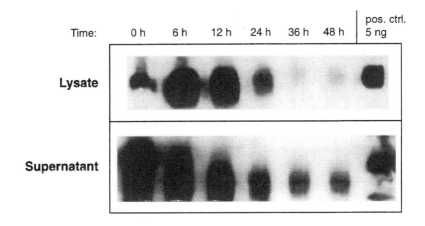

Peptide: Bio-Antp-SH3BP-4 [10 µM]
Bio-Antp-PPPALPPKRRR-amide

Precipitation: Streptavidin (top panel)

Blot: HRP-Streptavidin

FIGURE 2. Evaluation of the half-life of shuttling Bio-Antp-SH3BP-4 in PC12 cells. Cells were treated with 10 µM biotinylated peptide and then analyzed at different time points as indicated. Peptide from washed and lysed cells was precipitated with streptavidin beads and separated, together with peptide from the supernatants, by 16% SDS-PAGE. After semidry blotting and fixation with glutaraldehyde, peptides were detected with HRP-labeled streptavidin and ECL.

Uptake was confirmed by immunofluorescence of biotin-tagged peptides. The half-life of Antp-HACBPs is approximately 6–12 hours depending on the cell type analyzed (FIG. 2). Antp-HACBP, but not mutant control peptides, dramatically reduced the proliferation of Bcr-Abl transformed human chronic myelogenous leukemia (CML) cells. In a second generation of peptides, significant further increases in binding affinity under retention of binding specificity were obtained by elongating the termini of the core binding motif, allowing reduction in the working concentration of Antp-HACBPs into the low micromolar range. Analyses of downstream signal transducers of Bcr-Abl are currently ongoing to define in detail the effects of the HACBPs on these mediators of oncogenic Bcr-Abl signaling.

REFERENCES

1. FELLER, S.M. *et al.* 1998. Physiological signals and oncogenesis mediated through Crk family adapter proteins. J. Cell. Physiol. In press.

2. WU, X. *et al.* 1995. Structural basis for the specific interaction of lysine-containing proline-rich peptides with the N-terminal SH3 domain of c-Crk. Structure **3:** 215–226.
3. KNUDSEN, B.S. *et al.* 1995. Affinity and specificity requirements for the first Src homology 3 domain of the Crk proteins. EMBO J. **14:** 2191–2198.
4. POSERN, G. *et al.* 1998. Development of highly selective SH3 binding peptides for Crk and CRKL which disrupt Crk-complexes with DOCK180, SoS and C3G. Oncogene **16:** 1903–1912.
5. DEROSSI, D. *et al.* 1998. Trojan peptides: The penetratin system for intracellular delivery. Trends Cell Biol. **8:** 84–87.

Anti-HER2 Immunoliposomes for Targeted Drug Delivery

K. HONG,[a,c] D.B. KIRPOTIN,[a] J.W. PARK,[b] Y. SHAO,[a] R. SHALABY,[a]
G. COLBERN,[a] C.C. BENZ,[b] AND D. PAPAHADJOPOULOS[a]

[a]California Pacific Medical Center Research Institute, San Francisco,
California 94115, USA

[b]Division of Hematology/Oncology, University of California, San Francisco,
California 94143, USA

The pharmaceutical application of liposomes has been greatly advanced over the last decade by the introduction of long-circulating liposomes,[1,2] refinement of liposome preparation techniques,[3] and efficient loading of drug into liposomes.[4] The development of stable, long circulating liposomes has led to a new era in liposome drug delivery. For example, sterically stabilized liposomes (Doxil, Sequus Pharmaceuticals, Inc.) were generated by grafting polyethyleneglycol (PEG) onto the liposome surface. These liposomes display prolonged drug circulation and extravasate in solid tumors. However, these liposomes do not interact directly with tumor cells *in vitro* or *in vivo*, and instead they release drug for eventual diffusion into tumor cells.

Similarly, progress in monoclonal antibody (mAb)-based therapy of cancer has led to clinical validation after two decades of research (reviewed in ref. 5). A leading example has been the development of mAb directed against the p185HER2 (HER2) receptor tyrosine kinase, the product of the HER2 (erbB2, *neu*). HER2 is highly overexpressed in a significant proportion of cancers and HER2 overexpression is clearly associated with poor prognosis in breast cancer.[6]

Anti–HER2 immunoliposomes were developed to combine the tumor-targeting properties of mAbs such as rhuMAbHER2 (recombinant humanized anti-HER2 monoclonal antibody) with the drug delivery properties of sterically stabilized liposomes. We previously showed that anti-HER2 immunoliposomes efficiently bind to and internalize in HER2-overexpressing cells *in vitro*, resulting in intracellular drug delivery.[7,8] Here we show the therapeutic properties of anti-HER2 immunoliposomes containing doxorubicin (dox) in animal models (FIG. 1) and the novel mechanism of intracellular drug delivery of anti-HER2 immunoliposomes in these models (FIG. 2).

The antitumor efficacy of anti-HER2 immunoliposome–dox against human breast cancer xenografts was compared with control groups: saline and nontargeted liposome-dox + free rhuMAbHER2 (FIG. 1). Anti-HER2 immunoliposome-dox tested produced marked antitumor effects, including tumor growth inhibition, tumor regressions, and cures of mice and showed superior activity to the other treatment conditions.

---

[c]Address for correspondence: 2200 Webster Street, Room 209, San Francisco, CA 94115. Phone, 415-561-1777; fax, 415-923-3594.
e-mail, khong@cooper.cpmc.org

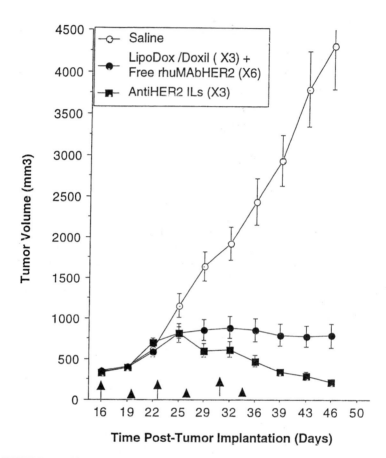

FIGURE 1. Efficacy of anti-HER2 immunoliposome-dox versus combination therapy in the BT-474 (HER2-overexpressing human breast cancer cells) tumor xenograft model. Dox-loaded anti-HER2 immunoliposomes containing rhuMAbHER2 Fab' covalently conjugated on the distal end of PEG-phosphatidylethanolamine (*square*) versus combination therapy (*circles*) of liposomal dox (Doxil) + free rhuMAbHER2 (Herceptin). Immunoliposomes and liposomal dox were administered iv at a total dox dose of 15 mg/kg on the indicated days posttumor implantation (*arrows*), and rhuMAbHER2 was administered at 0.3 mg/kg twice weekly over 6 doses (*arrows and arrowheads*).

Examination of tumors following iv treatment with gold-labeled immunoliposomes or liposomes revealed dramatic differences in intratumoral distribution and mechanism of delivery (FIG. 2). Immunoliposomes were observed dispersed throughout the tumor, and on higher magnification, they were predominantly seen within the cytoplasm of tumor cells. By contrast, liposomes accumulated extracellularly or within resident macrophages. These results have now confirmed that immunoliposomes, unlike nontargeted liposomes, achieved intracellular drug delivery *in vivo*. It is likely that this mechanism accounts for the significantly enhanced efficacy of immunoliposomes against HER2-overexpressing tumors.

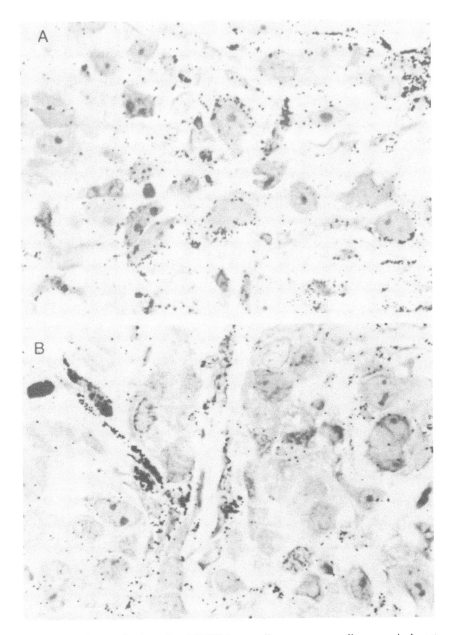

FIGURE 2. Localization of anti-HER2 immunoliposomes versus liposomes in breast cancer xenografts. Liposomes were loaded with colloidal gold and injected iv in nude mice bearing established sc BT-474 tumor xenografts. Twenty-four hours following the injection, mice were sacrificed and tumor was excised. Tissues were fixed and embedded and sections cut for silver enhancement. (**A**) Immunoliposomes were distributed diffusely throughout tumor tissue and had accumulated predominantly within tumor cells. (**B**) Control liposomes were predominantly concentrated in interstitial regions and especially within tissue macrophages.

We conclude that tumor-targeted drug delivery using anti-HER2 immunoliposomes enhances the therapeutic index of doxorubicin chemotherapy and therefore
may be a potent and useful therapy for cancers with HER2 overexpression. In addition, the strategy of immunoliposome delivery may have broad utility for targeted
delivery of other anticancer agents, such as those with narrow therapeutic indices,
pharmacokinetic limitations, or a requirement for intracellular delivery.

REFERENCES

1. ALLEN, T.M. & A. CHONN. 1987. Large unilamellar liposomes with low uptake into
   the reticuloendothelial system. FEBS Lett. 223: 42–46.
2. PAPAHADJOPOULOS, D., T.M. ALLEN, A. GABIZON, E. MAYHEW, K. MATTHAY. S.-K.
   HUANG, K-D. LEE, M.C. WOODLE, D.D. LASIC, C. REDEMANN & F.J. MARTIN. 1991.
   Sterically stabilized liposomes: Improvements in pharmacokinetics and anti-tumor
   therapeutic efficacy. Proc. Natl. Acad. Sci. USA 88: 11460–11464.
3. OLSON, F., C.A. HUNT, F.C. SZOKA, W.J. VAIL & D. PAPAHADJOPOULOS. 1979. Preparation of liposomes of defined size distribution by extrusion through polycarbonate
   membranes. Biochim. Biophys. Acta 557: 9š23.
4. HARAN, G., R. COHEN, L.K. BAR & Y. BARENHOLZ. 1993. Transmembrane ammonium
   sulfate gradients in liposomes produce efficient and stable entrapment of amphipathic weak bases. Biochim. Biophys. Acta 1149: 180–184.
5. SZNOL, M. & J. HOLMLUND. 1997. Antigen-specific agents in development. Semin.
   Oncol. 24: 173–186.
6. SLAMON, D.J., G.M. CLARK, S.G. WONG, W.J. LEVIN, A. ULLRICH & W.L. MCGUIRE.
   1987. Human breast cancer: Correlation of relapse and survival with amplification of
   HER2/neu oncogene. Science 235: 177–182.
7. PARK, J.W., K. HONG, P. CARTER, H. ASGARI, L.Y. GUO, G.A. KELLER, C. WIRTH, R.
   SHALABY, C. KOTTS, W.I. WOOD, D. PAPAHADJOPOULOS & C.C. BENZ. 1995. Development of anti-p185HER2 immunoliposomes for cancer therapy. Proc. Natl. Acad.
   Sci. USA 92: 1327–1331.
8. KIRPOTIN, D., J. W. PARK, K. HONG, S. ZALIPSKY, W.L. LI, P. CARTER, C.C. BENZ &
   D. PAPAHADJOPOULOS. 1997. Sterically stabilized anti-HER2 immunoliposomes:
   Design and targeting to human breast cancer cell in vitro. Biochemistry 36: 66–75.

Recombinant Cytotoxins Specific for Cancer Cells

WALDEMAR DEBINSKI[a]

Section of Neurosurgery/H110, Department of Surgery, Pennsylvania State University College of Medicine, 500 University Drive, Hershey, Pennsylvania 17033-0850, USA

Proteinaceous anticancer cytotoxins, when given systemically, showed limited promise in early trials in patients with solid tumors originating from peripheral organs.[1] One possible reason is insufficient specificity of targeting with the cytotoxins antigens/receptors. This insufficient specificity may prevent the therapeutic administration of relevant amounts of these candidate drugs that would well penetrate solid tumors. However, recent studies showed that local administration of cytotoxins of relatively low specificity for cancer cells showed promising efficacy in patients with malignant brain tumors, and clinical studies entered Phase II stage.[2] This finding provided one more encouragement for further preclinical development of antibrain tumor proteinaceous cytotoxins.

Glioblastoma multiforme (GBM) is an incurable brain malignancy. We discovered that GBM cells *in vitro* overexpress large amounts of a receptor (R) for interleukin 13 (IL13).[3] Of importance, the IL13R on GBM is also present clinically in large amounts, and it was detected in virtually all patients with this disease in situ.[4] IL13 is an immune regulatory cytokine and structurally homologous to IL4, but unlike IL4 it is not species-specific.[5,6] IL13 and IL4 are also functional homologs., and they compete for the shared physiologic signaling receptor, IL13/4R.[7,8] The GBM-associated receptor for IL13 is quantitatively and qualitatively different from its physiologic counterpart. This is because (a) the action of a cytotoxin composed of IL13 and either *Pseudomonas* exotoxin or *Diphtheria* toxin was not competed for by a wild-type IL4 on GBM cells, and (b) the binding of ^{125}I-labeled ILI3 was not neutralized by IL4 on GBM samples in situ.[3,4,9]

Even though overexpression of GBM-associated IL13R may provide pharmaceutically tractable specificity itself, we wished to further optimize the targeting of this receptor. To accomplish this goal, we took advantage of the fact that GBM-associated IL13R is not only quantitatively, but also qualitatively different from the shared physiologic IL13/4R. Therefore, to create a GBM-specific hILI3R, we designed (1) combination and (2) single reagent approaches. In a combination approach, the aim was to block the shared physiologic signaling IL13/4R of normal tissue without concomitantly impairing the binding of IL13 to the GBM-associated hIL13R. This would redirect the IL13 ligand, a new vector for delivery of anticancer drugs, much more specifically towards this GBM-associated receptor. To achieve it, we used an antagonist of all IL4 receptors, including the shared with IL13, human (h) IL4.Y124D.[10] hIL4.Y124D did counteract the low cytotoxic effect of hIL13-based

[a]Phone, 717/531-4541; fax, 717/531-5906.
e-mail, wdebinski@psghs.edu

NORMAL CELLS   CANCER CELLS

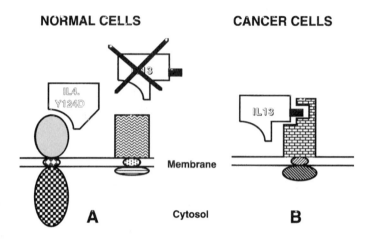

A   Cytosol   B

FIGURE 1. Schematic representation of the effect of hIL4.Y124D on the shared IL13/4 receptor (normal cells) and on the IL4-independent tumor-associated receptor (cancer cells). (**A**) 140-kD IL4R β–chain and a 45-kD IL13R α-chain; both chains are the principal elements of the heterodimeric IL13/4R. (**B**) A monomeric GBM-associated IL4-independent IL13R.

NORMAL CELLS   CANCER CELLS

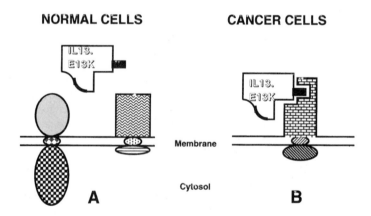

A   Cytosol   B

FIGURE 2. Schematic drawing of the effect of hIL13.E13K on the shared IL13/4 receptor (normal cells) and on the IL4-independent tumor-associated receptor (cancer cells). (**A and B**) As in FIGURE 1.

cytotoxin on, for example, normal human endothelial cells. Importantly, we observed a desirable lack of neutralization of the action of hIL13 cytotoxins on several GBM cell lines and GBM explant cells by hIL4.Y124D.[11] FIGURE 1 depicts the mode of action of the IL4 antagonist on normal and cancer cells.

Inherent in the combination approach, however, is the requirement of at least two therapeutic agents with all consequent pharrnacologic inconveniences. Therefore, we also developed a single reagent approach in which IL13 itself was re-engineered. We substituted an extraordinarily conserved and independent of species residue of a glutamic acid found in both IL13 and IL4. We changed this residue of glutamic acid to lysine in hIL13 (hIL13.E13K), because it was previously found that hIL4.E9K, an equivalent mutant to hIL13.E13K, lost its interaction with the principal chain of the IL4R and became ineffective in its binding to the receptor and signaling through this receptor.[12] We found that the proliferative activity of hIL13.E13K that is mediated by the shared hIL13/4R was obliterated as well. In addition, the low toxicity of hIL13.E13K cytotoxins to normal cells was further decreased. Unexpectedly, the hIL13.E13K cytotoxins became even more active on GBM tumors both *in vitro* and *in vivo*.[12] Thus, we achieved our goal to dissociate IL13 from its physiologic receptor and at the same time to preserve IL13 avidity towards the cancer-associated receptor (FIG. 2).

In summary, we identified new ways to increase receptor tumor specificity, which exploit both its overexpression and its dissimilarity to a physiologic receptor.

ACKNOWLEDGMENT

This work was supported by the Four Diamonds Fund Grant, Surgery Feasibility Grant, and National Institutes of Health Grant R01 CA74145.

REFERENCES

1. PAI, L. *et al.* 1996. Treatment of advanced solid tumors with immunotoxin LMB-1: An antibody linked to Pseudomonas exotoxin. Nature Med. **2:** 350–353.
2. LASKE, D.W. *et al.* 1997. Tumor regression with regional distribution of the targeted toxin TFCRM107 in patients with malignant brain tumors. Nature Med. **3:** 1362–1368.
3. DEBINSKI, W. *et al.* 1995. Human glioma cells over-express receptor for interleukin 13 and are extremely sensitive to a novel chimeric protein composed of interleukin 13 and Pseudomonas exotoxin. Clin. Cancer Res. **1:** 1253–1258.
4. DEBINSKI, W. *et al.* 1999. Receptor for interleukin 13 is a marker and therapeutic target for human high grade gliomas. Clin. Cancer Res. **5:** 985–990.
5. MCKENZIE, A.N.J. *et al.* 1993. Interleukin 13, a T-cell derived cytokine that regulates human monocyte and B-cell function. Proc. Natl. Acad. Sci. USA **90:** 3735–3739.
6. MINTY, A. *et al.* 1993. Interleukin-13 is a new human lymphokine regulating inflammatory and immune responses. Nature **362:** 248–251.
7. OBIRI, N.I, *et al.* 1997. The IL-13 receptor structure differs on various cell types and may share more than one component with IL-4 receptor. J. Immunol. **158:** 756–764.
8. DEBINSKI, W. *et al.* 1995. A novel chimeric protein composed of interleukin 13 and Pseudomonas exotoxin is highly cytotoxic to human carcinoma cells expressing receptors for interleukin 13 and interleukin 4. J. Biol. Chem. **270:** 16775–16780.
9. DEBINSKI, W. *et al.* 1996. Receptor for IL 13 does not interact with IL4 but receptor for IL4 interacts with IL13 on human glioma cells. J. Biol. Chem. **271:** 22428–22433.
10. ZURAWSKI, S.M. *et al.* 1993. Receptors for interleukin-13 and interleukin-4 are complex and share a novel component that functions in signal transduction. EMBO J. **12:** 2663–2670.
11. DEBINSKI, W. *et al.* 1998. Novel way to increase targeting specificity to a human glioblastoma associated receptor for interleukin 13. Int. J. Cancer **76:** 547-551.
12. DEBINSKI, W. *et al.* 1998. Novel anti-brain tumor cytotoxins specific for cancer cells. Nature Biotechnol. **16:** 449–453.

Index of Contributors